Pharmaceutical Statistics and Research Methodology :

Industrial and Clinical Applications

Pharmaceutical Statistics and Research Methodology :

Industrial and Clinical Applications

D. H. Panchaksharappa Gowda

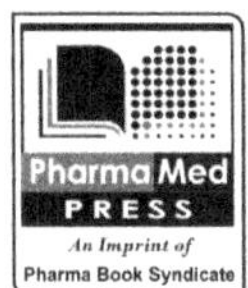

PharmaMed Press
An imprint of Pharma Book Syndicate
A unit of BSP Books Pvt. Ltd.
4-4-309/316, Giriraj Lane,
Sultan Bazar, Hyderabad - 500 095.

Pharmaceutical Statistics and Research Methodology : Industrial and Clinical Applications
by D. H. Panchaksharappa Gowda

Published by

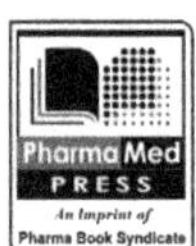

PharmaMed Press

An imprint of Pharma Book Syndicate
A unit of BSP Books Pvt. Ltd.
4-4-309/316, Giriraj Lane, Sultan Bazar, Hyderabad - 500 095.
Phone: 040-23445688, 23445600; Fax: 91+40-23445611
E-mail: info@pharmamedpress.com
www.pharmamedpress.com/pharmamedpress.net

ISBN: 978-93-89974-23-2

Foreword

It gives me an immense pleasure in introducing the text book **"Pharmaceutical Statistics and Research Methodology: Industrial and Clinical Applications"** authored by Mr. Panchaksharappa Gowda D.H. The book covers various topics mentioned in the syllabus of B.Pharm VIII-Semester and Fourth Year Pharm.D, which is prescribed by Pharmacy Council of India (PCI), New Delhi. The author has described the fundamental aspect of Biostatistics, with the application of statistical tools which are used for analyzing the data of formulation experiments and clinical trial problems. The book not only deals with the Pharmaceutical Statistics, but it also describes about the application of some statistical software's like Design of Experiment (DOE), SPSS & R online software and statistics for epidemiological studies with research methodologies. This book is not just theoretical, but also deals with the practical applications.

The author of this text book has written, with his expertise in teaching Biostatistics for more than thirty two years and Research methodology and Statistical software's for more than eleven years.

I am sure this book will be highly useful, informative and valuable for the students of B.Pharm VIII-Semester and Pharm.D.

It is my great pleasure to commend this textbook, as it covers the syllabus and supports learning the related aspects of Pharmaceutical Statistics and Research Methodology.

I do hope that students who read this book will get a good grasp of the subject, which may help them to understand theory and practical knowledge which is required to enhance their academic career.

Dr. B. Suresh
President, Pharmacy Council of India, New Delhi
Pro-Chancellor, JSS Academy of Higher Education & Research
Mysuru-570 015.

PREFACE

Pharmaceutical Statistics and Research Methodology has been given more importance in Pharmacy course to design the methodology and to analyze data of various experiments which are carried in preparing formulation and clinical trials. No students of these discipline cannot perform the statistical analysis without the knowledge of those topics which are explained in this book. The present text is designed to introduce students about the methods and how to apply and analyze the data after performing the experiments.

This book covers theoretical, Practical and applied aspects of statistics and research methodology in a clear and exhaustive way. The author has attempted to give as many illustrations as possible in order to make the students to understand various methods in analyzing using various statistical software's like SPSS, DOE and R. I claim that no originality for the matter presented in the text, however, the methods of presentation and arrangement of the subject matter is my own, which reflects an approach for statistical methods to solve and analyze the data and also understandability based on the long teaching experience of degree (B.Pharm, Pharm.D) and Post-graduate classes.

I hope that the book will be found more useful for the students. I invite suggestions from students as well as my teacher-friends for any improvement (addition or deletion) of the book in future. I would like to thank my colleagues for their encourage and suggestions.

The author accepts full responsibility for any typographical or subject-matter errors, which may be there in the book of this dimension and subject.

-Author

CONTENTS

1 Introduction

Statistics has its own vocabulary. We are frequently reminded about the fact that we are living in the information age. The subject statistics as it seems, is not a new discipline, but it is as old as the human society itself. It has been used right from the existence of life on this earth although the sphere of its utility was very much restricted. In the olden days statistics was regarded as the "science of Statecraft" and was the byproduct of the administrative activity of the state.

The word statistics seems to have been derived from the Latin word, status or the Italian word 'statista' or the German word, statistik or the French word 'statique' each of which means a political state.

In the ancient time the scope of statistics was primarily limited to the collection about

1. Age and sex-wise population of the county
2. Property and wealth of the Country.

Presently the statistics has been extended to Mechanical science, Pharmaceutical science, Medical science, life science and Paramedical science for collection and to analysis of data.

Historical evidences about the prevalence of a very good system of collecting vital statistics and registration of births and deaths even before 300 BC are available in Kautilya.

Sixteenth century saw the applications of the statistics for the collection of the data relating to the movements of heavenly bodies-stars and planets to know about their positioning and for the prediction of eclipses.

Seventeenth century witnessed the origin of vital statistics. Statistics was systematically applied to study of the birth and death statistics. The computation of mortality tables and the calculation of expectation of life at different ages led to the idea of "life insurance".

Modern stalwart in the development of statistics who contributed how to apply statistics in different fields to analyze the data. Francis Galton (1822-1921) who designed the regression analysis technique, Karl Pearson (1857-1936) developed the correlation analysis technique, also he developed Chi-square test (λ^2- test) of goodness of fit to analyze non-Parametric test.

RA Fisher is the real giant in the field of statistics, because he is pioneer in estimation of theory, sampling distribution, analysis of variance and design experiments. These are the statistical tools which are most frequently used in pharmaceutical calculation to analyze the experimental data and to verify the level of significance of the result.

Before RA Fisher, W.S.S Gosset one who developed the t-test to analyze the data of small size.

SOME BASIC CONCEPTS

Data: The raw material of statistics is data. Statistics are a set of numerical data, in fact only numerical data constitute statistics. Thus the raw material of statistics always originates from the operation of counting (enumeration) or measurements.

The person conducts the statistical measures are the characteristics under study to carry out further statistical analysis is known as investigator.

For our purpose we can define data as numbers - these data will be collected in two ways:

1. Measurement
2. Counts

When an Investigator measures the weights and temperatures of patients is measurement and counts is the total number of patients in different age Group is counting.

Another example is considered when hospital administrator counts the number of patients who have admitted and discharged in a day can be taken as count.

The entire structure of the statistical analysis for any enquiry is based upon systematic collection of data. When an investigator while doing clinical trials experiment, he has to collect data for every half an hour till the completion of clinical trial.

Distribution of concentration of drug in the blood and complete elimination of drug from the blood. That will become more accurate data to apply statistical tools to analyze and do draw inference about the results obtained.

STATISTICS

One can define the statistics as a field of study concerned with:

1. The collection, organization, summarization and analysis and
2. Drawing inferences about a body of data when only a part of the data is observed.

The field of utility of statistics has been increasing steadily in different field like, medical pharmaceutical, paramedical, life science and other different areas, people defined it in different ways.

Generally the Statistical methods embodying the theory and techniques used for collecting, analyzing and drawing inferences for the numerical data. Hence, statistics can be defined as the science of collection, presentation, analysis and interpretation of numerical data.

BIO STATISTICS

When the tools of statistics are applied to analyze the medical, biological and pharmaceutical sciences data, then it can be named as biostatistics.

Biostatistics is contraction of biology and statistics. Sometimes referred to as biometry or biometrics, is the application of statistics to a wide range of topics in biology.

PHARMACEUTICAL STATISTICS

Pharmaceutical statistics is the application of statistics, to the matters of concerning the pharmaceutical industry. The example is the design of experiments to analyze the product, to analyze the clinical trial experiments etc.

Example

1. To evaluate the activity of drug
   Ex: heat of caffeine on attention compare the analgesic effect of plant extract and NSAID
2. To explore whether the changes produced by the drug are due to the action of drug by chance
3. To compare the action of two or more different drugs or different dosages of the same drug are studied using statistical methods
4. To find an association between disease and risk factors such as coronary artery disease and smoking
5. Design and Analysis clinical trials in medicine

The science of biostatistics encompasses the design of biological experiments especially in medicine and pharmaceutical science.

VARIABLES

When we observe a characteristic we find that it takes on different values in different persons, places or things, we label those values are as a variable. The reason for doing this is that characteristic is not same when observed in different possessors of it. In general variables are termed as the measurements of the values which are the characteristics of data collected after performing the experiment.

Example: Blood pressure, sugar level, heartbeat, heights of patients, age of patients which area observed in clinic.

Types of Variables

Quantitative Variable

A quantitative variable is one that can be measures in the usual sense.

When we measure height of patients come to clinics, that variable can be called as quantitative variables. Measurements made on quantitative variable convey information regarding amount.

Qualitative Variables

Characteristic can be categorized only.

For example when a person with diseased diagnose, is designated as belongings to ethnic group of a person or object is said to possess or not to possess some characteristic of interest. In this case measurement consists of categorizing. These variables are termed as qualitative variables

Discrete Variable

Those variable which cannot take all the possible values within a given specified range are termed as discrete (discontinuous) variable. Discrete variable can take on a countable number of values. These variables are commonly observed in biological and Pharmaceutical experiments or clinical trial experiments. For example when patients are treated using a particular drug, then the different kinds of side effects of drugs will be measured. This type of measurement can be considered or can be included in discrete variable group.

Even the number of daily admissions to a general hospital in a day may be considered as discrete variable, because number of admissions each day must be represented by a whole number, such as 0, 1, 2 or 3.

The number of decayed, missing of filled teeth in a dental checkup camp in a village can be considered as a discrete variable.

Continuous Variable

Those variable which can take all the possible values (integral as well as fractional) within same range or interval can be termed as continuous variable (i.e., within a specified lower and upper limit). The limiting factor for the total number of possible observations or results is the sensitivity of the measuring instrument.

For Example, the age of patients in a hospital is a continuous variable because age can take all possible values (it can be measured to a nearest fraction)

Time: years, month, day, minutes, Seconds etc., in a certain range, say to 10 years or 10-20 years etc.,

More precisely a variable is said to be continuous if it is possible of passing from any given value to the next value by infinitely small gradation

Ex: Height, weight, temperature are continuous variable

FREQUENCY DISTRIBUTION

The organization of the data pertaining to a quantitative phenomenon. The frequency distribution can be defined as a table in which data's are grouped into classes and number of items which are falling in each class will be recorded.

It is an important function of statistics to facilitate the comprehension and meaning of large quantities of data by constructing simple data summaries.

The Frequency distribution can also be defined as a table or categorization of the frequency of occurrence of variables in various class intervals.

Sometimes it can also be defined set of data is simply called a distribution

For a sampling of continuous data, in general, a frequency distribution is constructed by classifying the observations.

A frequency distribution is constructed for three main reasons

1. To facilitate the analysis of data;

2. To estimate frequencies of the unknown population distribution from the distribution of sample data;

3. To facilitate the computation of various statistical measures.

Kind of Frequency Distribution

Frequency distribution can be classified into three types which area based on the methods of arranging data in the table. The three types of frequency distributions are named as

(a) Series of individual observations;

(b) Discrete series and;

(c) Continuous series.

a) Series of individual observations

The individual observations are a series, where items are listed singly after observation, as distinguished from listing them in groups. If height of 10 patients are given individually it will form a series of individual observation

Example: 1

Patient Number	Height (Inches)
1	62"
2	65"
3	68"
4	64"
5	60"
6	63"
7	67"
8	69"
9	70"
10	58"

This individual series data has to be arranged in either ascending or descending order for some statistical calculation purpose

Example: 2

B P of 10 Patients recorded in a hospital before including them in a clinical trial

Sl. No.:	1	2	3	4	5	6	7	8	9	10
BP	125	135	140	120	110	115	160	190	170	160

b) Discrete series: In case of discrete series data's are presented in a way that exact measurements of items or subjects are clearly mentioned and there will be a definite difference between the variables of different group of items.

Here each group is distinct and separate from other classes. There will be no continuity from one class to another

Example

Disease Type: Asthma   Heart Put   Diabetic   Cancer,   Arthritis

No. of Patients   25   70   120   30   100

(in Village with Particular diseases)

c) Continuous Series

Continuous series is one where measurements are taken in approximations and the data's are expressed in the form of class interval. In this case the variable can take any intermediate value between the lowest and highest value in the distribution. In case of continuous series the class intervals theoretically continues from the beginning of the frequency distribution to the end without having any break. Always it can be distinguished from the discrete frequency distribution of series, because here it contains two limits upper and lower limit of each class interval.

Example 1

Age of Diabetic Patients	Number of Patients
0 – 10	3
10 - 20	20
20 - 30	70
30- 40	100
40 - 50	200
50 - 60	75
60 - 70	12

Example 2

Weight interval (lb)	Frequency
10 - 20	5
20 - 30	19
30- 40	10
40 - 50	13
50 - 60	4
60 - 70	4
70 - 80	2
Net	**57**

The number of intervals chosen should result in a table that considerably improved the readability of the data. The following rules of them are useful to select or make the intervals for a frequency distribution table

1. Form the intervals, such that the intervals will have significance in relation to the nature of the data

2. While forming intervals, we should not have too many empty intervals or intervals without any frequency

3. Maximum number of intervals in a distribution can be taken up to eight to twenty

The width of all intervals in general should be the same and it helps the reader to read the data easily and allows for simple computation of statistical data or values.

Some Definition with Regard to Construction of Series

RANGE: The range of a frequency distribution may be defined as the difference between the lower limit of the first interval and the upper limit of last class interval. In the above example the range is 80-10 = 70

CLASS – INTERVAL: The class interval may be defined as the size of grouping of data. According to the example which is written above 10-20, 20-30, 30-40   - - - -   70-80, are class – intervals.

CLASS LIMITS: The class limits of frequency distribution are defined as the upper and lower limits of each class interval. Since each class interval contains all possible values ranging from the lower limit of the given class interval and infinitely approaching the lower limit of next higher class interval. In general lower limit one class interval and the upper limit of the next succeeding class interval as class limits. In the example mentioned above 10, 20, 30 40, 60, 70 are lower limits and 20, 30, 40, 50, 60, 70, 80 upper limits of class intervals. Together they are called as class limits. Lower limits are denoted as l1 and upper limits are written as l2.

MAGNITUDE OF A CLASS INTERVAL: The difference between the upper and lower limit of each class interval is called as magnitude of that class. Here in the above example 20-10 = 10 is the magnitude of the first class – interval.

MID-VALUE or MID-POINT: The central point of each interval is termed as mid-value or central value of an interval. Mid-value is written as M and it is obtained by using the equation
$$M = (l1 + l2)/2.$$

FREQUENCY: The number of items or observations which are falling within a particular class interval is termed as frequency of that class/class interval.

Methods of forming class Intervals:

There are two methods to form class intervals

1. Exclusive method
2. Inclusive method

Exclusive method: In case exclusive method, the upper limit of one class interval is the lower limit of the next class interval.

Exclusive Method		
Class-Interval		**Frequency**
0	10	5
10	20	12
20	30	18
30	40	22
40	50	40
50	60	19
60	70	13
70	80	8
80	90	4
Total		**141**

Inclusive method: In case inclusive method the ambiguity about items identical to a limit of the class interval is sought to be removed. Here upper limit need not be the lower limit of next interval and upper limit will be included in that interval.

Inclusive Method		
Class-Interval		Frequency
0	09	5
10	19	12
20	29	18
30	39	22
40	49	40
50	59	19
60	69	13
70	79	8
80	89	4
Total		**141**

Cumulative Series

Cumulative frequency distribution has a running total of the values. It is constructed by adding the frequencies of the first class interval to the frequency in the second class interval, the same totals is added to frequencies in the third class interval. This process continues until the final total appearing opposite the last class interval, that total will be equal to the total frequency of the frequency distribution. The cumulative frequency may be classified as downward and Upward.

The downward accumulation results in a list presenting the number of frequencies "less than" any given amount as revealed by the lower limit of succeeding class interval; and the upward accumulation results in presenting the number of frequencies "more than" and given amount as revealed by the upper limit of a preceding class interval.

DOWNWARD CUMULATION

Less Than	Frequency	Cf
10	5	5
20	12	17
30	18	35
40	22	57
50	40	97
60	19	116
70	13	129
80	8	137
90	4	141
	141	

UPWARD CUMULATION

More Than	Frequency	Cf
0	5	141
10	12	136
20	18	124
30	22	106
40	40	84
50	19	44
60	13	25
70	8	12
80	4	4
	141	

Measure of Central Tendency (Statistical Averages)

MEANING AND IMPORTANCE

An average reduces the whole distribution or large number of observation to a single figure or value. The average can be defined as **"Measures of central tendency"** because they describe the tendency of items to group around the Middle in a frequency distribution of numerical values or numbers.

This tendency of items to group around the middle is a characteristic which tends itself to measurement and the measurement of that tendency is called average. The averages plays an very important role in Biostatistics. Many statistical techniques which are applied in statistical analysis depend upon the average or central tendency. That may be the main reason for calling statistics as science of average

Ex:

1.   The average B P of the population can be called as central tendency
2.   Average weight of human being can also be taken as central tendency

OBJECTS AND FUNCTIONS OF AVERAGES

An average is the precise and a simple indicator of the central tendency of whole distribution. The main functions of an average are

1. **To present the salient features of a mass of complex data:** With the help of an average, it will be more convenient to express the data or information in a very abbreviated numerical form, in such a way that the salient features of the data collected in table are clearly brought out.

   Ex: when we measure the average height of the sample of a particular population, that single figure enable one to draw a general conclusion about characteristics of the phenomena under study.

   The purpose of an average is to represent a group of individual values in a simple and concise manner.

2. To facilitate comparison

An average will provide a common denominator for comparing the data of one group with data of other group and conclusion can be drawn about the characteristics of different groups.

Example: We can compare average amount the concentration drug in the plasma level between two samples or drugs which are used to treat same type of patients or subjects having same disease.

3. To know about Universe from a sample

Averages helps to know about a picture of complete group by means of sample data

4. **To help in decision making**: In the process of experimentation or in doing some research work it is most important to know the average value of variable. Averages are useful in setting standards estimating and planning in conducting research work in Pharmaceutical and medical science.

Various measures of averages or central tendency

The following are the measures of central tendency which are most often used in pharmaceutical and medical science to perform some statistical calculation and to analyze the experimental results.

- Arithmetic Mean
- Median
- Mode
- Geometric Mean
- Harmonic Mean

Among these five types of averages arithmetic, Geometric and Harmonic mean are included in mathematical average, because one has to do some arithmetic while finding that particular value.

Whereas median and mode are included in positional average, because these two averages can be obtained by looking at the position of the distribution.

Arithmetic Mean

The arithmetic is most often used and the most generally understood of all averages in Pharmaceutical calculation and medical science. The arithmetic mean of a given set observations which are recorded by doing clinical trial experiments or while doing any formulation experiments, the final the average of all the values are added and their sum is divided by number of trails or number of observations or data's recorded after performing experiment and obtaining result.

In general if X_1, X_2 .... X_n are n - observations or results obtained by performing an experiments, the their A.M., is usually denoted by $\overline{X}$ and obtained using equation

$$\overline{X} = \frac{X_1 + X_2 + X_3 - - - - - - + X_n}{n}$$

$$\bar{X} = \frac{\sum X}{n}$$

This method can be applied to all the series with different methods.

Arithmetic mean an individual series

The process of computing arithmetic mean of an individual series, there are two steps

1. All the observations are added up

2. Divide the sum of the values ($\sum X$) by the number of items (n)

$$\bar{X} = \frac{X_1 + X_2 + X_3 ------ + X_n}{n}$$

$$\bar{X} = \frac{\sum X}{n}$$

Example: Potency of 10 drugs as listed below

Potency: 195, 197, 198, 196, 200, 205, 201, 203, 200, 196

Solution:

X = 195, 197, 198, 196, 200, 205, 201, 203, 200, 196

$\sum X$ = 195 + 197+198+196+200+205+201+203+200+196

$\sum X$ = 1991

n = 10, $\quad \bar{X} = \frac{\sum X}{n}$

$$\bar{X} = \frac{1991}{10} = 199.1$$

Example 2:

An IV injection of 10 mg new drug was administered to a patient and urine volume and Urine drug concentration were measured for every one hour and results obtained are tabulated as follows. Compute mean of Urine volume and urinary drug concentration

Time	Volume of Urine (ml) X	Drug Concentration (µg /mL) Y
1	1225	1.8
2	1550	0.985
3	1750	0.545
4	1385	0.449
5	1625	0.224
6	1130	0.1
7	1000	0.036
	$\sum X$ = 9665	$\sum Y$ = 4.139

Mean of Urine Volume $= \dfrac{\Sigma X}{n} = \dfrac{9966}{7} = 1380.71$

Mean of Urinary Drug Concentration $= \dfrac{\Sigma Y}{n} = \dfrac{4.139}{7} = 0.59$

Arithmetic Mean of Discrete Series

To find A.M., one has to obtain the total number of observations considered or taken for study in the distribution, that is obtained by adding frequencies of all the classes, then we should obtain the total values of the distribution. To find total values of each distribution, frequency of each row is multiplied with the respective class size and then all values are totaled up. The total is then divided by the total of the frequencies to final out Arithmetic mean of the distribution

$\bar{X}$ = A.M., f = frequency

X = class - value of each group

$n = \Sigma f$ = Total number of items or subjects or observations

Steps

1. Multiply the frequency of each row with respective variable X and total them that total will be written as ΣfX

2. Finding the total number of observation add up all the frequencies and written Σf, that will be equal to $n = \Sigma f$

3. Finally divide the ΣfX by n to find A.M. $(\bar{X})$

4. $\bar{X} = \dfrac{\Sigma fX}{\Sigma f} = \dfrac{\Sigma fX}{n}$

Example: The blood pressure of 100 patients is recoded and find average B P of these 145 patients

X (B P)	No. of patients (f)	fx
100	50	500
105	08	840
110	20	2200
115	25	2875
120	12	1440
125	10	1250
130	9	1170
135	6	810
140	5	700
	$\Sigma f = n = 145$	$\Sigma Fx = 11785$

$$\bar{X} = \dfrac{\Sigma fX}{\Sigma f} = \dfrac{\Sigma fX}{n} \quad \dfrac{11785}{145} = 81.28$$

Arithmetic Mean of Continuous Series

In case of continuous frequency distribution the value of each individual frequency distribution is unknown. Hence the data's are expressed in the form of class-interval. Therefore to perform the average of the distribution, one has to take the mid-value of the class interval.

Steps

1. Mid-values of the class-intervals (m) are to be obtained
2. Mid values of each-intervals area multiplied by its corresponding frequency (fm) and product is written as fm
3. All the products of mid-value and frequency are added up to obtain $\sum$fm
4. Add up the number of frequency (n or $\sum$f)
5. Finally A M is obtained by using the equation

$$\bar{X} = \frac{\sum fm}{\sum f}$$

n = the total of the frequencies

$\sum$fm = Total of the product of mid-value and frequency of all the class intervals

$\bar{X}$ = A M

Example: obtain the average age of 100 patients who have been treated in a particular ward for a weak

Age :	0-10	10-20	20-30	30-40	40-50	50-60	60-70
(X) =	8	12	18	20	16	15	11

Age (x) (age of patients	No of Patients (t)	Mid Value (m)	fm
0-10	8	15	120
10-20	12	25	300
20-30	18	35	630
30-40	20	45	900
40-50	16	55	880
50-60	15	65	975
60-70	11	75	825
	$\sum$f = n = 100		$\sum$f m= 4630

$$\bar{X} = \frac{\sum fm}{\sum f} = \frac{\sum 4630}{100} = 46.30$$

Merits and demerits of arithmetic Mean ($\bar{X}$):

Merits

An ideal measure of central tendency arithmetic mean possesses the following merits:

1. Arithmetic Mean is simple to calculate and easy to understand

2. Arithmetic mean is rigidly defined value

3. It is a good basis of comparison

4. It is based on all the observations

5. It is suitable for further mathematical treatment

6. It is affected least by fluctuations of sampling. This property is explained by saying that arithmetic mean is a stable average.

Demerits

1. The stronger drawback of arithmetic mean is that it is very much affected by an extreme data or value

$$\text{Ex: When we calculate the average of 250, 249, 252, 249}$$
$$\bar{X} = \frac{250+249+252+249}{4} = 250$$

If 5000 is another extreme value which is included in the distribution then
$$\bar{X} = \frac{5000+ 250+249+252+249}{5} = 1200$$

2. Arithmetic mean which may not be an actual value of the series, then it is called as a fictitious average. It may not be a single value of the distribution

3. Arithmetic mean cannot be used if we are dealing with qualitative characteristics

    Ex: Severe, Intelligence, Honesty, Beauty, Mind

4. To obtain arithmetic mean, it is necessary to know the actual values of all the items in the distribution in an open end class distribution. The A M cannot be calculated without making assumptions regarding the magnitude of class intervals of the open end classes

5. Arithmetic mean cannot be computed by simply observing the series

Median

The median is another important and widely used statistical average in Pharmaceutical and medical science to perform some statistical calculation

It has the connotation of the middle most or most central value of a set of numbers. The median represents the center of a data set, without regard for the distance of each point from the center. The median is the value that divides the data into two halves, half the values beings less than and other half of the values greater than the median value. It is also called as positional average because it is that point on the number line, such that half of the scores are above and half below.

Median of Individual Series

To obtain or for calculating median of individual series of observations, the following steps are followed.

1. The observation in the series are arranged in either ascending or descending order. Both the way, we will get same result.

2. Median can be located by finding the size of $\left(\frac{N+1}{2}\right)^{th}$ item

$$M = \text{size of } \left(\frac{N+1}{2}\right)^{th} \text{ item}$$

$$M = \text{Median}$$

$$N = \text{Number of items}$$

Example 1: When N is Odd

The median of 5-items 35, 12, 40, 8, 60

Solution: Arrange them in Ascending order

8, 12, 35, 40, 60

$$M = \text{size of } \left(\frac{N+1}{2}\right)^{th} \text{ item}$$

$$M = \text{size of } \left(\frac{5+1}{2}\right)^{th} \text{ item} = \frac{6}{2} = 3^{rd} \text{ item}$$

$$M = 35$$

Here median is 35, because 35 is the value which divides the distribution into two equal parts.

Example 2: When N is Even

The median of 6 items 35, 12, 40, 8, 60, 50

Solution: Arrange them in Ascending order

8, 12, 35, 40, 50, 60

$$M = \text{size of } \left(\frac{N+1}{2}\right)^{th} \text{ item}$$

$$M = \text{size of } \left(\frac{6+1}{2}\right)^{th} \text{ item} = \frac{7}{2} = 3.5^{th} \text{ item}$$

$$M = \frac{3^{rd} + 4^{th}}{2} = \frac{35+40}{2} = \frac{75}{2} = 37.5$$

Median of Discrete Series: For the calculation of Median of discrete series or distribution, data need not be arranged either in ascending or descending order. The reason being that we have to find out the cumulative frequency, which automatically places the series in an ascending order only. Hence we need not go for arranging the data in the ascending or descending order.

STEPS INVOLVED IN CALCULATION OF MEDIAN:

1. Cumulative frequencies are computed (cf).

2. Median value is computed by applying the formula $\left(\frac{N+1}{2}\right)$

3. Median value is located in the frequency column and corresponding class value is considered as median.

Example: Obtain median height of patients who have been selected for clinical trial study.

Height (X)	58	59	60	61	62	63	64	65	66
Number of Patients	15	20	32	35	33	22	20	10	08

Solution:

Height (X)	Number of Patients (f)	Cumulative frequency (Cf)
58	15	15
59	20	35
60	32	67
61	35	102
62	33	135
63	22	157
64	20	177
65	10	187
66	08	195
	N = ∑f = 195	

$M = \text{size of } \left(\frac{N+1}{2}\right)^{th} \text{ item}$

$M = \text{size of } \left(\frac{195+1}{2}\right)^{th} \text{ item} = \frac{196}{2} = 98^{th} \text{ item}$

$= 98^{th}$ item lies in the 61st – class. Hence median M = 61

Median of Continuous Series: To calculate median of a continuous series, steps involved are

1. Cumulative frequencies are obtained (cf)

2. Median value is calculated by applying the formula $m = \left(\frac{N}{2}\right)^{th} \text{ item}$

3. Median value is located in cumulative frequency column and corresponding class interval is considered as median class-interval.

4. The median is computed by substituting the respective values in the equation

$$M = l_1 + \frac{i}{f}(m - c)$$

M = Median value

l_1 = Lower limit of the median class interval

I = Size of median class–interval

C= Cumulative frequency of a class–interval preceding median class interval

Example: Compute median age of 80 patients of different age group, who have been selected for clinical study and data's are represented in continuous series.

Age (X)	Number of Patients (f)
20-30	6
30-40	10
40-50	16
50-60	18
60-70	12
70-80	10
80-90	8

Solution:

Age (X)	Number of Patients (f)	Cumulative frequency (cf)
20 - 30	6	6
30 - 40	10	16
40 - 50	16	32
50 - 60	18	50
60 - 70	12	62
70 - 80	10	72
80 - 90	8	80

$$N = \sum f = 80$$

Median value = m = $\left(\frac{N}{2}\right)^{th}$ item = $\frac{80}{2}$ = 40

Median class interval is 50 – 60

L1 = 50, I = 10, f = 18 and c = 32

$$M = l_1 + \frac{I}{f}(L_1 - c)$$

$$M = 50 + \frac{10}{18}(50 - 32)$$

$$M = 50 + \frac{10 * 18}{18}$$

$M = 50 + 4.44$

$M = 54.44$

Merits and Demerits

Merits

1. It is very easy to calculate median and is readily understood.
2. Median can be obtained in case of open-end class – interval series.
3. It is not drastically affected by extreme values as is mean.
4. Uniqueness: as is true with median, there is only one median for a given set of data.
5. Median can be obtained or can be located graphically also
6. Very often it will the actual number of the series

Demerits

1. To compute median in certain cases, it requires the arraying of data in either ascending or descending order.
2. Since median is a positional average, it is not suitable for further mathematical treatment.
3. Median tends to be rather unstable value, if the size of the distribution is small.
4. Actual value of the median cannot be obtained, when group having even number of items in the series.
5. A substantial change in median will happen, when there is change in series. For example, if marks obtained by 7 seven students are 7, 12, 19, 52, 54 then the median is 19. If marks of two more students are 55 and 60 added to the series, then median will be 48.
6. Median is not amenable for further algebraic manipulation.

MODE

The mode is statistical average in the series, that occurs with the greatest frequency and thus is the most fashionable value.

"The mode in a distribution or series can be defined as the value which occurs most frequently".

If all the values are different, then there is no mode; on the other hand, a set of values may have more than one mode.

Example: The following are ages of 10 patients, in the OPD of a hospital. Obtain the mode

Age(X)	30	33	15	75	33	45	48	52	60	73

Age(X)	15	30	33	33	45	48	52	60	73	75

$M_0 = 33$

Mode of Individual Series

To obtain mode of an individual series, data in the distribution should be arranged in ascending or descending order, then the value which is repeated more number of times should be considered as mode.

Example: Obtain the mode of given individual series.

X: 27 3 21 32 22 43 52 47 32 35 32 31

Solution:

X: 21 22 27 31 32 32 3 35 43 52 47

Mode = 32

MODE OF DISCRETE SERIES: There are two methods to obtain mode of discrete series. They are a. Inspection b. Grouping method

a. Inspection Method:

If the given distribution is regular and homogeneous, mode can be located by observing or by inspecting the series. The class or size having the highest frequency will be considered as mode.

Example: Compute mode of age of the given distribution

Age (X)	10	12	14	16	18	20	22	24	26	28
Frequency (f)	01	02	04	08	14	10	07	04	02	01

Solution: The mode of the distribution is 18, because the distribution is regular and class 18 is having highest frequency 14.

b. GROUPING METHOD:

In case the frequency distribution is not being regular and homogeneous, then grouping method is applied to obtain mode. The procedure to obtain mode is as given below

1 For the given frequency distribution, in the frequency column, the highest frequency is noted and marked. That column is named as f_1.

2 The Second column is constructed by grouping two frequencies at a time, starting from top. Then totals are obtained taking two at a time and they are written in second frequency column. Highest frequency is marked in second column also.

3 Similarly third frequency column is constructed, by grouping two at a time, but grouping will start from second frequency. Here also highest value is marked.

4 In the fourth frequency column, frequencies are grouped three at a time, here grouping starts from the top. Their totals are obtained and highest frequency is marked.

5 To construct fifth frequency column, three frequencies are grouped at a time, grouping starts from second value (leaving the first frequency) . Totals are found out and highest frequency is marked.

6 To construct sixth, grouping starts from third frequency, here also three frequencies are grouped at a time leaving the first and second frequencies and the highest frequency is noted.

7 Analysis Column is constructed to find out, which class is mode, the grouping is analyzed.

Example:

Calculate the mode of given discrete series.

Age of Children (X)	2	3	4	5	6	7	8	9	10	11	12	13
Number of Patients (f)	3	8	10	12	16	14	10	8	17	5	4	1

Solution:

X	f_1	F_2	F_3	F_4	F_5	F_6	Analysis
2	3						
3	8	11					
4	10		18	21			I = 1
5	12	22			30		III = 3
6	16		**28**			**38**	IIIII =5
7	14	**30**		**42**			III = 3
8	10		24		**40**		I= 1
9	8	18				32	
10	**17**		25	35			I = 1
11	5	22			30		
12	4		9			26	
13	1	5		10			

$M_0 = 6$

Class 6 is repeated 5 – times for constructing frequency columns.

MODE OF CONTINUOUS SERIES:

For the computation of mode of a continuous series, the following steps are involved, they are:

1 Determine the modal class interval. If the distribution is regular, modal class-interval can be obtained by observing the (inspection method) and in case of irregular distribution, modal class-interval is obtained by grouping method, which is followed in discrete series.

2 Mode is obtained by using the formula

$$M_0 = l_1 + \left(\frac{f_1 - f_0}{2f_1 - f_0 - f_2}\right) * i$$

M_0 = Mode

l_1 = lower limit of modal class interval

f_1 = Frequency of Modal class interval

f_0 = Frequency of the class preceding modal class interval

f_2 = Frequency of the class following modal class interval

i = Size of the class – interval

Example: Inspection Method:

Obtain the mode of the given continuous series.

Class (X)	0-10	10-20	20-30	30-40	40-50	50-60	60-70	70-80
Frequency (f)	02	18	30	45	35	20	06	03

Solution: The given distribution is regular, hence the modal class interval is 30-40.

l_1 = 30

f_1 = 45, f_0 = 30, f_2 = 35 and i = 10

$$M_0 = l_1 + \left(\frac{f_1 - f_0}{2f_1 - f_0 - f_2}\right) \times i$$

$$M_0 = 30 + \left(\frac{45 - 30}{2*45 - 30 - 35}\right) \times 10$$

Example: Grouping Method:

Obtain the mode of the given continuous series.

Class (X)	04-08	08-12	12-16	16-20	20-24	24-28	28-32	32-36	36-40
Frequency (f)	10	12	16	14	10	08	17	05	04

Solution:

X	f_1	f_2	f_3	f_4	f_5	f_6	Analysis	
04-08	10						I	1
08-12	12	22					III	3
12-16	16		28	38			IIIII	5
16-20	14	30			42		III	3
20-24	10		24			40	I	1
24-28	08	18		32				
28-32	17		25		35		I	1
32-36	05	25				30		
36-40	04		09	26				

The modal class interval is 12-16

$l_1 = 12, i = 4, f_1 = 16, f_2 = 14$ and $f_0 = 12$

$$M_0 = l_1 + \left(\frac{f_1 - f_0}{2f_1 - f_0 - f_2}\right) \times i$$

$$M_0 = 12 + \left(\frac{16 - 12}{2*16 - 12 - 14}\right) \times 4$$

Merits and Demerits

Merits

1 Mode is inherently descriptive of the data, in such a way that its meaning is easily understood

2 Mode is the most probable value in the distribution

3 Mode can be found out for those quantitative data in which categorization or ranking is possible

4 Like the median, mode is unaffected by the dispersion of series

5 It is not affected by extreme items. It can be calculated even if extremes are not known.

6 Mode is more precise value

7 Mode can be obtained from graph.

Demerits

1. Mode is not suitable for further mathematical treatment.

Exercises

1. A formulation was prepared to optimize the rotation per minute. The ingredients used are lipid and surfactant with 2-level and results obtained are as listed below.

SL.No.	RPM
1	2500
2	300
3	2600
4	2500
5	3200
6	300
7	2400
8	3100

Compute the arithmetic mean of RPM

Answer: AM = 2112.5

2. A formulation was prepared to measure spreadability and optimize the result. The six trails were done using different levels of one ingredient. The experimental result is as listed below

1	71.66
2	83.33
3	56.66
4	76.66
5	66.66
6	65

Compute the arithmetic mean of spreadability

Answer: 69.995

3. A formulation was prepared to measure viscosity and optimize the result. The six trials were done using different levels of one ingredient. The experimental result is as listed below

Sl.No.	Viscosity
1	71.66
2	84.56
3	64.24
4	78.2
5	67.34
6	69.23

Compute the arithmetic mean of Viscosity

Answer: AM = 72.54

4. A formulation was prepared to measure pH and optimize the result. The six trails were done using different levels of one ingredient. The experimental result is as listed below

Sl.No	pH
1	4.79
2	5.2
3	4.68
4	5.02
5	4.82
6	4.74

Compute the arithmetic mean of pH.

Answer: 4.875.

5. A total of 100 mg of three factors stearic acid(A), starch(B) and DCP(C), are added to prepare a formulation. Dissolution time was measured in a simplex design with results as listed below.

Combination level of Ingredients	Dissolution time9Mins)
100 mg(A)	292
100 mg (B)	5.6
100 mg (C)	51.4
50 mg (A) and 50 mg (B)	24.6
50 mg (B) and 50 mg (C)	16.4
50 mg (A) and 50 mg (C)	125.6
33.33 mg (A), 33.33 mg (B, 33.33 mg (C)	38.00

Compute the arithmetic mean of dissolution time.

Answer: AM=73.66

6. A experiment performed using a composite design to prepare formulation using two drugs A and B such that three doses are at equally spaced. The levels of drug A are 5 and 10 mg & B are 50 and 100 mg . The centre point for the composite design is the combination are 7.5 mg of A and 75 mg of. B. The total number of formations prepared and results obtained listed below.

Combination level of Ingredients	Response rate
5 mg and 50 mg	9.7
5 mg and 75 mg	9.2
5 mg and 100 mg	8.5
7.5 mg and 50 mg	6.2
7.5 mg and 75 mg	5.1
7.5 mg and 100 mg	4.2
10 mg and 50 mg	8.0
10 mg and 75 mg	7.5
10 mg and 100 mg	4.2

Compute the arithmetic mean of response

Answer : AM = 6.96

7. Compute average age of patients, who have been suffering due to diabetic for the data listed below.

AGE (X)		Number of Patients (f)
0	10	5
10	20	12
20	30	18
30	40	25
40	50	50
50	60	18
60	70	10
70	80	6

Answer: 40.76

3 Measures of Dispersion

An average, as a significant value representing the central tendency of a statistical distribution. To understand a statistical distribution fully it very important to calculate the measures of dispersion. The measures of dispersion conveys information regarding the amount of variability in a set of data. The truth is that an average, being just a single figure representing a mass of values and thus serving an important use, conceals the variation among the values. If all the items in a distribution are widely spread and there is no tendency to concentrate around one value, then it indicates that no average can adequately describe the distribution. If all the values are same, then there is no dispersion. The amount of dispersion may be small, when the values are different, but all are close together.

Taking the measure of central tendency as base, the structure of the statistical distribution can be of two types.

1. The average of distribution may be same, but formation of the items may be very much different

Example:

The average of five values equal to 10 in two sets of value, but deviation is different.

$$X: 0 \quad 5 \quad 10 \quad 15 \quad 20$$

$$\sum X = 50, \quad \bar{X} = \frac{50}{5} = 10$$

$$d_x = (X - \bar{X}) = -10 \quad -5 \quad 0 \quad 5 \quad 10$$

$$Y: 5 \quad 10 \quad 10 \quad 10 \quad 15$$

$$\sum Y = 50, \quad \bar{Y} = \frac{50}{5} = 10$$

$$d_y = (Y - \bar{Y}) = -5 \quad 0 \quad 0 \quad 0 \quad 5$$

2. Average may be different, but the distribution of the items may be the same.

SLNO	A	B	C	$d_A=(A - \bar{A})$	$d_B=(A - \bar{A})$	$d_C=(C - \bar{C})$
1	10	30	100	-2	-2	-2
2	11	31	101	-1	-1	-1
3	12	32	102	0	0	0
4	13	33	103	1	1	1
5	14	34	104	2	2	2
	$\sum A = 60$	$\sum B = 160$	$\sum C = 510$			

$$\bar{A} = \frac{\sum A}{n} = \frac{60}{5} = 12, \quad \bar{B} = \frac{\sum B}{n} = \frac{160}{5} = 32, \quad \bar{C} = \frac{\sum C}{n} = \frac{510}{5} = 102,$$

In this example averages are different, but there is uniformity in the constitution of the three series.

This clears that the nature of statistical distribution and the average of the deviations of the values of the items from mean cannot be ascertained on the basis of the mean.

So in order to describe the characteristics of the experimental data, the measures of central tendency as well as measures of variation or dispersion are also important.

Definition of Dispersion

The dispersion is a measure of the extent to which the individual items vary

Or

The degree to which numerical data tend to spread about an average value is called the variation or dispersion of the data.

The extent of variability in a given set of data is measured by comparing the individual values of the variable with the average of all the values and then calculating the average of all individual differences.

PURPOSE OF MEASURING VARIATIONS: There are important purpose of measuring the dispersion, they are

1. **To gauge the reliability of an average:**

    The average will be a satisfactory measure, when it is derived from the data that are homogeneous. To summarize the characteristics of a series, both average and a measure of dispersion must be present. Without the average there would be no standard against which to compare the individual values and no useful way of measuring the amount of variation. Without an average of difference or deviations between the values and their average, there would be no basis for generalizing about the extent of variability.

    When dispersion is small, the average is a typical value, that closely represent the individual values and the values of the distribution are reliable. In that situation it is a good estimate of the corresponding average in the population.

    When the dispersion is very high, this indicates that the average may be quite unreliable.

2. **To Serve as a basis for control of variability itself:**

    Dispersion is used to determine the nature and causes of variation in order to control the variation. In case of medical problems, variations in body temperature, blood pressure and pulse rate are basic guidelines for diagnosis. Based on these facts, treatment will be prescribed to control the variability of temperature, blood pressure etc.

    In pharmaceutical industry in the production department, efficient operation requires control of quality variation, the causes of which are sought through inspection and quality control program.

3. **To Compare two or more series with regard to their variability:**

   After the measurement of dispersion, the extent of variability between two or more series can be compared.

   Types of Measures of Dispersion:

   There are three important types of measures of dispersion, they are:

   a. Range

   b. Mean deviation

   c. Standard deviation

Range: One way to measure the variation in a set of values is to compute the range. This is one of the simplest measures of dispersion. To determine the range two extreme values of the distribution are required.

The range is the difference between the largest and the smallest value in a set of observations.

If R is notation for range and x_l and x_s denotes largest and smallest values in the distribution. Then the range can be obtained by using the formula $R = x_L - x_S$.

Example: Obtain the range for the age of 10 patients or subjects who participated in a study on smoking cessation.

AGE: 32   35   48   47   52   55   60   39   42   46

Solution: $X_L = 55$ and $X_S = 32$ then

Range $= X_L - X_S = 55 - 32 = 23$

Coefficient of Range:

The coefficient of range is a relative measure of range. It can be obtained by using the formula

$$\text{Coefficient of Range} = \frac{Largest\ value\ -Smallest\ value}{largest\ value\ +Smallest\ value}$$

$$\text{C.R} = \frac{L-R}{L+R}$$

Merits and Demerits

Merits

1. It is a simplest measure of dispersion or it is very easy to calculate and understand.
2. Ranges gives a broad picture of the data in that, it include limits within which all of the items occurs.
3. Range can be used to prepare control chart in the quality control department to control the quality of products.
4. It gives us total picture of the problem with a single glance.

Demerits

1. It is very much affected by extreme items.

2. The range provides no measures of the dispersion of other, except that they lie between two extreme values.
3. Range is influenced very much by fluctuation of sampling.
4. Range is not a reliable measure, because it depends only on extreme values.

Mean Deviation

The mean deviation is a measure of dispersion that is based upon all the items in a distribution.

The mean deviation is the arithmetic mean of the deviations of the data from a measure of central tendency. Average deviation is the average amount of scatter of items in a distribution from either the mean or Median or mode, ignoring the signs of the deviations.

The mean deviation can be defined as sum of the absolute deviations is divided by the number of items N

$$\text{M.D} = \frac{\Sigma |d|}{N}$$

Mean deviation can be denoted by symbols as

$\delta \bar{X}$ (Mean deviation from Mean)

δ_M (Mean deviation from Median)

δ_{M0} (Mean deviation from Mode)

Coefficient of Variation:

For the purpose of comparing variation among different sets of data, relative measures are required.

A relative measure of dispersion can be obtained by dividing the absolute measure of mean deviation by the average from which deviations were obtained.

(i)   Coefficient of mean deviation from Mean $= \dfrac{\delta \bar{X}}{\bar{X}}$

(ii)   Coefficient of mean deviation from median $= \dfrac{\delta M}{M}$

(iii)   Coefficient of mean deviation from median $= \dfrac{\delta M0}{M_0}$

Mean Deviation of Individual Series

Steps involved to obtain mean deviation are:

1. Compute arithmetic mean of the distribution
2. For each individual absolute deviation are obtained from mean
3. Summation of the absolute deviation is obtained
4. Mean deviation is obtained using the equation $\delta \bar{X} = \dfrac{\Sigma |d|}{N}$

Example:

SL NO	X	$|dx| = |X - \bar{X}|$
1	45	11
2	47	9
3	52	7
4	54	4
5	57	2
6	57	1
7	71	1
8	57	15
9	47	16
	$\sum X = 487$	$\sum |dx| = 66$

$$\bar{X} = \frac{\sum X}{N} = \frac{504}{9} = 54.1$$

$$\delta\bar{X} = \frac{\sum |d|}{N} = \frac{66}{9} = 7.33$$

Coefficient of mean deviation from Mean $= \dfrac{\delta\bar{X}}{\bar{X}} = \dfrac{7.33}{54.1} = 0.13\sum$

Mean Deviation – Discrete Series

To find the mean deviation of a discrete series, following steps are involved.

1. The mean of the distribution is computed

2. Absolute deviations of each individual values are obtained from mean

3. Total frequency of the distribution is obtained and that is written $N = \sum f$

4. Absolute deviations are multiplied with the corresponding frequencies and their products are added up $\sum f|dx|$

5. Mean deviation is obtained using the equation $\dfrac{\sum f|dx|}{\sum f}$

6. Coefficient of mean deviation is obtained by using the equation $\dfrac{\delta\bar{X}}{\bar{X}}$

Example:

Class (X)	Frequency (f)	fX	$|dx| = |X - \bar{X}|$	$f*|dx|$
4	2	8	6.2	12.4
6	1	6	4.2	4.2
8	3	24	2.2	6.6
10	6	60	0.2	1.2
12	4	48	1.8	7.2
14	3	42	3.8	11.4
16	1	16	5.8	5.8
	$N = \sum f = 20$	$\sum fX = 204$		$\sum f|dx| = 48.8$

$$\bar{X} = \frac{\Sigma fx}{N} = \frac{204}{20} = 10.2$$

$$\delta\bar{X} = \frac{\Sigma f|dx|}{\Sigma f} = \frac{48.8}{20} = 2.44$$

Coefficient of mean deviation $= \dfrac{\delta\bar{X}}{\bar{X}} = \dfrac{2.44}{10.2} = 0.239$

Mean Deviation of Continuous Series

To obtain mean deviation in a continuous series, the following steps are to be followed

1. The mean (AM) is obtained
2. Absolute deviation $|dx|$ are obtained for every mid values of the interval.
3. Later absolute deviations are multiplied with their respective frequencies and products are added up and sum of the product is obtained using the formula $\Sigma f|dx|$
4. Mean deviation is obtained using the formula $\delta\bar{X} = \dfrac{\Sigma f|dx|}{\Sigma f}$
5. Coefficient of mean deviation is obtained by using the equation $\dfrac{\delta\bar{X}}{\bar{X}}$

Example:

Class (X)	Frequency (f)	m	fm	$|dx| = |X - \bar{X}|$	$f*|dx|$
0-10	3	5	15	37.6	112.8
10-20	8	15	120	27.6	220.8
20-30	15	25	375	17.6	264.0
30-40	20	35	700	7.6	152.0
40-50	25	45	1125	2.4	60.0
50-60	10	55	550	12.4	124.0
60-70	9	65	585	22.4	201.6
70-80	6	75	450	32.4	194.4
80-90	4	85	340	42.4	169.4
	$N = \Sigma f = 100$		$\Sigma fm = 4260$		$\Sigma f|dx| = 1499.2$

$$\bar{X} = \frac{\Sigma fm}{N} = \frac{4260}{100} = 42.6$$

$$\delta\bar{X} = \frac{\Sigma f|dm|}{\Sigma f} = \frac{1499.2}{100} = 14.992$$

Coefficient of mean deviation $= \dfrac{\delta\bar{X}}{\bar{X}} = \dfrac{14.992}{42.6} = 0.351$

Standard Deviation

The concept of standard deviation was first introduced in the year 1893 by Karl Pearson. The term "standard" is assigned to this measure of variation probably, because it is the most flexible in terms of variety of applications of all measures of variation.

Standard deviation is also calculated using arithmetic mean of the distribution.

It is defined as the square root of the average of the squared deviations which is obtained from mean or arithmetic mean.

To compute standard deviation of a distribution, the deviation of the different values from the mean are found out. The deviations will be positive as well as negative. Then the individual deviations are squared up.

The standard deviation is denoted using symbol Greek letter (σ) small sigma.

The standard deviation of a sample is an estimate of the true standard deviation. The true standard deviation is a constant and does not change with the change in sample size, however, we can say that the estimate of the true standard deviation as observed in a sample is more reliable and less variable as the sample size increases. But on the average, the standard deviation of a small or large sample will approximate the true standard deviation.

Coefficient of Standard Deviation

To compare the variability between two groups of series or two groups of treatment, the relative measures of standard deviation is obtained. It is named as **"Coefficient of Standard deviation"**.

It is calculated using the equation $= \dfrac{\sigma}{\bar{X}}$

Standard Devaition of Individual Series

The steps involved in computations of standard deviation are

1. The arithmetic mean of distribution is obtained
2. The deviation of each items from mean is obtained.
3. Deviation of the distributions are squared up (d^2)
4. The sum of the squared deviations is obtained
5. Standard deviation is obtained using the equation $\sigma = \sqrt{\dfrac{\Sigma d^2}{N}}$

Example: Compute standard deviation of glucose level between five patients

Patient No	Glucose level (mg/dl)(X)	$d = (X - \bar{X})$	d^2
1	88	-2	4
2	92	2	4
3	89	-1	1

Patient No	Glucose level (mg/dl)(X)	$d = (X - \bar{X})$	d2
4	90	0	0
5	91	1	1
	$\Sigma x = 450$		$\Sigma d^2 = 10$
SD			

$$Mean = \bar{X} = \frac{\Sigma X}{N} = \frac{450}{5} = 90$$

$$\sigma = \sqrt{\frac{\Sigma d^2}{N}} = \sqrt{\frac{10}{5}} = 1.41$$

Standard Deviation of Discrete Series

To obtain the standard deviation of discrete series, following steps are considered.

1. The arithmetic mean ($\bar{X}$) of the series is calculated.

2. The deviations of each class values are found out from mean

3. Deviations are squared up ((d^2)

4. Squared value of deviations are multiplied with their respective frequencies and the total of the product is determined.

6. The standard deviation is obtained or determined using the formula $\sigma = \sqrt{\dfrac{\Sigma f d^2}{N}}$

Example: Estimate the mean duration and also standard deviation of post-partum amenorrhea from the following data. The data given below gives the month of resumption of menstrual cycle from the month of termination of pregnancy.

Month(X)	No. of Women (f)	fX	$d = (X - Mean)$	d^2	fd^2
1	15	15	-3.78	14.29	214.3031
2	51	102	-2.78	7.73	394.0911
3	107	321	-1.78	3.17	338.9419
4	92	368	-0.78	0.61	55.94381
5	81	405	0.22	0.05	3.927603
6	43	258	1.22	1.49	64.0224
7	30	210	2.22	4.93	147.8789
8	31	248	3.22	10.37	321.4607
9	22	198	4.22	17.81	391.8223
10	14	140	5.22	27.25	381.5071
11	7	77	6.22	38.69	270.8364
12	2	24	7.22	52.13	104.2626
	$N = \Sigma f = 495$	$\Sigma f x = 2366$			2688.998

$$Mean = \bar{X} = \frac{\Sigma fX}{N} = \frac{2366}{495} = 4.78$$

$$Standard\ Deviation = \sigma = \sqrt{\frac{\Sigma fd^2}{N}} = \sqrt{\frac{2688}{495}} = 2.33$$

Standard Deviation of Continuous Series

In case of continuous series, mid-values of class intervals are obtained, then Arithmetic Mean is obtained.

Then the procedure to calculate standard deviation is same as the discrete series procedure.

Example: Estimate the Average age and Standard deviation of the patients who are suffering due diabetic problem of the given distribution.

Age (X)		No. of patients (f)	mid value (m)	fm	$d=(m-\bar{X})$	d^2	fd^2
0	10	10	5	50	-34	1156	11560
10	20	19	15	285	-24	576	10944
20	30	34	25	850	-14	196	6664
30	40	100	35	3500	-4	16	1600
40	50	122	45	5490	6	36	4392
50	60	29	55	1595	16	256	7424
60	70	10	65	650	26	676	6760
70	80	6	75	450	36	1296	7776
		N =Σf = 330		Σf m=12870			57120
Mean	39						
SD	13.16						

$$Mean = \bar{X} = \frac{\Sigma fm}{N} = \frac{12870}{330} = 39$$

$$Standard\ Deviation = \sigma = \sqrt{\frac{\Sigma fd^2}{N}} = \sqrt{\frac{57120}{330}} = 13.16$$

VARIANCE: The Square of the standard deviation is called as variance. It is denoted as σ^2

COEFFICIENT OF VARIATION: The coefficient of standard deviation multiplied by 100 gives the coefficient of variation. It is written as $CV = \left(\frac{\sigma}{\bar{X}}\right) \times 100$

It indicates the relationship between the standard deviation and arithmetic mean expressed in terms of percentage. The coefficient of variation is also considered as relative standard deviation, it is denoted as RSD.

According to Professor Karl Pearson who recommended this measure "coefficient of variation is the percentage variation in mean, standard deviation considered as the total variation in the mean".

Coefficient of Variation plays very important role to compare the variability, stability, homogeneity, uniformity and consistency between two results which are carried out by applying two treatments.

Since the coefficient of variation is independent of the scale measurement, it is useful statistic for comparing the variability of two or more variables measured on different scales.

Example: The reduce in weight of 10- patients, by practicing two diets is recorded below.

Diet (A) (Kg): 5 2 5 3 4 4 3 5 6 6

Diet (B) (Kg): 5 3 7 10 5 6 7 9 12 13

Which diet is more variable and why?

Solution:

Diet A	Diet B	d_a=(A-Mean(A))	d_b=(B-Mean(B))	da^2	db^2
5	5	0.7	-2.7	0.49	7.29
2	3	-2.3	-4.7	5.29	22.09
5	7	0.7	-0.7	0.49	0.49
3	10	-1.3	2.3	1.69	5.29
4	5	-0.3	-2.7	0.09	7.29
4	6	-0.3	-1.7	0.09	2.89
3	7	-1.3	-0.7	1.69	0.49
5	9	0.7	1.3	0.49	1.69
6	12	1.7	4.3	2.89	18.49
6	13	1.7	5.3	2.89	28.09
ΣA43	ΣB77			16.1	94.1

$$\bar{A} = 43/10 = 4.3, \quad \bar{B} = 77/10 = 7.7$$

$$\sigma_A = \sqrt{\frac{16.1}{10}} = 1.27, \quad \sigma_B = \sqrt{\frac{94.1}{10}} = 3.07$$

$$CV_A = \left(\frac{\sigma}{\bar{A}}\right) \times 100 = 29.51, \quad CV_B = \left(\frac{\sigma}{\bar{B}}\right) \times 100 = 39.84$$

$CV_A > CV_B$, then diet(A) is more consistent than diet(B)

Determination of the range of the spread of items and verifying the normality of distribution.

The normal distribution is the most important and most widely used distribution in pharmaceutical calculation and also in clinical trial experiments. It is sometimes called the bell curves, although the total qualities of such bell would be less than the pleasing. It is also called as the Gaussian Curve.

The limits for the distribution of items are

$\bar{X} \pm \sigma$ Covers 68.27% of total items.

$\bar{X} \pm 2\sigma$ Covers 95.45% of total items.

$\bar{X} \pm 3\sigma$ Covers 99.33% of total items.

The distribution of data can be shown in graph.

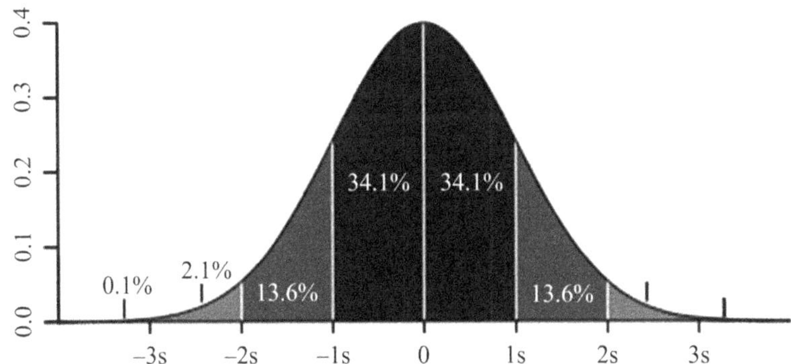

Example: Find the mean and standard deviation for the data listed below. What percentage of values lies on either side mean at la distance of $\pm\sigma$, $\pm2\sigma$, $\pm3\sigma$, where σ denotes standard deviation. On the basis of this, can it be inferred that the distribution is normal?

X	d = (X-Mean(X))	d^2
92	3	9
94	5	25
95	6	36
93	4	16
86	-3	9
78	-11	121
72	-17	289
68	-21	441
67	-22	484
66	-23	529
77	-12	144
81	-8	64
82	-7	49

Table contd...

88	-1	1
94	5	25
102	13	169
107	18	324
116	27	729
126	37	1369
96	7	49
1780		4882
$\bar{X}$	89	
σ	15.62	

$\bar{X} \pm \sigma = 89 \pm 15.62 = 104.62 - 73.38$

The items which are falling within this limits are 92, 94, 95, 93, 86, 78, 77, 81, 82, 88, 94, 102, 96

Total number of items equal to 13

Hence $(13/20)*100 = 65\%$ of the items fall within $\bar{X} \pm \sigma$

$\bar{X} \pm 2\sigma = 89 \pm 2*15.62 = 120.24 - 57.96$

The number of items falling within this limits are 92, 94, 95, 93, 86, 78, 77, 81, 82, 88, 94, 102, 96, 72, 68, 67, 66, 107, 116

Total number of items equal to 19

Hence $(19/20)*100 = 95\%$ of the items fall within $\bar{X} \pm 2\sigma$

$\bar{X} \pm 2\sigma = 89 \pm 2*15.62 = 120.24 - 57.96$

The number of items falling within this limits are 92, 94, 95, 93, 86, 78, 77, 81, 82, 88, 94, 102, 96, 72, 68, 67, 66, 107, 116, 126

Total number of items equal to 20

Hence $(20/20)*100 = 100\%$ of the items fall within $\bar{X} \pm 3\sigma$

Hence the distribution is almost normal

Merits and Demerits of Standard Deviation

Merits

1. The standard deviation makes use of all the information found in the set of observations. The meaning of that is, it includes every items of the experimental data.

2. Deviations are calculated from arithmetic mean and deviations are squared up, so that they automatically become positive. Being based on correct mathematical process, it is amenable to further statistical analysis.

3. It is a significant measure for making comparison between variability of two sets of observation, to test the significance of various statistical measures of random samples, correlation and regression analysis.

4. It provides the unit of measurement for the normal distribution.

Demerits

1. It is difficult to understand and compute the standard deviation

2. The extreme values are given more weight, because values are squared up.

Example 1: Compute standard deviation for the data given below

Patient No	Glucose level (mg/dl)(X)	D = (X - Mean)	d2
1	88	-2	4
2	92	2	4
3	89	-1	1
4	90	0	0
5	91	1	1
	450		10
5			
Mean	90		

Mean = 90,   SD = 1.41

Example 2: Compute standard deviation for the women patients who suffered due to cholera for the data as listed per month in the year 2012-13 due to water problem in a slum area of a particular city.

Month(X)	No. of Women (f)	fX	d = (X - Mean)	d^2	fd^2
1	15	15	-3.78	14.29	214.3031
2	51	102	-2.78	7.73	394.0911
3	107	321	-1.78	3.17	338.9419
4	92	368	-0.78	0.61	55.94381
5	81	405	0.22	0.05	3.927603
6	43	258	1.22	1.49	64.0224
7	30	210	2.22	4.93	147.8789
8	31	248	3.22	10.37	321.4607
9	22	198	4.22	17.81	391.8223
10	14	140	5.22	27.25	381.5071
11	7	77	6.22	38.69	270.8364
12	2	24	7.22	52.13	104.2626
	N = $\sum$f = 495	$\sum$f x = 366			$\sum$f d^2 = 2688.998

Answer: Mean = 4.78, SD = 2.33

4 Correlation and Regression

CORRELATION

Correlation refers to the relationship between the variables. Some relationship found in certain type of variables, for example the measure of relationship between time interval and concentration of drug that distributes in the body.

"WHEN THE RELATIONSHIP IS OF QUANTITATIVE IN NATURE, THE APPROPRIATE STATISTICAL TOOL FOR DISCOVERING AND MEASURING THE RELATIONSHIP AND EXPRESSING IT IN A BRIEF FROMULA IS KNOWN AS CORRELATION".

Two variables are said to be correlated, if the change in one variable results in a corresponding change in the other variables.

Correlation is a statistical technique which measures and analyzes the degree or extent to which two variables or phenomenon fluctuates with reference to each other. The correlation also denotes the interdependence between two variables.

Correlation methods are used to measure the association between two or more variables. Here one will be concerned with observations for each sampling unit. Here investigator will be interested in finding, if two values are related, in the sense that one variable may be predicted from a knowledge of the other. Better is the prediction, the better is the correlation.

Example: It is possible to find or predict the dissolution of a tablet based on tablet hardness. After obtaining the coefficient of correlation, we can say what type of correlation exits between dissolution and hardness.

Types of Correlation

On the basis of nature of relationship between the variables, i.e., the direction in which change takes place in them or the ratio by which they change, correlation can be classified as:

1. Positive or negative

2. Simple, Partial or Multiple correlation

3. Linear or Non-linear correlation

Positive or Negative Correlation

POSITIVE: Positive or direct correlation refers to the movement of the variables in the same direction. As one variable increases, the other variable also increases. Then this is called as positive correlation.

Example: In the distribution phase, the amount of drug that distributes in the body increases as the time increases. Vice versa is also true.

NEGATIVE: Negative or inverse correlation refers to, when one variable increases or decreases, as the other variable moves in the reverse direction. Such type of correlation is found between decrease in concentration of drug in body as time increases in elimination phase.

SIMPLE, PARTIAL or MULTIPLE CORRELATION: This refers to the number of variables involved in the study and the technique involved in measuring the correlation. When the study of relation involves only two variables the analysis of relationship between items is named as simple correlation. In this case the independent variable is named as **subject series** and the dependent variable is called as **relative series**.

In Pharmaceutical study or analysis, more than two variables are involved, then it is named as **multiple correlation**.

Example: The study of relationship between physical fitness, food habits and Physical exercises of a subject he practices.

LINEAR OR NON-LINEAR CORRELATION: Here the linear and non-linear correlation is based upon the consistency of the ratio of changes between the variables or factors which are considered in the study of experimental analysis.

If the ratio of change between two variables is uniform, then there will be linear correlation between them. This type of relationship is best described by a straight line.

In case of non-linear or curvilinear, the amount of change in one variable due to change in other variable, does not bear a constant ratio.

Example: The concentration of drug against time in body

Time	0	2	4	6	8
Concentration of drug (mg)	0	20	40	60	80

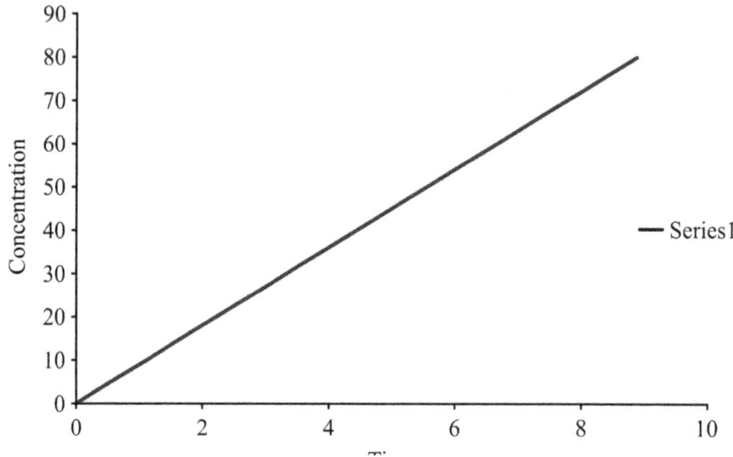

Time	0	2	4	6	8
Blood Pressure After treatment	180	140	120	112	110

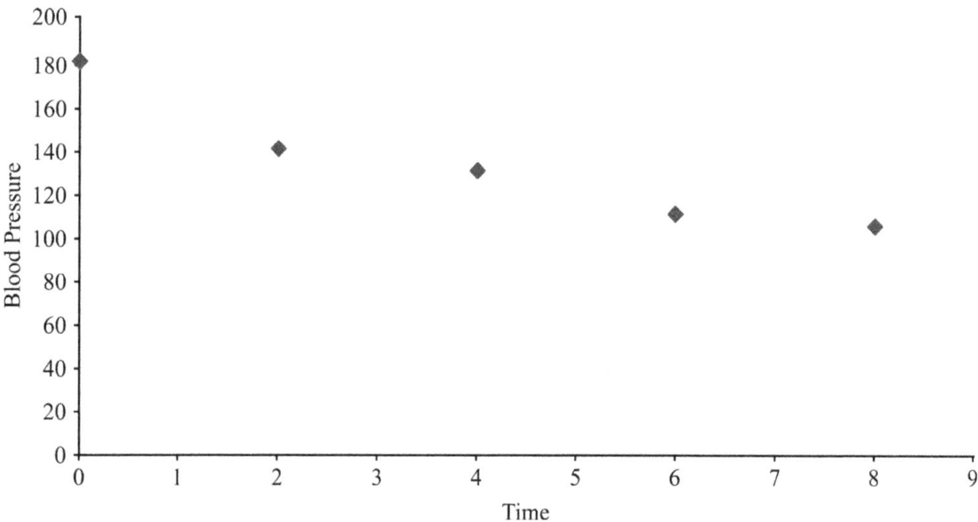

Degree of Correlation

The intensity of relationship between two variables can be ascertained by the quantitative value of coefficient of correlation which can be found out by computation.

Perfect Correlation

When changes between two variables are exactly proportional, there is perfect correlation between them. If the proportion of changes is in the same direction, then there is perfect positive correlation between two sets of variables. If equal proportional changes are in the opposite direction, then there is perfect negative correlation.

Absence of Correlation

If interdependence between the two variables does not exists, then it refers, the absence of correlation between the variables.

Karl Pearson has contributed an equation for measuring correlation. The result of that value will be denoted by r, that varies between ±1.

In case of Perfect +ve correlation, the value of r will be +1 and in case of Perfect negative correlation r will be -1.

If r is ± 0.9, this indicates that there is high degree correlation between two variables.

Degree of Correlation	Positive	Negative
Perfect correlation	+1	-1
Very High degree of correlation	+0.9 or more	-0.9 or more
Sufficiently high degree of correlation	+0.75 to +0.9	-0.75 to -0.9
Moderate degree of Correlation	+0.6 to +0.75	-0.6 to -0.75
Only the possibility of correlation	+0.3 to +0.6	-0.3 to -0.6
Possibly No correlation	<+0.3	<-0.3
Absence of correlation	0	0

OR

Strength of correlation	Size of r Interpretation
0.90 to 1.00	Very high correlation
0.70 to 0.89	High correlation
0.50 to 0.69	Moderate correlation
0.30 to 0.49	Low correlation
0.00 to 0.29	Little if any correlation

Methods of Studying Correlation

The commonly used methods for studying the correlation between two variables are:

(i)   Scatter diagram method

(ii)   Karl Pearson's coefficient of correlation (Covariance Method)

(iii)   Rank difference method.

Scatter Diagram Method

Scatter diagram is one of simplest tool of ascertaining the correlation between two variables.

For example the variable X-denotes height and variable Y-denotes weight respectively, then pairs, (x_1, y_1), (x_2, y_2) ----(x_n, y_n) may represent the heights and weights in pairs. The diagram of dots so obtained is known as scatter diagram.

a. If the points are very close to each other, that indicates a fairly good amount of correlation may be expected.

b. If the points on the scatter diagram explains any trend (dots moving upward or downward) the variables are said to be correlated and if no trend is explained, the variables are uncorrelated.

c. If there is an upward trend rising from lower left corner and moving upward to the right corner, then correlation is said to be +ve correlation.

   On the other hand, if the points, depict a downward trend from the upper left hand corner to lower right corner, then the correlation is said to be −ve correlation

d. If all the points lie on a straight line, moving upward then the correlation is perfect +ve correlation.

e. If all the points lie on a straight line, moving downward, then the correlation is said to perfect −ve correlation.

   The data below are heart rates of students. Students measured their heart rates (in beats per minute), then took a brisk walk and measured their heart rates again.

Before	After		Before	After		Before	After
86	98		58	128		60	70
62	70		64	74		80	92
52	56		74	106		66	70
90	110		76	84		80	92
66	76		56	96		78	116
80	96		72	82		74	114
78	86		72	78		90	116
74	84		68	90		76	94

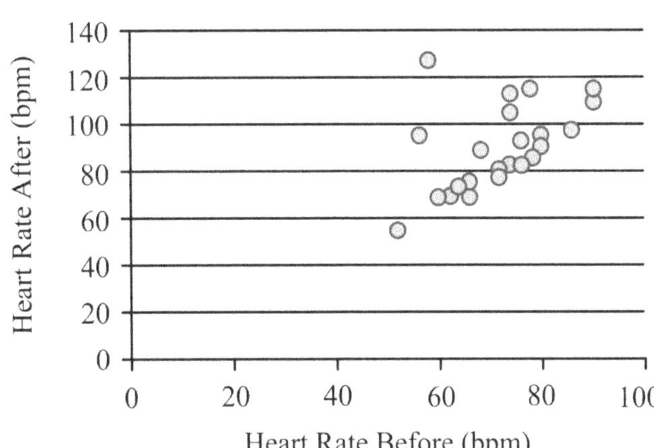

KARL PEARSON'S COEFFICIENT OF CORRELATION (COVARIANCE METHOD)

The correlation coefficient is a quantitative measure of the relationship of two variables. This will measure the intensity of linear relationship between two variables. This method was designed by Karl Pearson. This is the most widely used method to measure the relationship between two variables.

If X and Y are two variables, then the relationship between them is denoted by the symbol or notation r_{xy} or r.

The equation is $r = \dfrac{\sum d_x d_y}{N\sigma_x \sigma_y}$

$\sum d_x d_y$ = Covariance of X & Y

σ_x = Standard deviation of X- series

σ_y = Standard deviation of Y- series

N = Number of subjects or items of both the series

Example 1: Compute the coefficient of correlation Age and Bilirubin level of 10 patients for the data listed below

AGE X	Bilirubin (mg/dl) Y	$d_x=(X-\bar{X})$	$d_y=(Y-\bar{Y})$	d^2_x	d^2_y	$d_x \times d_y$
70	11	12.4	1.71	153.76	2.92	21.204
68	12.3	10.4	3.01	108.16	9.06	31.304
81	14.7	23.4	5.41	547.56	29.27	126.594
59	9.1	1.4	-0.19	1.96	0.04	-0.266
64	7.8	6.4	-1.49	40.96	2.22	-9.536
48	6	-9.6	-3.29	92.16	10.82	31.584
50	9	-7.6	-0.29	57.76	0.08	2.204
44	7	-13.6	-2.29	184.96	5.24	31.144
50	8	-7.6	-1.29	57.76	1.66	9.804
42	8	-15.6	-1.29	243.36	1.66	20.124
ΣX 576	ΣY 92.9			Σd^2_x 1488.4	Σd^2_y 62.989	$\Sigma d_x \times d_y$ 264.16

$$\bar{X} = \frac{\Sigma X}{N} = \frac{576}{10} = 57.6 \qquad \bar{Y} = \frac{\Sigma Y}{N} = \frac{92.9}{10} = 9.29$$

$$\sigma_x = \sqrt{\frac{d^2_x}{N}} = \sqrt{\frac{1488.4}{10}} = 12.20 \qquad \sigma_y = \sqrt{\frac{d^2_y}{N}} = \sqrt{\frac{62.989}{10}} = 2.509$$

$$r = \frac{\Sigma d_x d_y}{N \sigma_x \sigma_y} = \frac{264.16}{10*12.2\times.2509} = 0.863$$

Example 2: A single dose of 500 mg drug was administered by a rapid IV injection to the patient who is weighing 75 kg. Plasma sample were obtained from 0 hour to 7 hours and assay of the drug as tabulated below. Compute the co-efficient correlation.

Time (t)	Concentration (mg/L) (X)	Dt = (t-Mean(t))	Dx = (X-Mean(x))	dt^2	dx^2	Dt×dx
0	69	-2.58	43.54	6.66	1895.73	-112.33
0.25	54.8	-2.33	29.34	5.43	860.84	-68.36
0.5	43.2	-2.08	17.74	4.33	314.71	-36.90
0.75	35.1	-1.83	9.64	3.35	92.93	-17.64
1	29	-1.58	3.54	2.50	12.53	-5.59

Time (t)	Concentration (mg/L) (X)	Dt = (t-Mean(t))	Dx = (X-Mean(x))	dt^2	dx^2	dt*dx
1.5	21.3	-1.08	-4.16	1.17	17.31	4.49
2	17	-0.58	-8.46	0.34	71.57	4.91
2.5	14.2	-0.08	-11.26	0.01	126.79	0.90
3	12.7	0.42	-12.76	0.18	162.82	-5.36
4	10.5	1.42	-14.96	2.02	223.80	-21.24
5	9	2.42	-16.46	5.86	270.93	-39.83
6	8.2	3.42	-17.26	11.70	297.91	-59.03
7	7	4.42	-18.46	19.54	340.77	-81.59
$\sum t$= 33.5	$\sum X$ = 331			63.05	4688.63	-437.59

$$\text{Mean(t)} = \frac{\sum t}{n} = \frac{33.5}{13} = 2.58$$

$$\text{Mean(x)} = \frac{\sum x}{n} = \frac{331}{13} = 25.46$$

$$\text{SD(t)} = \sqrt{\frac{\sum dt^2}{n}} = \sqrt{\frac{63.05}{13}} = 2.20$$

$$\text{SD(X)} = \sqrt{\frac{\sum dx^2}{n}} = \sqrt{\frac{4688.63}{13}} = 18.99$$

$$r = \frac{\sum d_t d_x}{N \sigma_t \sigma_x} = \frac{-437.59}{13 \times 2.20 \times 18.99} = -0.80$$

PROBABLE ERROR

After computing the value of the correlation coefficient, the next step is to find, to what extent to which it is dependable. Probable error of correlation coefficient, denoted as PE(r) , a method is used to verify the level of reliability of an observed value of correlation coefficient in so far as it depends upon the condition of random sampling.

If r is coefficient of correlation and N is Number of subjects or observations in each group, then standard error of r is written as SE(r) and it is obtained by the equation $SE(r) = \frac{1-r^2}{\sqrt{N}}$ .Then the probable error of r is obtained by the equation $P.E(r) = 0.6745 \times SE(r)$.

The 0.6745 is taken, because that in a normal distribution 50% of the observations or results obtained from an experiments lie in the range of $\mu \pm 0.6745 \times \sigma$.

μ = Mean of the population

σ = Standard deviation

The probable error of correlation coefficient may be defined as an amount which is added to and subtracted from the mean correlation coefficient, gives the values within which the chances are even that a coefficient of correlation from a series selected at random will fall.

USES OF PROBABLE ERROR

1. It will be used to determine the limits within which the population correlation coefficient would lie. The limit is obtained by the equation $r \pm PE(r)$

2. The Probable error can be used to test the significance of r.

3. If r< PE(r) , r is less than its P.E(r) , then r is not significant

4. If r>6×PE . If r is greater than 6 times of PE , then r is definitely significant..

5. In some situation, nothing can be concluded with certainty.

ASSUMPTION UNDERLYING KARL PEARSON'S CORRELATION COEFFICIENT

i. Two variables X and Y which are considered for study are linearly related.

ii. Every variables or series is being affected by large number of independent contributory, causes of such a nature so as to produce normal distribution.

Example: The variables like Ages, heights, weights, BP, sugar etc., conform to this assumption.

iii. The forces so operating on each of the variable of the series are not independent of each other, but are related in a causal fashion.

Example: Cause and effect relationship exists between with different types of forces, which are operating on the items of the two variable series.

1. Intelligence and Income

2. Health condition and Income.

INTERPRETATION OF r

The observed or computed value of r can be interpreted as:

i. If r = +1, this indicates, there is a perfect positive correlation between the variables

ii. If r = -1, this implies that there is perfect negative correlation between variables.

iii. If r = 0 indicates, that there is no correlation or the absence of correlation between the variables which are taken for study.

iv. If r lies between +1 and -1 , then this indicates, there will be set guidelines to give interpretation. At the most one can conclude, if r is nearer to 1 , then closer is the relationship between the variables.

v. The r is significant, can be decided by computing probable error.

MULTIPLE CORRELATION

To study the relationship of more than two dependent variables with one independent variables, multiple correlation method is applied.

The multiple correlation is a measure of combined relationship of two or more dependent variables.

The multiple correlation can be calculated using equations

$$r_{x.yz} = \sqrt{\frac{r_{xy}^2 + r_{xz}^2 - 2\,r_{xy}\,r_{yz}\,r_{zx}}{1 - r_{yz}^2}}$$

Similarly

$$r_{y.xz} = \sqrt{\frac{r_{yz}^2 + r_{yx}^2 - 2\,r_{xy}\,r_{yz}\,r_{zx}}{1 - r_{xz}^2}}$$

$$r_{z.xy} = \sqrt{\frac{r_{zx}^2 + r_{zy}^2 - 2\,r_{xy}\,r_{yz}\,r_{zx}}{1 - r_{xy}^2}}$$

Example:

For the given data, obtain the multiple correlation between Height(X), radius length(Y) and Femur length (Z) as listed below.

Height (X)	Radius Length (Y)	Femur Length (Z)	d_x	d_y	d_z	dx^2	dy^2	dz^2	dx*dy	dy*dz	dz*dx
149	21	42	-14.8	-2.441	-5.34	219.04	5.96	28.52	36.13	13.03	79.03
152	21.79	43.5	-11.8	-1.651	-3.84	139.24	2.73	14.75	19.48	6.34	45.31
155	22.4	44	-8.8	-1.041	-3.34	77.44	1.08	11.16	9.16	3.48	29.39
159	23	46.4	-4.8	-0.441	-0.94	23.04	0.19	0.88	2.12	0.41	4.51
162	24	47.5	-1.8	0.559	0.16	3.24	0.31	0.03	-1.01	0.09	-0.29
166	24.3	48	2.2	0.859	0.66	4.84	0.74	0.44	1.89	0.57	1.45
172	24.92	49	8.2	1.479	1.66	67.24	2.19	2.76	12.13	2.46	13.61
174	25	50	10.2	1.559	2.66	104.04	2.43	7.08	15.90	4.15	27.13
176	26	51	12.2	2.559	3.66	148.84	6.55	13.40	31.22	9.37	44.65
173	22	52	9.2	-1.441	4.66	84.64	2.08	21.72	-13.26	-6.72	42.87
$\sum X = 1638$	$\sum Y\ 234.41$	$\sum Z$ 473.4				$\sum dx^2$ 871.6	$\sum dy^2$ 24.25569	$\sum dz^2$ 100.704	$\sum dxdy$ 113.762	$\sum dy \times dz$ 33.1756	$\sum dz \times dx$ 287.68
$\bar{X} = 163.8$	$\bar{Y} = 23.441$	$\bar{Z} = 47.34$									

$$\bar{X} = \frac{\sum X}{N} = \frac{1639}{10} = 163.8 \qquad \bar{Y} = \frac{\sum Y}{N} = \frac{234.41}{10} = 23.441 \qquad \bar{Z} = \frac{\sum Z}{N} = \frac{473.4}{10} = 47.34$$

$$\sigma_x = \sqrt{\frac{\sum dx^2}{N}} = \sqrt{\frac{871.6}{10}} = 9.34, \quad \sigma_y = \sqrt{\frac{\sum dy^2}{N}} = \sqrt{\frac{24.255}{10}} = 1.56, \quad \sigma_z = \sqrt{\frac{\sum dz^2}{N}} = \sqrt{\frac{100.704}{10}} = 3.17$$

$$r_{xy} = \frac{\sum d_x d_y}{N \sigma_x \sigma_y} = \frac{113.762}{10 \times 9.34 \times 1.56} = 0.78, \quad r_{yz} = \frac{\sum d_y d_z}{N \sigma_y \sigma_z} = \frac{33.1756}{10 \times 1.56 \times 3.17} = 0.67$$

$$r_{xz} = \frac{\Sigma d_x d_z}{N \sigma_x \sigma_z} = \frac{287.68}{10 \times 9.34 \times 3.17} = 0.97$$

$$r_{x.yz} = \sqrt{\frac{r_{xy}^2 + r_{xz}^2 - 2\, r_{xy}\, r_{yz}\, r_{zx}}{1 - r_{yz}^2}} = 0.99$$

Partial Correlation

The partial correlation will be considered, when tow variables may be correlated partly on account of the fact, that each of them is correlated with third variable.

The equation used for computing coefficient of partial correlation are

$$r_{xy.z} = \frac{r_{xy} - r_{yz} * r_{xz}}{\sqrt{(1 - r_{xz}^2)(1 - r_{yz}^2)}}$$

$$r_{xz.y} = \frac{r_{xz} - r_{xy} * r_{yz}}{\sqrt{(1 - r_{xy}^2)(1 - r_{yz}^2)}}$$

$$r_{yz.x} = \frac{r_{yz} - r_{xy} * r_{xz}}{\sqrt{(1 - r_{xy}^2)(1 - r_{xz}^2)}}$$

The purpose of partial correlation coefficient is to measure the intensity of the relationship between any two variables when the influence of all other variable has been removed.

REGRESSION ANALYSIS

Regression means to revert or return back. This term was first introduced by Sir Francis Galton in 1877, who was a British Biometrician.

But today the word regression is used in statistics has a much wider perspective without any reference to Biometry.

In general sense, the regression analysis means the estimation or prediction of one unknown value of one variable from the known value of the other variable. It is one of the most widely used method in pharmaceutical science to analyze the experimental results of formulations and clinical trial problems.

Regression Analysis also is a mathematical measure of the average relationship between two or more variables in term of the original unit of data".

Simple linear regression analysis is a statistical technique that defines the functional relationship between two variables X and Y by the best fitting straight line. The straight is described by the equation Y = a + bX. Here Y is considered as dependent variable (ordinate) and X is independent variable (abscissa), and a and b are the y-intercept and slope of the regression line.

This technique is commonly used to:

1. To establish the functional relationship between optical density against drug concentration.

2. When the functional form of a response is unknown, but here one wish to represent a trend or rate as characterized by the slope.

   Example: Pharmacological action of drug with respect to time

3. When a process is described by relatively simple equation, that will establish a relation of response Y to a fixed value of X.

   Example: Stability Prediction.

   Concentration of drug against time, can be measured or predicted using simple regression function or equation.

SIMPLE REGRESSION ANALYSIS

The regression analysis when it is confined to the study of only two variables at a time, is named as simple regression.

The regression analysis when it is applied for establishing a functional relationship between more than two variables, at a time is known as multiple regression.

Linear and Non-linear Regression

When the given bivariate data plotted on a graph, the scatter diagram will be more or less will be around a curve, that is termed as curve of regression.

If the regression curve is straight line, we say that there is linear regression between the variable under study.

However, if the curve of regression is not a straight line or linear, regression can be called as non-linear regression or curved regression.

MULTIPLE REGRESSION: Multiple regression involves more than two independent variables and one dependent variable.

OBJECT OF REGRESSION ANALYSIS: There are some objectives of regression

1. To provide a procedure to estimate of values of the dependent variable from the values of independent variables. The estimation of values can be done by applying the regression line. This line describes the average relationship existing between X and Y variables.

2. The second objective is to obtain a measure of the error involved in using the regression line as a basis for estimation.

REGRESSION LINES: Line of regression is the line which gives the best estimate of one variable from any value of other variable.

When there are two variables under study, then there will be two lines of regression, they are Y on X and X on Y. These two regression lines show the average relationship between the variables. These two equations can be written as

1. $Y = a + bX$ where Y is dependent and X-is independent.
2. $X = a + bY$ where X is dependent and Y is independent.

Here a – Intercept and b – slope.

These two equations can be compared with the equation of the straight line $Y = mX + C$ or $Y = C + mX$ and $X = mY + C$ or $X = C + mY$.

The equations $y = a + bx$ and $x = a + by$ cut each other at the point of mean of X and Y.

If the correlation between X and Y is (± 1) is perfect, then these two lines will coincide, i.e., there will be only one line.

If the correlation between X and Y is zero ($r = 0$), these two lines will be perpendicular to each other. The perpendicular drawn from the point of intersection touch the X-axis at the mean value of X and other one touch Y-axis at the mean value of Y.

FORMATION OF REGRESSION EQUATION

1. Normal Equation form

The normal equation, for finding the values of constants a and b in the regression equation y on x ($y = a + bx$) are

$$\sum y = Na + b\sum x \qquad .....1$$

$$\sum xy = a\sum x + b\sum x^2 \qquad .....2$$

For the equation x on y ($x = a + by$) the normal equations used are

$$\sum x = Na + b\sum y \qquad .....1$$

$$\sum xy = a\sum x + b\sum x^2 \qquad .....2$$

Example: A drug seems to decompose in a manner, such that appearance of degradation of product is linear with time ($c_d = kt$)

X(t) :	1	2	3	4	5
Y(Cd) :	3	9	12	17	19

Solution:

X	Y	X^2	y^2	xy
1	3	1	9	3
2	9	4	81	18
3	12	9	144	36
4	17	16	289	68
5	19	25	361	95
$\sum x = 15$	$\sum y = 60$	$\sum x^2 = 55$	$\sum y^2 = 884$	$\sum xy = 220$

$$\sum y = Na + b\sum x$$

$$60 = 5a + b15$$

$$60 = 5a + 15b \qquad .....(1)$$

$$\sum xy = a\sum x + b\sum x^2$$

$220 = a15 + b\,55$

$220 = 15a + 55b$ $\qquad$ .....(2)

Solve 1 and 2

$(60 = 5a + 15b)*3$

$220 = 15a + 55b$

$180 = 15a + 45b$

Subtract these two equations

$220 = 15a + 55b$

$180 = 15a + 45b$

$40 = \qquad 10b$

$10b = 40$

$b = 4$

Substitute $b = 4$ in equation $60 = 5a + 15b$

$60 = 5a + 15\times4$

$60 = 5a + 60$

$5a = 0$

$a = 0$

The Equation is y a + bx is written as $y = 0 + 4x$

$y = 4x$

in this equation $a = 0$ and $b = 4$

FORMATION OF REGRESSION EQUATION BY MATRIX METHOD

Example:

X	Y
5	3
8	4
7	5
6	2
4	1

Solution:

$$X = \begin{bmatrix} 1 & 5 \\ 1 & 8 \\ 1 & 7 \\ 1 & 6 \\ 1 & 4 \end{bmatrix} \quad Y = \begin{bmatrix} 3 \\ 4 \\ 5 \\ 2 \\ 1 \end{bmatrix} \text{ and } \alpha = \begin{bmatrix} a \\ b \end{bmatrix}$$

$$X^T = \begin{bmatrix} 1 & 1 & 1 & 1 & 1 \\ 5 & 8 & 7 & 6 & 4 \end{bmatrix}$$

$$X^T X = \begin{bmatrix} 1 & 1 & 1 & 1 & 1 \\ 5 & 8 & 7 & 6 & 4 \end{bmatrix} \begin{bmatrix} 1 & 5 \\ 1 & 8 \\ 1 & 7 \\ 1 & 6 \\ 1 & 4 \end{bmatrix}$$

$$= \begin{bmatrix} 1+1+1+1+1 & 5+8+7+6+4 \\ 5+8+7+6+4 & 25+64+49+36+16 \end{bmatrix}$$

$$X^T X = \begin{bmatrix} 5 & 30 \\ 30 & 190 \end{bmatrix}$$

Find Co-factor Matrix of $X^T X$

$$\left. \begin{array}{l} \text{Cofactor of } 5 = +(190) \\ \textit{Cofactor of } 30 = -(30) \end{array} \right\} \text{- First row elements}$$

$$\left. \begin{array}{l} \text{Cofactor of } 30 = -(30) \\ \textit{Cofactor of } 30 = +(5) \end{array} \right\} - \text{Second row elements}$$

Cofactor Matrix $X^T X = \begin{bmatrix} 190 & -30 \\ -30 & 5 \end{bmatrix}$

adjoint$(X^T X) = \begin{bmatrix} 190 & -30 \\ -30 & 5 \end{bmatrix}$ (Transpose of Co-factor Matrix)

$$\left| X^T X \right| = \begin{vmatrix} 5 & 30 \\ 30 & 190 \end{vmatrix} = 950 - 900 = 50$$

$$[X^T X]^{-1} = \frac{1}{\left| X^T X \right|} \text{ adjoint } (X^T X)$$

$$= \frac{1}{50} \begin{bmatrix} 190 & -30 \\ -30 & 5 \end{bmatrix}$$

Find the product of $X^T Y = \begin{bmatrix} 1 & 1 & 1 & 1 & 1 \\ 5 & 8 & 7 & 6 & 4 \end{bmatrix} \begin{bmatrix} 3 \\ 4 \\ 5 \\ 2 \\ 1 \end{bmatrix}$

$$= \begin{bmatrix} 3+4+5+2+1 \\ 5+8+7+6+4 \end{bmatrix}$$

$$= \begin{bmatrix} 15 \\ 98 \end{bmatrix}$$

Find the product of $[X^T X]^{-1}\ X^T Y = \alpha = \begin{bmatrix} a \\ b \end{bmatrix}$

$$\begin{bmatrix} a \\ b \end{bmatrix} = \frac{1}{50} \begin{bmatrix} 190 & -30 \\ -30 & 5 \end{bmatrix} \begin{bmatrix} 15 \\ 98 \end{bmatrix}$$

$$= \frac{1}{50} \begin{bmatrix} 2850 - 2940 \\ -450 + 490 \end{bmatrix}$$

$$= \frac{1}{50} \begin{bmatrix} -90 \\ 40 \end{bmatrix}$$

$$\begin{bmatrix} a \\ b \end{bmatrix} = \begin{bmatrix} -1.8 \\ 0.8 \end{bmatrix}$$

$a = -1.8$

$b = 0.8$

$Y = a + bX$

$Y = -1.8 + 0.8X$

MULTIPLE REGRESSION

Multiple regression is the extension of simple regression, it is applied to measure the effect of more than one independent variable X on the dependent variable Y. The principles involved between multiple and simple regression are same.

In the multiple regression ,we assume that a linear relationship exists between k-independent variables of X $(x_1, x_2, x_3\text{-------------}x_k)$ and dependent variable Y. Very often the independent variables referred as explanatory variables, because of their use in explaining the variation in Y. These independent variables can also be called as predictor variables, because of their use in predicting. Very often the independent variables referred as explanatory variables, because of their use in explaining the variation in Y. These independent variables can also be called as predictor variables, because of their use in predicting Y or Y can be predicted with the use of the variables x_1, $x_2, x_3\text{-------------}x_k$ independent variables.

This multiple regression equation measures the simultaneous effect of a number of independent variables.

The general equation of multiple regression can be written in the form as

$$Y = a + b_1x_1 + b_2x_2 + \ldots\ldots\ldots + b_kx_k$$

FORMATION OF REGRESSION EQUATION BY MATRIX METHOD

If the independent variables are x_1, x_2 and x_3 and dependent variable is Y, then the regression equation will be $Y = a + b_1x_1 + b_2x_2 + b_3x_3$. The regression coefficients and intercept can be obtained by matrix method, as explained below.

$$X = \begin{bmatrix} 1 & x11 & x21 \\ 1 & x12 & x22 \\ 1 & x13 & x23 \\ . & . & . \\ . & . & . \\ 1 & x1k & x2k \end{bmatrix} \qquad Y = \begin{bmatrix} y1 \\ y2 \\ : \\ yk \end{bmatrix} \quad \text{and} \quad \alpha = \begin{bmatrix} a \\ b1 \\ b2 \end{bmatrix}$$

1. Obtain the transpose of X, X^T

2. Obtain the product of $X^T X$

3. Obtain cofactor matrix of $X^T X$

4. Obtain the value of determinant $|XT\ X|$

5. Obtain the adjoint of $(X^T X)$

6. Obtain the inverse of $X^T X$, $[X^T X]^{-1} = \dfrac{1}{|X^T\ X|}$ adjoint$(X^T X)$

7. Obtain the product of X^T with Y, i.e., $X^T Y$

8. Then to find the regression coefficients, obtain the product of $[X^T X]^{-1}$ and $X^T Y$
   i.e., $[X^T X]^{-1} X^T Y$

$$\alpha = [X^T X]^{-1} X^T Y$$

$$\begin{bmatrix} a \\ b1 \\ b2 \end{bmatrix} = [X^T X]^{-1} X^T Y$$

After obtaining the values a, b_1, b_2 then the equation can be written as $Y = a + b_1 x_1 + b_2 x_2$

With the help of this multiple regression, we can estimate the predicted values of dependent variable (Y) , which is influenced by two independent variables x1 and x2 using the equation

$Y = a + b_1 x_1 + b_2 x_2$

Example: The following table shows the weight and total cholesterol and triglyceride level in 10 patients just before treatment. Find the multiple regression equation which describes the relationship between the variables.

Y Weight (Kg)	X1 (Total Cholesterol (mg/100ml)	X2 (Triglyceride (Mg/100ml)
76	301	130
78	370	102
89	420	57
70	346	67
52	376	112
67	321	42
78	423	78
73	345	60
80	370	67
81	325	80

PARTIAL REGRESSION COEFFICIENT

The partial regression coefficient can be obtained with the help of standard deviation and correlation coefficients.

The formulae used for calculation of partial regression coefficients are

$$b_{12.3} = \frac{\sigma_1}{\sigma_2} \times \frac{r12 - r13 * r23}{1 - r_{23}^2}$$

$$b_{13.2} = \frac{\sigma_1}{\sigma_3} \times \frac{r13 - r12 * r23}{1 - r_{13}^2}$$

$$b_{21.3} = \frac{\sigma_2}{\sigma_1} \times \frac{r21 - r23 * r13}{1 - r_{13}^2}$$

STANDARD ERROR ESTIMATE OF REGRESSION

The line of best fit is really a line of average relationship, since for each x-value it represents the various Y-values on an average y-values, and by connecting the points for these average values a straight line is formed. Here each value on the line is like an average that used to represent the central tendency of many values. Just like an average, each point on the line conceals the variation that exists around it. If the variation around an average is very small, the average may be used to estimate with a high degree of accuracy of any of the values around it.

The variation around the line of the best fit found out by standard error of estimate. The measure is the standard deviation of the errors of estimating Y for X or X for Y.

If the actual and estimated values are the same, then the standard error of estimate will be zero. In this case correlation coefficient r = 1 and correlation must be perfect and all estimates made from the regression equation must be perfect.

The equation used for computing standard error estimate is $S_{yx} = \sqrt{\frac{(y - y^1)}{N - k}}$, $S_{xy} = \sqrt{\frac{(x - x^1)}{N - k}}$ where S_{yx} is standard error of estimate for y on x and S_{xy} is standard error of estimate for x on y .

$y - y^1$ = deviation between actual value and computed value of x-variables and $x - x^1$ = deviation between actual and computed value of y-variables.

N = Number of items

K = Number of constants in the regression equation

K = 2 when one dependent and one independent variables are considered.

In case of multiple regression (three variables are considered), then the standard error estimate is obtained by the equation $S_{yx} = \sqrt{\frac{(y - y^1)}{N - k}}$. In this case K = 3

CONFIDENCE INTERVAL FOR SLOPE (b) and INTERCEPT (a)

To construct a confidence interval for slope – b the standard error of b, $S_b = \dfrac{Syx}{\sqrt{\Sigma(X-\bar{X})^2}}$ is estimated and t- is computed us ing equation $t = \dfrac{b-0}{s_b}$.

The value of t for degree of freedom N – K at the level of significance (95% or 99%) will be compared with calculated value (computed value) of t. If the computed value of t is greater than the table value, the relationship will be linear with the computed value of standard error, then the confidence limits of b can be obtained us ing the equation b±1.96S$_b$ at 95% level of significance for the corresponding degree of freedom (N – K)

Problem:

X	Y	dx= (X-Mean(x))	dy= (Y-Mean(y))	dx^2	dy^2	dx*dy	y^1 = 7.6*x +32	(y-y^1)	(y-y^1)^2
3	40	-2	-30	4	900	60	54.8	-14.8	219.04
3	55	-2	-15	4	225	30	54.8	0.2	0.04
4	55	-1	-15	1	225	15	62.4	-7.4	54.76
4	60	-1	-10	1	100	10	62.4	-2.4	5.76
4	75	-1	5	1	25	-5	62.4	12.6	158.76
5	70	0	0	0	0	0	70	0	0
5	80	0	10	0	100	0	70	10	100
5	75	0	5	0	25	0	70	5	25
6	90	1	20	1	400	20	77.6	12.4	153.76
6	80	1	10	1	100	10	77.6	2.4	5.76
7	75	2	5	4	25	10	85.2	-10.2	104.04
8	85	3	15	9	225	45	92.8	-7.8	60.84
60	840			26	2350	195	840		887.76

$\bar{X} = 5$

$\bar{Y} = 70$

$\sigma_x = 1.47$

$\sigma_y = 13.99$

$r = 0.8$

Regression Equation Y on X

$(Y - \bar{Y}) = (r\dfrac{\sigma x}{\sigma y}(X - \bar{X}))$

(Y-70)= 0.8×14/1.47(X - 5)

Y- 70 = 7.6X - 38.0

Y = 7.6X+32

Standard Error of Estimate:

$$S_{yx} = \sqrt{\frac{(y-y^1)}{N-k}} \quad = \quad \sqrt{\frac{(887.76)}{12-2}} = 9.42$$

Standard of b:

$$Sb = \frac{Syx}{\sqrt{\Sigma(X-\bar{X})^2}} = \frac{9.42}{\sqrt{26}} = 1.85$$

$$t = \frac{b-0}{S_b} = \frac{7.6-0}{1.85} = 4.1$$

The table value of t at 10 degree of freedom at 5% level of significance = 2.228, at 1% level of is 3.169. The calculated value of t = 4.1 > 3.169 and also 4.1 > 2.228, hence b differ significantly from 0, hence the relationship between X and Y is significant at 5% as well as at 1% level of significance.

Hence the value of b at 95% level of confidence (or 5% level of significance)

b ± 1.96 × s_b = 7.6 ± 1.96 × 1.85 = 7.6 ± 3.626

Exercise

1. The data listed in gives age (x – in years) and the systolic pressure (y in mmHg) of 10 women. Obtain the regression and find the predicted value of systolic pressure of 50 year old woman.

PATIENT NUMBER	Age(x-Years)	Systolic Blood Pressure (y-mmHg)
1	42	132
2	45	126
3	43	142
4	70	100
5	82	155
6	76	162
7	72	150
8	78	156
9	85	162
10	73	158

PARTIAL REGRESSION COEFFICIENT

The partial regression coefficient can be obtained with the help of standard deviation and correlation coefficients.

The formulae used for calculation of partial regression coefficients are

$$b_{12.3} = \frac{\sigma_1}{\sigma_2} \times \frac{r12 - r13 * r23}{1 - r_{23}^2}$$

$$b_{13.2} = \frac{\sigma_1}{\sigma_3} \times \frac{r13 - r12 * r23}{1 - r_{13}^2}$$

$$b_{21.3} = \frac{\sigma_2}{\sigma_1} \times \frac{r21 - r23 * r13}{1 - r_{13}^2}$$

Polynomial Regression

In statistics, polynomial regression is a form of regression analysis in which the relationship between the independent variable x and the dependent variable y is modelled as an nth degree polynomial in x.

Polynomial regression fits a nonlinear relationship between the value of x and the corresponding conditional mean of y, denoted $E(y \,|x)$, and has been used to describe nonlinear phenomena such as the growth rate of tissues, the distribution of carbon isotopes in lake sediments and the progression of disease epidemics. Although *polynomial regression* fits a nonlinear model to the data, as a statistical estimation problem it is linear, in the sense that the regression function $E(y \,|x)$ is linear in the unknown parameters that are estimated from the data. For this reason, polynomial regression is considered to be a special case of multiple linear regression.

The explanatory (independent) variables resulting from the polynomial expansion of the "baseline" variables are known as higher-degree terms. Such variables are also used in classification settings.

The goal of regression analysis is to model the expected value of a dependent variable y in terms of the value of an independent variable (or vector of independent variables) x. In simple linear regression, the model $y = a_0 + b_1x + \varepsilon$ is used, where ε is an unobserved random error with mean zero conditioned on a scalar variable x. In this model, for each unit increase in the value of x, the conditional expectation of y increases by b_1 units.

In many settings, such a linear relationship may not hold. For example, if we are modelling the yield of a chemical synthesis in terms of the temperature at which the synthesis takes place, we may find that the yield improves by increasing amounts for each unit increase in temperature. In this case, we might propose a quadratic model of the form, which will be in the form of $y = a_0 + b_1x + b_2x^2$. The polynomial model with an independent variable present in higher powers than second order, will not be use in pharmaceutical calculation. There are two important uses of quadratic models, they are:

1. When true relation between the variables unknown, this second degree polynomial provides best fit than the linear model.

2. More often the quadratic model is used for the purpose of establishing the linearity.

The most potential drawback of this model is that x and x^2 are strongly related and x is restricted to a narrow range; then we will find standard error will be more. This polynomial model is most ideal to analyze the result of formulation.

LOGISTIC REGRESSION: DICHOTOMOUS

INDEPENDENT VARIABLE

Logistic regression is a statistical method for analyzing a dataset in which there are one or more independent variables that determine an outcome. The simplest situation in which the logistic regression is applicable is one in which both the dependent and independent variables are dichotomous. In general dependent variable (outcome) indicate whether or not a subject acquired a disease or whether or not the subject died.

In logistic regression contains data coded as 1 (TRUE, success, pregnant, etc.) or 0 (FALSE, failure, non-pregnant, etc.).

The goal of logistic regression is to find the best fitting (yet biologically reasonable) model to describe the relationship between the dichotomous characteristic of interest (dependent variable or response or outcome variable) and a set of independent (predictor or explanatory) variables. Logistic regression generates the coefficients (and its standard errors and significance levels) of a formula to predict a *logit transformation* of the probability of presence of the characteristic of interest.

In case of regression the simple regression analysis involves only two variable and the equation can be written $y = a + bx + \varepsilon$. Here y is an arbitrary observed value of the continuous dependent variable. When the ε, the difference between observed and predicted value. If the difference is zero, then the equation can be written as $y = a + bx$. This model not appropriate when Y is dichotomous variable, because the expected value may 0 or 1.

If we take $p = P(Y = 1)$, then the ratio $p/(1-p)$ can take values between 0 and plus infinity. When we apply the, natural logarithm (ln) of $p/(1-p)$ is taken, then it can take values between minus infinity and plus infinity. Then the equation can be written as $\ln\left[\dfrac{p}{1-p}\right] = a + bx$. This equation is called logistic regression model, because it transforms the simple regression equation into $\ln\left[\dfrac{p}{1-p}\right]$ is called as logit transformation also it can be written as $p = \dfrac{e^{a+bx}}{1+e^{a+bx}}$, here e is inverse function of ln. The p is obtained by simplifying the equation $\ln\left[\dfrac{p}{1-p}\right] = a + bx$.

Take e both side, then we get

$$\frac{p}{1-p} = e^{a+bx}.$$

$p = e^{a+bx}(1\text{-}p)$

$p = e^{a+bx} - e^{a+bx}p$

$p + e^{a+bx}p = e^{a+bx}$

$p(1 + e^{a+bx}) = e^{a+bx}$

$$p = \frac{e^{a+bx}}{1+e^{a+bx}}$$

Example: For the given data obtain the logistic regression model. The data listed in following table is about infant mortality by mothers marital status.

Infant Mortality	Unmarried	Married	Total
Death	16,712	18,784	35,496
Alive for 1 Year	1,197,142	2,878,421	4075563
Total	1,213,854	2,897,205	4,111,059

$p_1 = 16{,}712/1213854 = 0.0138$

$p_0 = 18784/2897205 = 0.0065$

$a = \ln(p0) = -5.0385$

$b = \ln(p1/p0) = 0.7531$

$p = -5.0385 + 0.7531$

$a = \ln(p_0/(1-p_0)) = -5.0320$

$b = \ln(p_1/(1-p_1)) - \ln(p_0/(1-p_0)) = 5.0321$

Then $\ln(p/(1-p)) = -5.0320 + 0.7604x$

Then
$$p = \frac{e^{-5.0320+0.7604x}}{1+e^{-5.0320+0.760x}}$$

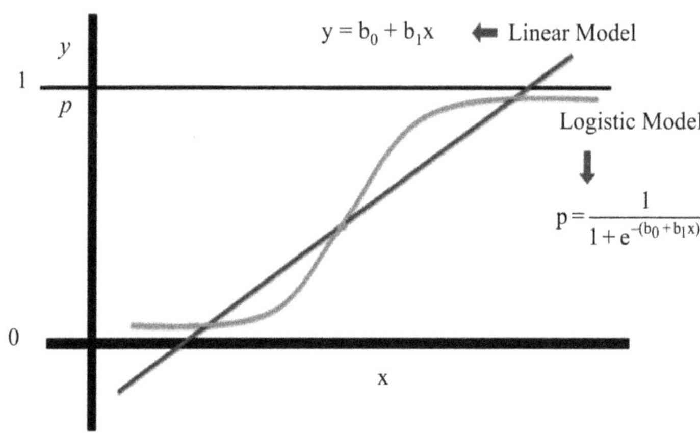

$\hat{p}$ — *the predicte value can be obtained by substituting the value in the equation*

Then
$$\hat{p} = \frac{e^{-5.0320+0.7604x}}{1+e^{-5.0320+0.760x}}$$

5 Probability

Some Important Definitions

Random Experiment

Any experiment is said to random experiment, when same experiment is conducted repeatedly under some homogeneous conditions, the result will be not unique, but may have any one of the possible outcomes.

Trial: Performing of a random experiment is called or termed as trial.

Ex: Treating a patient with a new drug to measure the efficacy of the drug.

Event: Outcome or combination of outcomes are called events.

Example:

a. When a patient is treated with a new drug, the possible outcomes may be cure or death.

b. When two patients are treated with a new drug, the possible outcomes are Cure cure, cure death, death cure and death death.

Simple Event: An event is said to simple event, if it corresponds to single possible outcome of the experiment or trial.

Composite Event: An event is said to be composite, if it does not corresponds to a single possible outcome of the experiment or trial.

Example: When two patients are treated at a time using same drug, getting either cure or death is simple event, but when both patients are cured can be considered as composite event.

Exhaustive Cases or Event: The total number of possible outcomes of random experiment is called as the exhaustive event or cases for the experiment one has done.

Example:

1. When a patient is treated using a new drug, the possible outcomes of this experiment are cure or death. These two are exhaustive cases.

2. When a coin is tossed, the possible exhaustive events are head or tail.

Favourable Cases or Events

The number of outcomes of a random experiment, which are favourable to an investigator are termed as favourable event or events.

Example: When two patients are treated, then the favourable events are both the patients are cured.

Mutually Exclusive Events

Two or more events are said to be mutually exclusive, if the occurrence or happening of any of the event excludes or prevents the occurring or happening of any other events in the same random experiment is termed as mutually exclusive event or events.

Example: Cure of a patient prevents the occurrence of death. Here cure and death are mutually exclusive events.

Equally Likely Cases: The outcomes are said to be equally likely or equally probable, if none of them is expected to occur in preference to other.

Example: When a patient is treated, both the outcomes are equally likely, if the treatment is unbiased.

Independent Events: Two events are said to be independent, if the occurrence of one event, does not prevent the occurrence of the other event is termed as independent events.

Example: When two patients are treated for the same type disease using same drug, then the cure of first patient does not prevent the cure of second patient.

Sample Space

The set of all possible outcomes of an experiment is termed as sample space.

Example:

1. When a coin is tossed, then the sample space S is   S = {H, T}

2. When a patient is treated, then the sample space is S = {C, D} C = Cure, D = Death.

Introduction: For some statistical inference the theory of probability, provides some foundation. The objectives this chapter are to make the investigator or students to understand mathematical ability in the area of probability and to understand the concepts.

The concept of probability is including the health professional also. For example, when a doctor performs an operation, after the operation, the chances of survival of a patient may be 50:50.

Permutation: In general the permutation means arrangement

Example:

1. When three subjects or volunteers A, B and C are selected for a clinical trial study, then the number of possible arrangements of these subjects are

   ABC, ACB, BAC, BCA, CAB, CBA – Six possible arrangements

2. When three subjects or volunteers A, B and C are selected for a clinical trial study, then the number of possible arrangements of these subjects when two are taken at a time are

AB, AC, BA, BC, CA, CB - $2 \times 3 = 6$ possible arrangements

Definition: A permutation of n= different objects, taking 'r' at a time, without any repetition is written $^nP_r = n(n-1)(n-2) \qquad ....(n-r+1)$

$^5P_2 = 5(5-1) = 5.4. = 20$

$^4P_3 = 4.3.2 = 24$

$^nP_n = n(n-1)(n-2) \qquad .....3.2.1$

$^nP_n = n!$

Factorial

The product of n-natural numbers viz 1, 2, 3 - - - n is called factorial of n or n-factorial and it is written as n!

$n! = 1.2.3 ----- (n-1)\, n$

$\qquad = n(n-1)(n-2)$

$5! = 5.4.3.2.1 = 120$

In general $^nP_r = \dfrac{n!}{(n-r)!}$

$^3P_2 = \dfrac{3}{(3-2)!} = \dfrac{3.2.1.}{1!} \dfrac{3.2.1.}{1} = 6$

Note : $0! = 1$

Combination

A combination of an n-different objects taken r at a time , is denoted as ^nc_r or $\binom{n}{r}$ is a selection of r-objects in a group of n-objects. The combination is written as $^nc_r = \dfrac{n!}{(n-r)!\,r!}$

Note: 1) $^nc_0 = 1$

2) $^nc_n = 1$, 3) $^nc_r = {^nc_{n-r}}$ $r = 0, 1, 2, 3----n$

Probability

If a random experiment results in N exhaustive, mutually exclusive and equally likely outcomes (Cases) out of which m events are favourable to the happening of an event A, then the probability of occurrence of A , usually denoted by P(A) is given by

$$P(A) = \dfrac{Number\ of\ favourable\ cases\ of\ A}{Exaustive\ number\ of\ cases}$$

OR it can be defined as the ratio of the number of favourable events to the total number of possible events of a random experiment.

In general P is written as probability of success and q is written as probability of failure.

Example: When two patients are treated, then the sample space S can be written as

$S = \{CC, CD, DC, DD\}$

Here the number of favourable events equal to 1 and non-favourable events are 3, then

Probability of success $P = \dfrac{1}{4}$ and Probability of failure $q = \dfrac{3}{4}$

Note:

1. If number of events which are favourable to success are n, and N is total number of possible events, then the number of non-favourable events are (N-n) . Then $q = \dfrac{N-n}{N}$

2. If P is the probability of success and q is probability of failure, then $p + q = 1$

3. Since n and N are non-negative integer, then $p \geq 0,$ since the favourable number of event are always less than the total number of possible events, $(n \leq N)$, then $p \leq 1$. This indicates that $0 \leq P \leq 1.$

4. If $p + q = 1$ then $q = 1 - p$

Example: In a group of eight patient's, 3 are women, 5 are men. What is the probability of selecting only 2-women patient for study.

Solution: Total number of Patients in the sample is 8

2 Patients should be selected at a time

Total number of possible ways to select 2 from $8 = {}^8C_2$

Selecting 2 women patients from $3 = {}^3C_2$

Then probability of selecting only two women patients is $P = {}^3C_2 / {}^8C_2$

$$P = \frac{\dfrac{3.2}{1.2}}{\dfrac{8.7}{1.2}} = 3/28$$

ADDITIONAL THEOREM: If A, B, C are mutually exclusive events, then the probability of observing A or B or C ... is the sum of the probabilities of each event A,B,C,----

$$P(A \text{ or } B \text{ or } C) = P(A) + P(B) + P(C)$$

This property holds good when events are mutually exclusive

Example: In a group of 1000 tablets, 5% are specked, 3% are chipped edges and 4% are discoloured. If these defects are mutually exclusive, then the probability of selecting an defectable tablets is $P(SUCUD) = P(S) + P(U) + P(D)$

$$= 0.05 + 0.03 + 0.04$$

$$= 0.12$$

Then the probability of choosing an acceptable tablet is $= 1 - 0.12 = 0.88$

This indicates 88% are acceptable and 12% are non-acceptable.

If A and B are two events not mutually exclusive, then

$$P(A \text{ or } B) = P(A) + P(B) - P(A \cap B)$$

Example:

In a group of 3000 subjects 5% patients are suffering from cancer, 3% are suffering from heart problem and 6% are suffering from both cancer and heart problems. Compute the probability of healthy patients.

Solution: In a group of 3000 subjects,   P(cancer Patients) = P(C) = 0.05

$$P(\text{Heart Patients}) = P(H) = 0.03 \text{ and}$$

$$P(\text{Both Heart and Cancer}) = P(C \cap H) = 0.06$$

Hence $P(C \cup H) = P(C) + P(H) - P(C \cap H)$

$$= 0.05 + 0.03 - 0.06$$

$$= 0.02$$

Then the probability of healthy subjects is $= 1 - P(C \cup H) = 1 - 0.02 = 0.98$

$$= 98\%$$

The total number of healthy patients or subjects is 98%

The total number healthy patients out of 3000 patients/ subjects $= 0.98 \times 3000$

$$= 2940 \text{ subjets}$$

Independent Events

Two events A and B are said to be independent events, if the occurrence of one does not prevent the occurrence of other event is termed as independent event.

Then $P(A \cap B) = P(A)\, P(B)$

When two patients are treated by a physician, then the cure of one patient, does not prevent the cure of second patient, then these two events are said to independent events.

If $P(A) = \frac{1}{2}$ and $P(B) = \frac{1}{2}$

Then $P(A \cap B) = \frac{1}{2} \times \frac{1}{2} = \frac{1}{4}$

Theoretical Distribution

Binomial Distribution

The Binomial distribution is one of the most widely encountered probability distribution which is used in statistics. Binomial distribution is also known as "Bernoulli distribution" after the Swiss mathematician James Bernoulli (1654 – 1705) who discovered in the year 1700 and the same published in the year 1713.

The Binomial distribution used under the condition that when:

(i)   The random experiment is performed repeatedly in a finite and fixed number of time. Here we consider n is finite and fixed number of trials.

(ii)   The outcome of the random experiment (trial) results in the dichotomous classification of events. The dichotomous events are classified as success (the occurrence of the event) and failure (the non occurrence of the event).

(iii)   All the trials which are performed by an investigator are independent.

(iv)   If p is the probability of success for one trial and $q = 1 - p$, is the probability of failure and that will be constant for each trial.

Definition: If P is probability of success and q is probability of failure for one trial. If N is total number of trial (repeated N-times), X- is number of success in N-trial. Then N-X is total number of failure, then $P(X) = {}^{N}C_X \, p^X \, q^{(N-X)}$

Example:

A group of 4 – patients who are treated with an antibiotic, if the probability of cure for one trial is 0.75, and there are five possible outcomes in a trial, they are

(i)   0-Patient is cured

(ii)   1 – Patient is cured

(iii) 2. – Patients are cured

(iv) 3 – Patients are cured

(v)   4 – Patients are cured

Apply Binomial distribution and Compute the probability of success for five possible outcomes.

Solution:

i. 0-Patient is cured

Here p=0.75 for one trial, then $q = 1 - p = 1 - 0.75 = 0.25$

$X = 0$ and $N = 4$ then

$P(X) = {}^{N}C_X \, p^X \, q^{(N-X)}$

$P(0) = {}^{4}C_0 \, (0.75)^0 \, (0.25)^{(4-0)}$

$\qquad = 1.1 \,.(0.25)^4$

$\qquad = 0.00391$

Similarly $P(1) = 0.04628$

$\qquad\qquad P(2) = 0.21094$

$\qquad\qquad P(3) = 0.42188$

$\qquad\qquad P(4) = 0.31641.$

Properties of Binomial Distribution

1. The shape and location of Binomial distribution changes as p changes for given n. When $p = 0.1$, the probability distribution is quite positively skewed, with the probabilities of small values. As the value of p increases, the skew becomes less pronounced. When $p = 0.5$, the

distribution is symmetrical, the probability p for one trial will be equal q = (1 −p). As the value increases (p > 0.5), then the distribution becomes negatively skewed. The distribution between p = 0.1 and p = 0.9 are identical, but in reverse sequence.

2.   The probability p for one trial is considered as fixed, and size n is varied, the distribution becomes very close to each other.

3. The mean of the Binomial distribution will increase, for corresponding increase of n, when p is fixed or remaining constant.

4. Standard deviation is obtained by the equation $\sqrt{npq}$

5. The mean is obtained by the equation np

Poisson Distribution

Poisson distribution was derived in 1837 by a French mathematician Simeon D. Poisson (1781-1840). Poisson distribution may be obtained as limiting case of Binomial probability distribution under the following conditions:

1. n, the number of trial we perform on subjects or animals must be very large or indefinitely large i.e., n$\longrightarrow \infty$.

2. p, the constant probability of success for each trial becomes very small , it may tend to zero p$\longrightarrow$ 0

3.   np = λ will be finite one

With all the three conditions mentioned above, the Poisson distribution is defined as

$$P(x) = \frac{\lambda^{x} e^{-\lambda}}{x!}$$

Where e = 2.7183

Generally Poisson distribution is applicable where there are number of random situations, where the probability of a success on a single trial is small and the number of trials is very large.

Example 1.

In a pharmaceutical industry, there is a chance of manufacturing 1/500 defective tablets. The strip pack consists of 10 tablets. Apply Poisson distribution to obtain the approximate number of strip packets containing zero defective, one defective and two defective tablets in a consignment of 10,000 strip packets.

Solution: N = 1000

   n = 10

   p = 1/500=0.002

   λ = np = 0.02

   $e^{-\lambda}$ = 0.9802

$$P(x) = \frac{\lambda^x e^{-\lambda}}{x!}$$

$10000 \times P(0) = \qquad 10000*0.9802 = 9802$

$10000 \times P(1) = \quad 10000* \ 0.019603973 = 196$

$10000 \times P(2) = \ 10000 *0.00019604 = 2.0$

Example 2: If the proportion of defectives in a bulk is 4%, obtain the probability of not more than 2 defectives in a sample of 10.

Solution:

$n = 10$

$p = 4/100 = 0.04$

$\lambda = np = 10 \times 0.04 = 0.4$

$e^{-\lambda} = 0.6703$

$$P(x) = \frac{\lambda^x e^{-\lambda}}{x!}$$

$P(0) = 0.6703$

$P(1) = 0.26813$

$P(2) = 0.053626$

$P(\text{not more than } 2) = P(0) + P(1) + P(2)$

$\qquad = 0.992$

$\qquad = 99.2$

Example 3: Fit a Poisson distribution to the following data and calculate the theoretical frequencies

Number patients cured(Success) X	Number times success happened Frequency (f)	f*X
0	123	0
1	59	59
2	14	28
3	3	09
4	1	04
	$\sum f = 200$	$\sum fx = 100$

$p = 1/2 = 0.5$

$\lambda = \text{mean} \ = \sum fx / \sum f = 0.5$

$e^{-\lambda} = 0.6065$

$$P(x) = \frac{\lambda^x e^{-\lambda}}{x!}$$

POISSON DISTRIBUTION

X P(X)	N*P(X)	Expected frequencies
0 0.6065	N*P(0)	121
1 0.30327	N*P(1)	61
2 0.075816	N*P(2)	15
3 0	N*P(3)	0
4 0	N*P(4)	0

NORMAL DISTRIBUTION

Normal Probability distribution commonly is called as normal distribution. This is one of most important continuous theoretical distribution in statistics.

Normal distribution was first discovered by an English Mathematician De-Moivre (1667-1754) in 1733, who obtained the mathematical equation for distribution while dealing with problems arising in the game of chance. This Normal distribution is also called as Gaussian distribution, because it was used by Karl Friedrich Gauss, who used this distribution to describe the theory of accidental errors of measurements involved in the calculation of orbits of heavenly bodies.

A variable is said to be normally distributed or have a normal distribution if its distribution has the shape of a normal curve - a special bell-shaped curve. The graph of a normal distribution is called the normal curve, which has all of the following properties: The mean, median, and mode are equal.

Normal Probability Curve

If X is a continuous random variable following normal probability distribution with mean μ, standard deviation σ, then its probability density function is by the equation

$$P(x) = \frac{1}{\sqrt{2\pi}\sigma} e^{-\frac{1}{2}\left(\frac{x-\mu}{\sigma}\right)^2} \qquad -\infty < x < \infty$$

This equation can also be written as

$$y = \frac{1}{\sigma\sqrt{2\pi}} e^{\frac{-(x-\mu)^2}{2\sigma^2}}$$

$$-\infty < x < \infty$$

where $\pi = 3.14$, $e = 2.7183$ (base of Natural logarithms)

From the above formula for normal distribution, it can be inferred that about 68% of all values lie within one standard deviation from the mean; 95.4% of all values lie within two standard deviations from the mean and 99.7% of all values lie within three standard deviations from the mean.

From the basic bell shaped curve, there can be many special cases derived that become meaningful under different situations.

Properties of a Normal Distribution

1. The graph of the p(x) is the in the form of bell shaped curve. The top of the bell is directly above the mean;
2. The normal curve is symmetrical about the mean μ;
3. The mean is at the middle and divides the area into halves;
4. Since the distribution is symmetrical, mean, median and mode coincide. Thus Mean = Median = Mode;
5. The total area under the curve is equal to 1;
6. It is completely determined by its mean and standard deviation σ (or variance σ^2)
7. No portion of curve lies below the x-axis, since p(x) being the probability can never be negative.
8. Theoretically, the range of the distribution is between $-\infty\ and\ \infty$, practically , Range = 6σ
9. Near the mean value, the normal curve is concave, while near $\pm3\ \sigma$, the curve is convex to the horizontal axis. The points of inflection, i.e., the points where the change in curvature occurs are $\pm1\sigma$;
10. Within a range 0.6745 of the σ on both sides of the mean 50% of the frequencies occur. This is probable error;
11. The area lying between the normal curve and horizontal axis is said to be the area under curve and is equal to the number of frequencies in the distribution. The standard deviation distributes the area under the normal curve as given below.

    (i) Mean $\pm1\sigma$ covers 68.268% area. 34.134% area will lie on either side of the mean.

    (ii) Mean $\pm2\sigma$ covers 95.725% area. 47.725% area will lie on either side of the mean.

    (iii) Mean $\pm3\sigma$ covers 99.73% area. 49.865% area will lie on either side of the mean. It covers almost all the area, leaving only 0.27% area outside the curve

A graph of this standardized (mean 0 and variance 1) normal curve is shown

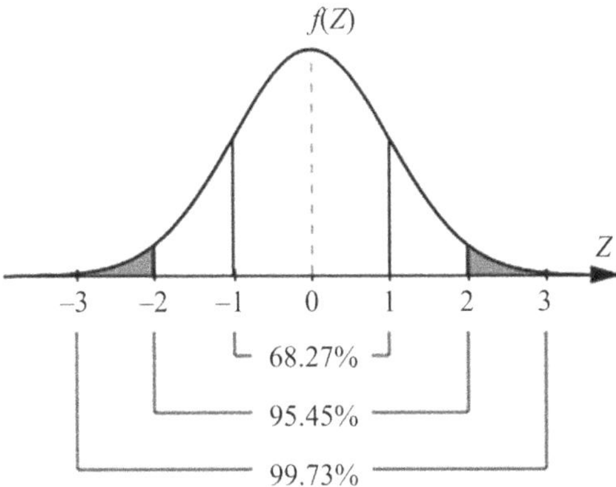

Standard Normal Curve showing percentages $\mu = 0$, $\sigma = 1$

Area under Normal Distribution using Integration

The probability of a continuous normal variable X found in a particular interval (a, b) is the area under t bounded by x = a and x = b and is given by

$$P(a < x < b) = \int_{a}^{b} f(x)\,dx$$

and the area depends upon the values of μ and σ.

In order to compute the probability of a random variable lying between two specified values, we need to know the area under the normal curve between two specified values. The equation of the normal distribution involves two parameters, they are mean (μ) and standard deviation (σ). Since μ and σ can assume an infinite number of values, it is impossible to tabulate the areas under the curve for different values of μ and σ. A normal distribution with $\mu = 0$ and $\sigma = 1$ is called the standard normal distribution or the unit normal distribution, as given by the equation. Such curve with $\mu = 0$ and $\sigma = 1$ is called as the standard normal curve.

For our convenience, it is useful to transform a normally distributed variable into such a form that a single table of areas under the normal curve would be applicable regardless of the units of the original data. We need to know the area between the mean and a point above the mean some specified distance measured in standard deviations. That variable is treated as a variable and it is denoted by Z, sometimes the value of Z is referred as a normal deviate. The distance Z that separates a possible normal random variable value x from its mean may be determined from the following expression for normal deviate:

$Z = \dfrac{x - \mu}{\sigma}$ where Z = z transformation, x = the value of the observation, μ = the mean the distribution and σ = the standard deviation of the distribution.

Areas Under Standard Normal Curve

Distance from the mean ordinates in terms of $\pm\sigma$	Area under the curve
$Z = \pm 0.6745$	$50\% = 0.50$
$Z = \pm 1.00$	$68.26\% = 0.6826$
$Z = \pm 1.96$	$95\% = 0.95$
$Z = \pm 2.00$	$95.44\% = 0.9544$
$Z = \pm 2.58$	$99\%\ 0.99$
$Z = \pm 3.0$	$99.73\%\ 0.9973$

Example 1: The hourly wages of 1000 workers in pharmaceutical industry are normally distributed around mean of Rs. 70 and with a standard deviation of Rs. 5. Estimate the number of workers whose hourly wages will be

(a) Between Rs 69 and Rs. 75

(b) More than Rs. 80

(c) Less than 65

Solution:

(a) Between Rs 69 and Rs. 75

$$Z = \frac{x - \mu}{\sigma}$$

When x = 69 $\mu = 70$, then $Z = \frac{69 - 70}{5} = -0.2$

When x = 75 $\mu = 70$, then $Z = \frac{75 - 70}{5} = 1$

$P(69<x<75) = P(-0.2<Z<1) = P(-0.2<Z<0)+(P(0<Z<1)$

$$= P(0<Z<0.2)+(P(0<Z<1)$$

$$= 0.0793 + 0.3413 = 0.4206$$

Hence the numbers of workers required = 1000*0.4206 = 420

(b) More than Rs. 80

$$Z = \frac{x - \mu}{\sigma}$$

When x = 69 $\mu = 70$, $Z = \frac{80 - 70}{5} = 2$

$P(x>80) = P(Z>2) = 0.5 - P(0<Z<2) = 0.5 - 0.4772 = 0.0228$

Hence the numbers of workers required = $1000 \times 0.0228 = 23$

(c) Less than 65,

$$Z = \frac{x - \mu}{\sigma}$$

When x = 65 $\mu = 70$, $Z = \frac{65 - 70}{5} = -1$

$P(x<65) = P(Z<-1) = 0.5 - P(0<Z<1) = 0.5 - 0.3643 = 0.1357$

Hence the numbers of workers required = $1000 \times 0.1357 = 136$

Example 2: Suppose tablet potencies mean is 50 mg and standard deviation is 5 mg . When these two parameter are given, what proportion of tablets in a batch would be expected to have more than 58.25 mg of drug?

Solution: First we have to calculate the transformation $Z = \dfrac{x-\mu}{\sigma}$

Here $\mu = 50$, $\sigma = 5$ and x = 58.25

Then $Z = \dfrac{x-\mu}{\sigma} = \dfrac{58.25 - 50}{5} = 1.65$

According to the standard table, the area between the points Z = -∞b and Z = 1.65 is 0.95

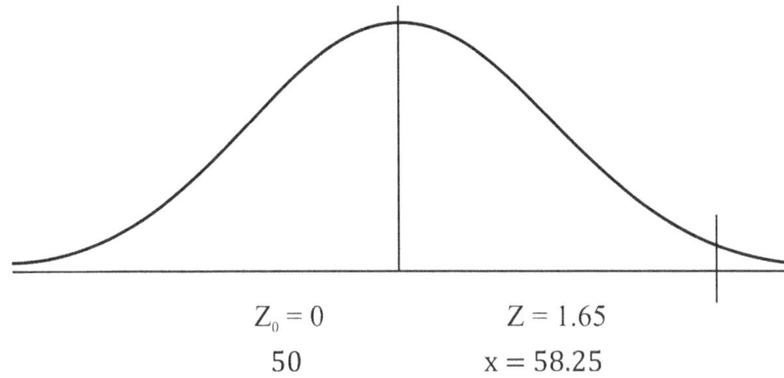

The area above 58.25 is 1 – 0.95 = 0.05.

This implies that 5% of the tablets have at least 58.25 mg drug in the particular batch of tablets.

Example 3: If the total cholesterol value for a normally distributed population is found to be 200 mg/ 100 ml mean and 20 mg / 100 ml standard deviation. What is the probability that an individual will have cholesterol value?

a) 180 and 200 mg/100 ml

Solution:

Here we have calculate P(180≤x≤200).

To find that, transform both the variables to Z

When x = 180 and μ = 200, $Z = \dfrac{x-\mu}{\sigma}$, $Z = \dfrac{180 - 200}{20} = -20/20 = -1$

When x = 200 $Z = \dfrac{200 - 200}{20} = 0$

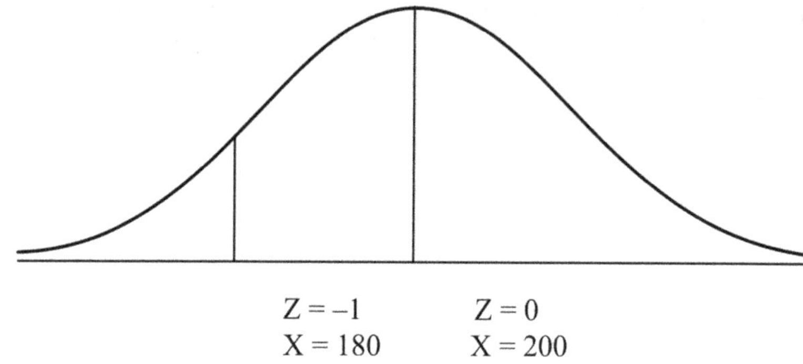

Here we have to calculate area between z = 0 and z = −1

$P(180 \leq x \leq 200) = P(-1 \leq Z \leq 0) = P(0 \leq Z \leq 1) = PZ0 = 0.3413 = 34.13\%$

Example 4:

IQ Scores for college graduates are normally distributed with a mean of 120 (as compared to 100 for general population) with a standard deviation of 12. What is the probability of randomly selecting graduate student with an IQ score

(a) Between 110 and 130

(b) Above 140?

(c) Below 100?

Solution: a) Given that $\mu = 120$ and $\sigma = 12$, $Z = \dfrac{120 - 120}{12} = 0$

$$x = 110 \text{ and } \sigma = 12, \ Z = \dfrac{110 - 120}{12} = -0.83$$

$$x = 130 \text{ and } \sigma = 12, \ Z = \dfrac{130 - 120}{12} = 0.83$$

$P(110 \leq x \leq 130 = P(-0.83 - 1 \leq Z \leq 0.83) = P(0 \leq Z \leq 0.83) + P(-0.83830 \leq Z \leq 0)$

$= P(0 \leq Z \leq 0.83) + P(0 \leq Z \leq 0.83)$ (After taking absolute value)

$= 0.2967 + 0.2967 = 0.5934$

Exercises

1. Suppose the average length of stay of patient of chronic disease in a hospital is 60 days with a standard deviation of 15. Assume the length of stay in the hospital is normal, find the probability that a randomly selected patient from this group will have a length of stay.

    (a) Greater than 50 days
    (b) less than 30 days
    (c) Between 30 and 60 days
    (d) Greater than 90 days

2. What is the probability that a normal patient has cholesterol value below 180 when population mean $\mu = 215$ and standard deviation $\sigma = 35$.

3. Obtain the probability of 3-success in 100 trials if P = 0.01.

4. The mean height of patients of a particular population is 68.22 inches and standard deviation is 3.286. How many patients in a regiment of 10000 would you expect to be

   (a) Over six feet tall and

   (b) Below 5.5 feet?

5. Serum sodium value for normal persons have a mean 140 m eq / L and standard deviation is 2.5. What is the probability that a persons serum sodium will be between 137 and 142 mEq/L?

6. What is the probability that a normal person has a B.P value between 150 and when $\mu = 120$ and standard deviation $\sigma = 25$?

6 Sampling Theory and Design of Sampling Survey

The study of statistics of Biostatistics broadly studied under two methods, they are

1. Descriptive
2. Inductive

Descriptive Statistics: Descriptive statistics mainly focuses on describing some characteristics of the numerical data, which are recorded after performing experiments on human beings or animals.

Inductive Statistics: It is also named as statistics of inference. It helps us to draw statistically valid conclusions about the totality of cases or samples selected from population for study.

This process of studying on the sample and generating the results to the population, for which we will be selecting subjects for study.

This generalizing involves an element of risk, that is making a wrong decisions. In this chapter we are going to discuss various techniques of drawing samples from the population.

Population

Statistical investigation lies in studying various characteristics relating to items or subjects who have been selected from a particular group.

The group of individuals under study is known as the population or Universe.

"In Biostatistics, population is the entire universe with a particular characteristics"

"In statistics , population is the aggregate of objects, animate or inanimate, under study in any statistical investigation".

In general the population means, the larger group from there the samples are drawn for study or selected for clinical trials or experimental study.

A population containing a finite number of objects or subjects so large as appears to be practically infinite, is named as an infinite population.

Sampling

Sampling is a process of selecting sample from population for experimental study is termed as sampling.

A major purpose of doing research is to infer or generalize research objectives from a sample to a larger population. The process of inference is accomplished by using statistical methods based on probability theory. A sample is a subset of the population selected, which is an unbiased representative of the larger population. Studies that use samples are less expensive, and study of the entire population is sometimes impossible. Thus, the goal of sampling is to ensure that the sample group is a true representative of the population without errors. The term error includes sampling and non-sampling errors. Sampling errors that are induced by sampling design include selection bias and random sampling error. Non-sampling errors are induced by data collection and processing problems, and include issues related to measurement, processing and data collection errors.

Types of Sampling

The choice of an appropriate sampling design is of paramount importance in the execution of a sample survey.

The sampling system may be classified into three types:

(i)   Purposive or subjective or judgment sampling
(ii) Probability sampling
(iii) Mixed sampling

Purposive or Subjective or Judgment Sampling

In case of purposive or subjective or judgment sampling, a required number of subjects are selected purposely depending upon the subjects or items which are representing the true characteristics of the population which will be selected for study.

The important drawback of this sampling system is that, it is highly subjective in nature, because the selection of the sample depends on the personal convenience and prejudices of the investigator. The main goal of purposive sampling is to focus on particular characteristics of the population that are of interest, which will enable to answer the research questions which have been selected.

Example: Selecting sample from the population, with a particular characteristics like cancer, diabetic and heart problem etc.

Here the investigator select the sample of their choice, which can match the population.

Probability Sampling

A probability sampling method, which will give scientific procedure or technique of selecting samples from the population according to some form of random selection. In case of probability sampling, there are three important methods of selecting samples for study, they are:

(i) Each sampling units have an equal chances of being selected.

(ii) Each sampling units have varying probability of being selected.

(iii) Probability of selection of subjects or items will be proportional to the sample size.

The following sampling methods are example of probability sampling

1. Simple random sampling
2. Stratified random sampling
3. Systematic sampling
4. Multistage sampling
5. Cluster sampling
6. Quota sampling

Simple Random Sampling

Simple random sampling is a technique in which every member or subject or items which are taken from the population has an equal and independent chances of being included in the sample.

In this case, if any subject or patient or item selected for study is not replaced in the population before we go for the next draw. Then it is known as simple random sample without replacement and if it is replaced back in the population before making the next selection or before next draw, then sampling is called as simple random sampling with the replacement.

Selection of subjects in simple random sample: In this case proper care must be taken to ensure that sample or patient or subject selected for study is random and that is the representative of the population. A random sample may be selected by:

(a) Lottery method

(b) Random numbers table method

Lottery Method

This method consists of identifying each and every subject of patients or every members or unit of the population which is recorded with a distinct number on a slip or on a card. The slip selected to write numbers must be as homogeneous as possible in shapes, size, colour etc., to control the human bias. These slips are placed in a container and shuffled thoroughly. Finally a sample of 10 or 20 are drawn out one by one. The individual patients of items bearing the number on these selected slips will be taken as a sample for study.

Random Number Table

The lottery method is quite time consuming and cumbersome to use, if the population is very large. The most practical and inexpensive method for selecting randomly is random number table. This method is most frequently used as a device to choose samples, which will be included in a survey, a quality control department for the inspection of samples or to assign experimental items or subjects for the treatment, that is assigning patients for drug treatment. The numbers are assigned consecutive manner from 1 to N, where N is the number of units under consideration. When we have to select sample from a population of size $N \leq 99$, then can be combined two by two pairs from 00 to 99. Similarly if $N \leq 999$ or $N \leq 9999$ and so on, then the combining of digits three by three or four by four and so on can be formed in random number table.

Example 1: A sample of 20 bottles is to be selected from a universe of 900 medicine bottles. Here the bottles will be numbered from 1 to 900, that include 900 also.

Example 2: Random numbers can be used to assign patients randomly for treatments in clinical trials, when a drug for the treatment of diabetics is to be compared with Placebo treatment.

In a clinical trial studies patients are usually selected by an investigator (doctor) and all the patients who meet the inclusive criteria and are willing to participate will be included in clinical trials.

The method of drawing samples in a random order includes:

(i)   Identify N subjects from the population by numbering as 1 to N.

(ii) Select any number from random number table in a row, column or diagonal in a random way.

Stratified Sampling

Thus, apart from increasing the sample size, the only way to increase the precise of sample estimate of the population mean and also can be treated as a device to reduce the variability in the population. This also can be achieved by applying stratified sampling technique.

When the population is heterogeneous with a particular characteristic under study, then the stratified sampling technique will be applied. The stratified sampling is procedure in which the population will be divided into different layers or into subsets or strata and random samples are selected from each strata. Stratified sampling is a recommended way of sampling, when the strata are very different from each other, but objects within which each stratum are alike.

In this stratified random sampling

1. The sampling units or items or subjects within each stratum are homogeneous to the maximum extent possible.

2. The differences between various strata can be marked.

3. Various strata are non-overlapping.

Example: In clinical study, when diabetic patients are selected, the stratification could be accomplished by dividing the diabetic patients into subsets or subgroups or strata depending on the age, duration of disease, severity of illness etc. Then the patients will be assigned to treatments randomly within each strata of subgroups or subsets.

This stratified sampling results in better precision in mean of the population, from which the sample has been drawn for study.

Stratification of clinical trials, is the partitioning of subjects and results by a factor other than the treatment given.

Stratification can be used to ensure equal allocation of subgroups of participants to each experimental condition. This may be done by gender, age, or other demographic factors. Stratification can be used to control for confounding variables (variables other than those the researcher is studying), thereby making it easier for the research to detect and interpret relationships between variables. For example, if doing a study of fitness where age or gender was expected to influence the outcomes, participants could be stratified into groups by the confounding variable. A limitation of this method is that it requires knowledge of what variables need to be controlled

Example: To treat trauma in a hospital, trauma centers are given rating, depending on their capability to treat various traumas.

The level1 trauma centre is the highest level of available trauma care and a level4 trauma centre is the lower level of trauma care.

Merits and Demerits

Merits

1. *More representative sample.* A stratified random sample gives adequate representation to each strata and eliminate the possibility of any important group of the population being completely ignored. In case of stratified sampling method, result obtained is more accurate, because random sampling provides a more representative sample of the population.

2. Greater precision, Due to the reduction in the variability within each stratum, this sampling method provides more, effective result or outcome as compared with simple random sampling.

3. Stratified random sampling enables us to obtain the results of known precision for every individual stratum.

4. The problem can be tackled effectively through stratified sampling.

Demerits

1. The success of this sampling depends on

(i) Effective stratification of the universe into homogeneous group.

(ii) Appropriate size of the sample to be drawn from each of the stratum.

Systematic Sampling

A systematic method that is most widely used in healthcare research system. Medical records which contain raw data used in healthcare research, are generally stored in a file system or on a computer and hence are easy to select in a systematic way.

In case of systematic sampling subject or item or patient is selected at random and the remaining units are automatically selected in a definite sequence at an equal spacing from one another.

Example: Suppose that N – sampling units in the population are arranged in some systematic order and they are numbered as I to N and if one wish to draw a sample of size n from it, such that $N = nk \rightarrow k = \dfrac{N}{n}$ where k is called as sample interval.

If n = 50 and N = 1000, then $k = \dfrac{N}{n} = \dfrac{1000}{50} = 20$

If an investigator select any number between 1 to 20 at random, then the corresponding number in the list is selected.

If the selected number is 6, then item or subject number 26 will be selected, after that 46, 66, 86----------------- 986 are selected . This systematic sample consists of 50 subjects for study. In general if i is the first subject selected from the first group, then the sequence will be.

i, i+k, i+2k, ------ $\rightarrow$ -------------------- i+(n-1)k.

Merits and Demerits

Merits

1. It is very easy to operate and verifying can be done very quickly.
2. It is more time saving.
3. Systematic sampling may be more efficient than simple random sampling, provided the frame is complete and up-to-date.

Demerits

1. This method is well only if the complete and up-to-date frame is available and subjects or items are arranged in randomly.
2. This method gives a biased results, when there are periodic features in the frame and the sampling interval (k) is equal to or multiple of the period.

Cluster Sampling

In case of cluster sampling, entire population is divided into some sub-divisions, depending upon the problem under investigation, that is named as cluster.

A simple random sample is selected for study. This method is most ideal for observational study to collect the information about a particular area. To do these type of study, whole city will be divided into N – different blocks or localities, that is considered as cluster. That cluster will be selected for a particular type study, then the investigator is going to perform two stage cluster sampling, when there are many primary units, each of which can be considered as subsamples.

Suppose that, one wish to inspect tablets, packaged in a final labeled container. The batch of 20,000 bottles of 200 bottles each sample.

Here the primary units are the bottles, and subsample units are the tablets within each bottles.

Cluster sampling, might consists of randomly selecting a sample of 200 bottles, and then inspecting a random sample of 20 tablets from each of these bottles and this can be called as stage sampling.

Clusters are commonly based on geographic areas or districts and, therefore, this approach is used more often in epidemiologic research than in clinical studies.

Multistage Sampling

This is a better estimating by resorting to sub-samples within the clusters. This method is named as two-stage sampling, here cluster being termed as primary units or subjects and the subjects or units within the clusters is considered as secondary units.

This can be generalized and that can be called as multistage sampling.

Here population selected for study is considered as primary stage, this population can further be composed of number of secondary stage units and so on, till we finally reach the desired sampling unit.

Examples: Cancer patients in this country is primary stage, then the cancer patients selected from a particular state is secondary and district, taluk, village etc.

These stages may be added to arrive at a sample of the desired sampling subjects or items or units.

Quota Sampling

Quota sampling is a non-probability sampling technique in which researchers search for a particular characteristic in their subjects, who have been selected for study, and then take a tailored sample that is in proportion to a population of interest.

Choosing a quota sample can be done in four steps.

Step 1: First, the researcher must divide the population of interest into strata, or groups of individuals that are similar in some way, that is important to the response.

These strata should be exclusive, meaning that participants in the study only belong to one strata.

For example, you could create strata from a population of diabetic patients.

Step 2: Second, the researcher must then determine the proportion of subgroups in the population.

For example, diabetic patients, can be divided into subgroup depending of number of years they are suffering. (1year, 2 years, and so on).

Step 3: Next, the researcher must choose their sample size.

For example, if you are sampling 1,000 people you might choose a quota sample of 100.

Step 4

Finally, the researchers must then choose participants to take part in their study. It's imperative to adhere to the subgroup to population proportion.

Researchers must then continue this process until their quotas are filled, or in the case of our example, until we have 1,000 participants.

Quota sampling is very similar to stratified random sampling, with one exception.

In quota sampling, the samples from each stratum do not need to be random samples.

For this reason, stratified random sampling is a preferable method over quota sampling, as the random selection in stratified random sampling ensures a more accurate representation of the larger population.

However, researchers use quota sampling when stratified random sampling is not possible.

The Advantages and Disadvantages of Quota Sampling

Quota sampling comes with both advantages and disadvantages.

Merits

Relatively easy to administer

Can be performed quickly

Cost-effective

Accounts for population proportions

A useful method when probability sampling techniques are not possible.

Demerits

Sample selection is not random

There is a potential for selection bias, which can result in a sample that is unrepresentative of the population.

Theory Estimation and Testing of Hypothesis

Introduction

The inductive inference can be called as a logic of drawing a valid conclusion about the population characteristics, on the basis of a sample selected or drawn from that population, after performing statistical analysis by applying some statistical tools. The technique which we apply to analyze the data, enables us to generalize the results of the sample to the population, to find and also estimate the population parameters along with the degree of confidence. The answer for all these types of problems are obtained by a very important branch of statistics, known as statistical inference. This can be classified as:

(i) Theory of estimation

(ii) Testing of hypothesis

"In general statistical inference is defined as the procedure by which we reach a conclusion about a population on the basis of the information contained in a sample drawn from that population.

Estimation Theory

Estimation of population parameter like mean, Variance, proportion, correlation coefficient etc., from the corresponding sample statistics is one of the most valuable problem for statistical inference.

The rationale behind estimation in the health science field, rests on the assumption that workers in this field have an interest in the parameters, such as means and proportions of various populations. Many populations of interest, although finite, are so large that a 100 percent examination would be prohibitive from the standpoint of cost.

If one wants to know the average or the mean age of patients admitted to a hospital during that given year. It will be more expensive to refer all the records of the patients admitted, during that particular year and overcome this problem, select to examine a samples of records, from which the concerned authority can estimate the mean age of patients who were admitted during that year.

When the doctors in general may be interested to know, what proportion of patients who suffered due to side effect after taking a part in clinical study.

To get solution for the above mentioned problems, theory of estimation was founded by Prof. F. A. FISHER in the year 1930 and that was divided into two groups, they are termed as:

(i)   Point Estimation

(ii) Interval Estimation

In case of point estimation, a sample statistics like, mean, standard deviation etc., are used to provide an estimate of the population parameter. Whereas that interval estimation, that will provide a range within which the true value of the parameter might be expected to lie.

Point Estimation

A particular value of a statistics which is used to estimate a particular parameter is called as point estimator or estimator of the parameter. A good parameter is one which will be very close to the true value of parameter. Nevertheless a sample statistics like Mean and standard deviation are best estimate of the true parameter.

Example: The computation mean ($\bar{X}$) and standard deviation(σ) for the potencies of 200 tablets from a batch of 10000 tablets, one may very well inquire about true mean potency of the batch. If mean potency is 50mg, then the best estimate of the true batch can be considered as 50 mg.

But in many cases, a parameter may be estimated by more than one estimator. The decision will be based on an objective measure or set of criteria that reflect some required property of a particular estimator. When measured against these criteria, some estimator are better than others, one of these criteria is the property of unbiasedness. The estimator say, T of the Parameter θ is said to be unbiased estimator of θ if $E(T) = \theta$. $E(T)$ – Estimated statistics or expected value of T. In general $E(T) = \mu$. For an infinite population , $E(T)$ is defined in terms of calculus.

Interval Estimation

Since most of the problems that we will encounter are concerned about normal distribution, specially for the sampling means, here we are interested in confidence interval for means. This interval estimation consists in the determination of two constants C1 and C2, such that $P[C1 < \theta$ C2] for any given value of t =1-α. t-statistics are mean ($\bar{X}$) and standard deviation(S) and α – is level of significance. (Which is discussed in the chapter hypothesis). If t is the statistics used to estimate the parameter θ, then confidence limit for $\theta = t \pm S.Et_{(\alpha/2)}$, where $t_{(\alpha/2)}$ is the significant or critical value of t at the level of significance α for a two- tailed test. Where S.E is the sampling distribution of statistics t. $1 - \alpha$ appropriate confidence coefficient.

Interval Estimation for Large Sample

1. Confidence Limits for Mean μ:

When a large random sample size of n chosen from an infinite population, whose mean is μ and standard deviation is σ or variance is σ^2, then

$$Z = \frac{\bar{X}-\mu}{\frac{\sigma}{\sqrt{n}}} \qquad .....(1)$$

When the sample is greater than 30 will be considered as large sample, for our practical purpose.

When areas under normal probability curve is considered, then

$$P(-1.96 \leq Z \leq 1.96) = 0.95$$

i.e.,
$$P(-1.96 \leq \frac{\bar{X}-\mu}{\frac{\sigma}{\sqrt{n}}} \leq 1.96) = 0.95$$

i.e
$$P(\bar{X}-1.96\frac{\sigma}{\sqrt{n}} \leq \bar{X} - \mu \leq X + 1.96\frac{\sigma}{\sqrt{n}}) = 0.95$$

where σ – assumed to be known. Then the confidence interval can be written as

$$[\bar{X}-1.96\frac{\sigma}{\sqrt{n}}, \quad X + 1.96\frac{\sigma}{\sqrt{n}}]$$

This is the 95% confidence interval for estimating μ (Population mean).

Similarly the confidence interval for 99% level of significance can be obtained , here

$$P(-2.58 \leq Z \leq 2.58) = 0.99$$

i.e.,
$$P(-2.58 \leq \frac{\bar{X}-\mu}{\frac{\sigma}{\sqrt{n}}} \leq 2.58) = 0.99$$

i.e.,
$$P(\bar{X}-2.58\frac{\sigma}{\sqrt{n}} \leq \bar{X} - \mu \leq \bar{X} + 2.58\frac{\sigma}{\sqrt{n}}) = 0.99$$

Hence the confidence interval is $[\bar{X}-2.58\frac{\sigma}{\sqrt{n}}, \quad \bar{X} + 2.58\frac{\sigma}{\sqrt{n}}]$

This confidence interval changes depending on the sample chosen, because although σ and N remains same, $\bar{x}$ varies from sample to sample. A confidence interval using the mean from any sample taken population may or may not contain the true mean. Without the knowledge of the true mean, one cannot decide whether or not any given interval contains the true mean.

Confidence Limits for Proportion

To find confidence interval for proportional, the statistics value t $=$ p for large sample size, then

$$Z = \frac{p-E(p)}{SE(p)} = = \frac{p-P}{\sqrt{\frac{pq}{n}}}$$

When sample is taken from infinite population, then for $100(1-\alpha)\%$ confidence limits for P are given by

$$p \pm Z_{\alpha/2}SE(p) = p \pm Z_{\alpha/2}\sqrt{\frac{pq}{n}}$$

For large sample $Z_\alpha = 1.96$ at 95% confidence and $Z_\alpha = 2.58$ at 99% confidence. Then confidence interval can be written as

$$p \pm 1.96 \sqrt{\frac{pq}{n}} \quad \text{and} \quad p \pm 2.58 \sqrt{\frac{pq}{n}}$$

Example 1: The labelled potency of a tablet dosage form is 100 mg. Then tablets from that group are assayed according to a quality control specification. The assay results are as listed below and assumption is that the distribution is normal. If average of this sample is 103 and standard deviation is 2.2. Construct a 95% confidence interval for the true batch mean.

Solution:

Tablets	1	2	3	4	5	6	7	8	9	10
Assay (X)	101.8	102.6	99.8	104.9	103.8	104.5	100.7	106.3	100.6	105.0

Here Mean $= \bar{X} = 103$ and $S = 2.22$ then $= [\bar{X} - 1.96 \frac{\sigma}{\sqrt{n}}, \quad X + 1.96 \frac{\sigma}{\sqrt{n}}]$

$$= [103 - 1.96 \frac{2.22}{\sqrt{10}}, \quad 103 + 1.96 \frac{2.22}{\sqrt{10}}$$

$$= 101.41, 104.59$$

when σ (SD) is known. Here if $\sigma = 2$ then for large sample confidence interval is

$$[\bar{X} - 1.96 \frac{\sigma}{\sqrt{n}}, \quad \bar{X} + 1.96 \frac{\sigma}{\sqrt{n}}]$$

$$= [103 - 1.96 \frac{2}{\sqrt{10}}, \quad 103 + 1.96 \frac{2}{\sqrt{10}}]$$

$$= 101.76 \quad \text{to} \quad 104.24$$

Example 2: The average percentage saturation of bile for 31 male patients is 84.65 and the standard deviation $S = 24.00$, then obtain the confidence interval of 95% level.

Solution: The confidence interval is $[\bar{X} - 1.96 \frac{\sigma}{\sqrt{n}}, \quad \bar{X} + 1.96 \frac{\sigma}{\sqrt{n}}]$

$$[84.65 - 1.96 \frac{24}{\sqrt{31}}, \quad 84.65 + 1.96 \frac{24}{\sqrt{31}}]$$

$$76.2, 93.1$$

Confidence Limits for Difference of Means

If $\bar{x_1}$ and $\bar{x_2}$ are the means of two samples selected randomly from two infinite populations whose means μ_1 and μ_2 and their standard deviations are $\sigma 1$ and $\sigma 2$ then the confidential limits can be obtained by the equation

$$(\bar{x_1} - \bar{x_2}) \pm Z_{\alpha/2} \text{SE}(\bar{x_1} - \bar{x_2})$$

where
$$\text{SE}\overline{(x_1 - x_2)} = \sqrt{\frac{\sigma 1^2}{n1} + \frac{\sigma 2^2}{n2}}$$

n1 = Size of sample1, n2 = Size of sample2

When sample are taken large population and sample is also large, then $Z_{\alpha/2} = 1.96$ for 95% confidence limits and $Z_{\alpha/2} = 2.58$ for 99% confidence limits.

Confidence Limits for Difference of Proportion

If p_1 and p_2 are the proportions of two large sample, which are randomly chosen from infinite populations with their proportions P1 and P2 , then Q1 = 1- P1 , Q2 = 1 – P2 of populations and q1 = 1 – p1 and q2 = 1 –p2 for two large samples, then the confidence limits for the difference of proportion P1 and P2 at 95% confidence level is

$$(p1 - p2) \pm 1.96 \sqrt{\frac{P1Q1}{n1} + \frac{P2Q2}{n2}}$$

when P1 and P2 are known.

When P1 and P2 are unknown then, confidence limits is

$$(p1 - p2) \pm 1.96 \sqrt{\frac{p1q1}{n1} + \frac{p2q2}{n2}}$$

Example 1: A public health officials educated the people to make them to understand the side effect of smoking. Before educating a sample of size n1 =100 males were interviewed and found that 51 are smokers. Again after 2 years, second random sample of n2 = 100 males were chosen, survey showed that n2 = 43 were smokers. Obtain the confidence limits before and after two years.

Solution:

Before 2 years p1 $= \dfrac{x1}{n1} = \dfrac{51}{100} = 0.51$ and q1 = 1- p1 = 1 – 0.51 = 0.49

$$SE(p1) = \sqrt{\frac{p1\,q1}{n1}} = \sqrt{\frac{0.51*0.49}{100}} = 0.05$$

Confidence limits at 95% level is   p1 $\pm$ 1.96 (SE(p1))

0.51 $\pm$ (1.96)(0.05)

0.41, 0.61

41%, 61%

After 2 years p2 $= \dfrac{x1}{n1} = \dfrac{43}{100} = 0.43$ and q2 = 1- p2 = 1 – 0.43 = 0.57

$$SE(p2) = \sqrt{\frac{p2\,q2}{n2}} = \sqrt{\frac{0.43*0.57}{100}} = 0.05$$

Confidence limits at 95% level is   p2 $\pm$ 1.96 (SE(p2))

0.43 $\pm$ (1.96)(0.05)

0.33, 0.53

33%, 53%

Testing of Hypothesis

When an health investigator seeks to understand the effect of a new drug, investigator formulates research question in the form of a Hypothesis. To study these things, the modern theory of probability plays a very important role to make any decision and the branch of statistics which supports the investigator in arriving at the criterion for such decisions is known as testing of Hypothesis. This testing of hypothesis was first introduced by J. Neyman and E. S. Pearson to give conclusion about the experimental results.

Statistical Hypothesis

A statistical Hypothesis is some assumption or statement, which may or may not be true about a population or equivalently about the probability distribution characterizing the given phenomenon, which we are interested to test on the basis of some evidence from a random sample chosen from that particular population.

In context of sampling from a normal population $N(\mu, \sigma^2)$, then the hypothesis can be written as;

$$H: \mu = \mu_0 \text{ and } \sigma^2 = \sigma_0^2$$

The test of a statistical Hypothesis is a two way action of taking decision, after observing the experimental results of a random sample taken from the known population. The two way action may be the acceptance or rejection of the Hypothesis under consideration.

Example: A physician may make statement hypothesize that a certain drug will be effective in 90 percent of the cases for which it has been tested. That hypothesis is one determines whether or not such statement are true or not with the available experimental result or data.

Tests of Significance

By using the statistics of the sampling distribution, investigator can find the probability that a sample statistics ($\bar{x}$, σ^2 etc) would differ from a given hypothetical value of the parameter or from another sample value, by more than a certain amount and hence to answer the question of significance.

Accordingly, a procedure which has been followed to assess the significance of a statistics or difference between the two or more independent statistics is termed as or known as tests of significance.

To perform these tests of significance, depending on the type of clinical or interventional study or based on the problem in which investigator doing experiments, different statistical tests like t-test, ANOVA, Chi-Square test etc., will be applied to test the significance of the parameter of population with sample statistics.

Types of Hypothesis

After selecting the random sample from the given population with a particular characteristic, makes the tests of significance valid for an investigator, who will be doing experiments on animals or patients.

Before applying any test of significance, investigator must set up a hypothesis, that is a definite statement about the population parameter(s) like mean, standard deviation.

Null Hypothesis (H_0)

Such a statistical hypothesis, which is under test, is usually considered as hypothesis of no difference and it is named as null hypothesis. It is denoted as H_0.

In General null hypothesis can be defined as "Hypothesis which is tested for possible rejection under the assumption that is true".

OR

Hypothesis to be tested for possible rejection or acceptance is also named as Null Hypothesis.

Alternative Hypothesis

Any hypothesis which is against to the hypothesis or hypothesis which is complementary to the null hypothesis is called as alternative hypothesis. It is very important to explicitly state the alternative hypothesis in respect of any null hypothesis H_0.

Rules for Stating Statistical Hypothesis

When hypothesis are considered in any study, then the indication of equality (either $=$, $\leq$ or $\geq$) must appear in the null Hypothesis.

Example : Average height for certain population is not 66", then null Hypothesis is

1. $H_0 : \mu = 64$" and the alternative Hypothesis $H_1 : \mu \# 64$"
2. Suppose , if we want to conclude that population average is greater than 64" then
   $H_0 : \mu \leq 64$" then $H_1 > 64$"
3. If we conclude that the population mean is less than 64", then hypothesis can be written as
   $H_0 : \mu \geq 64$" then $H_1 < 64$"

Example :

1. When we say that a patient is free from any disease, that is H_0 is true.

2. After conducting or performing pathological test, doctor gives conclusion that patient is free from the disease, then H_0 is true, then H_0 will be accepted, that there is no difference between population mean and sample mean. i.e., $\mu = \mu_0$.

3. If patient is having any disease, conclusion will be against to the null hypothesis, then alternative hypothesis is true. H_1 is accepted. Population mean is not equal to H_0, $\mu \# \mu_0$.

Types of Error in Testing Hypothesis

In any experimental study, the inference consists of coming to the conclusion to accept or reject null Hypothesis (H_0) after observing the result obtained from a random sample taken from the population. There are chances of taking wrong decisions about the result obtained or on the Hypothetical statement. There are four possibilities to make decision about the result obtained from the random sample. The decisions are:

(i) Reject H_0 when H_0 is true is false

(ii) Accept H_0 when H_0 is true is true

(iii) Reject H_0 when H_0 is true is true

(iv) Accept H_0 when H_0 is true is false

Example:

1. When patient is not free from disease, H_0 is not true, reject H_0 – decision is correct.

2. When patient is free from disease, H_0 is true, accept H_0 – decision is correct.

3. When patient is not free from disease, H_0 is true , but the investigator reject H_0 – decision is incorrect.

4. When patient is not free from disease, H_0 is not true, but the investigator or test result says, he is free from the disease, accepts H_0 – decision is incorrect.

There are two possible errors which will be committed by the investigators, they are named as Type-I and Type-II error.

TYPE-I – Error: The error of rejecting H_0 when H_0 is true is known as Type-I error.

TYPE-II – Error: The error of accepting H_0 , when H_0 is false or rejecting H1 , when H1 is true is known as Type-II.

Those decision can be shown in the table form

Condition of Null Hypothesis

		True	False
Possible Actions	Reject H1 when H1 - true	Correct Action	Type – II Error
	Reject H0 when H0 - True	Type-I Error	Correct action

Note:

Investigator makes Type-I Error by rejecting H_0 and Type-II-Error by rejecting H_1 when H_0 and H_1 are true. These two errors can be written as

$P[Reject\ H0\ when\ H0\ is\ true] = P[Type - I\ Error] = \alpha$

$P[Reject\ H1\ when\ H1\ is\ true\ or\ Accepting\ H0\ when\ H0\ in\ not\ true]$

$= P[Type - II - Error] = \beta$

In the terminology of clinical trial

$\alpha = P[Rejecting\ healthy\ patients]$

$\beta = P[Accepting\ diased\ patients]$

and in the terminology of Pharmaceutical industrial problems, quality control department , when they go to inspect the quality of manufactured drugs in lot

$\alpha = P[Rejecting\ a\ good\ lot\ of\ drugs]$

$\beta = P[Accepting\ a\ bad\ lot\ of\ items].$

In general the Type-I, Error is known as producer's risk and the Type-II, Error is known as Consumer's risk

Power of Test

According to the hypothetical statement β can be written as

$\beta = P[Type - II - Error]$

$= P[\,Accepting\ H0\ when\ H0\ is\ not\ true]$

But according to theory of probability, if p is probability of success and q – is probability of failure, then $p + q = 1$

$\therefore P[\,Accepting\ H0\ when\ H0\ is\ not\ true] + P[\,Accepting\ H0\ when\ H0\ ist\ true] = 1$

$\beta + \alpha = 1$

$\alpha = 1 - \beta$

$1 - \beta = P[\,Accepting\ H0\ when\ H0\ ist\ true]$ is called as the power of tests

Hence, minimizing β, results in maximizing $(1 - \beta)$, which is called as power of test. In the usual practice of the study or testing the hypothesis, the α will be fixed and then try to obtain a criterion to minimize β.

Level of Significance

The maximum size of type-I error, where the investigator prepared to risk is known as the level of significance. The level of significance is denoted as α. In statistical analysis the commonly used level of significance are 5% (0.05) and 1% (0.01).

When we say 5% level of significance, it implies that 5 samples out of 100, we are likely to reject. In other way, that the investigators are 95% confident, that the decision taken to reject H_0 is correct. In any statistical calculation or analysis that is always fixed in advance, before collecting the information about the sample which we are going to select for experimental study.

Critical Region

When an investigator takes several samples of same from a particular population, on which experimental study has to be performed and compute some statistics t (say $\bar{x}$, p etc) for each samples. The statistics of each samples $(t_1, t_2, t_3\text{-----}t_k)$ may be used to test some null hypothesis. Some statistics of these samples may lead to rejection of H_0 and other may lead to acceptance of H_0. The statistics which leads to the rejection of H_0 is called as critical region (C) or rejection region (R), and statistics which leads to the acceptance of H_0 can be called as Acceptance region (A).

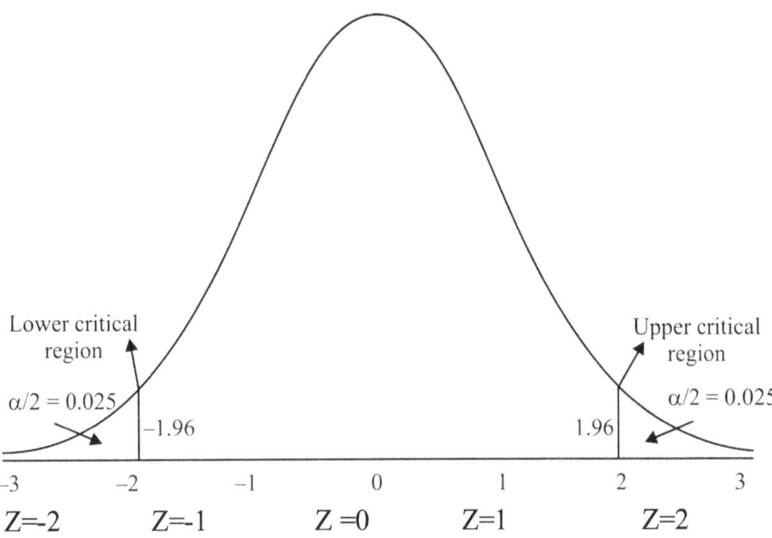

The critical region for two tailed test at the level of significance α is given by $Z > Z_{\alpha/2}$ or $Z < -Z_{\alpha/2}$

Right tailed test

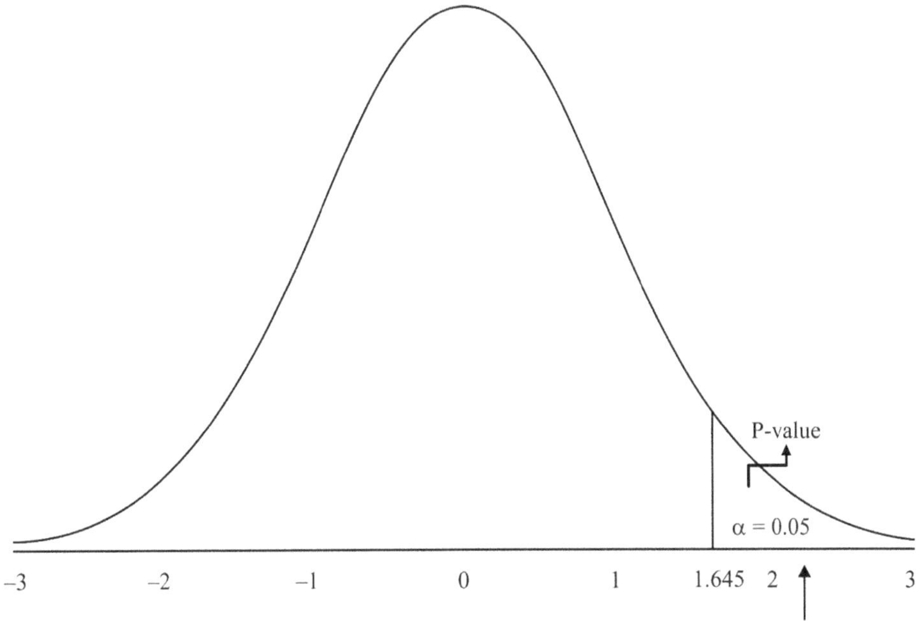

Left tailed test

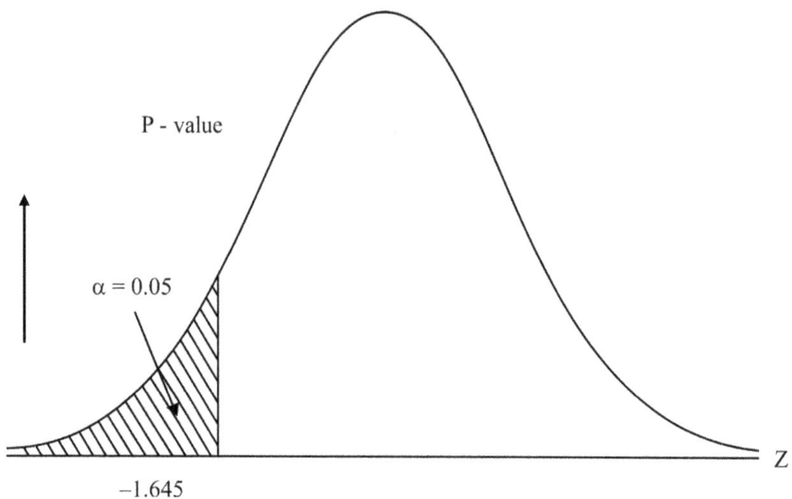

The critical (rejection) region at the level of significance α is

(i) $Z > Z\,\alpha$ for right tailed test

(ii) $Z < -Z\,\alpha$ for left tailed test

P-Values

Instead of making a statement on the experimental or observed value of the test – statistics is significant or not, many investigator writes in their research paper report of the result in terms P value. The **P-value** is the level of marginal significance within a **statistical** hypothesis test representing the probability of the occurrence of a given event. The **p-value** is used as an alternative to rejection points to provide the smallest level of significance at which the null hypothesis would be rejected.

Probability of getting values of the test statistics as extreme as or more extreme than, that observed if the null hypothesis is true.

When $P < \alpha$, H_0 is rejected

$P \geq \alpha$, H_0 is not rejected.

However, the reporting of P-values as part of the results of an investigation is more informative to the readers than statements such as "the null Hypothesis is rejected at the level of 0.05 or 5%" or "the results are not significant at the level of 0.05 or 5%".

Steps involved for Testing Hypothesis

There are two methods to perform hypothesis testing, they are:

1. Rejection region method

2. P-Value testing Method

Rejection Region Method

Step 1: Set/state null Hypothesis

Step 2: Set the alternative Hypothesis

Step 3: Select the appropriate level of significance (α) (5% or 1% level in advance)

Step 4: Define the appropriate sample statistics to be used

Step 5: Define test statistics and calculate test statistics for defined hypothesis (H_0 or H_1)

(The test statistics may be t-test, F-test, Chi-square test etc)

Step 6: Select or obtain the critical value and critical region for the particular test statistics which will be computed

Step 7: If the computed value of test statistics lies in the rejection region, then H_0 will be rejected, the H_1 will be accepted at a particular level of significance α (5% or 1%)

Step 8: Draw inference of the test.

If the calculated value of test statistics is less than the difference is significant, then H_0 – null hypothesis will be accepted at the level of significance α.

If the calculated value of test statistics is greater than the standard value, then the difference is significant. Here H_0 – Null hypothesis will be rejected at the level of significance α.

P-Value testing Method

Step 1: Compute from the observations the observed value t_{obs} of the test statistic T.

Step 2: Calculate the p-value. This is the probability, under the null hypothesis, of sampling a test statistic at   least as extreme as that which was observed.

Step 3: Reject the null hypothesis, in favour of the alternative hypothesis, if and only if the p-value is less than the significance level (the selected probability) threshold.

The two processes are equivalent. The former process was advantageous in the past when only tables of test statistics at common probability thresholds were available. It allowed a decision to be made without the calculation of a probability. It was adequate for class work and for operational use, but it was deficient for reporting results.

The latter process relied on extensive tables or on computational support not always available. The explicit calculation of a probability is useful for reporting. The calculations are now trivially performed with appropriate software.

8   Parametric Tests

Standard error is the approximate standard deviation of a statistical sample population. Standard error is a statistical term that measures the accuracy with which a sample represents a population. In statistics, a sample mean deviates from the actual mean of a population; this deviation is the standard error.

The standard error (SE) of a statistic (usually an estimate of a parameter) is the standard deviation of its sampling distribution or an estimate of that standard deviation. The standard error of mean measure only sampling error. The sampling errors are those, which are involved in estimating a population parameter from a sample instead of including all the information in the population. The standard error of mean gives the range of deviation from the population mean within which means of infinite number of large sample would lie. If the parameter or the statistic is the mean, it is called the standard error of the mean (SEM).

The sampling distribution of a population mean is generated by repeated sampling and recording of the means obtained. This forms a distribution of different means, and this distribution has its own mean and variance. Mathematically, the variance of the sampling distribution obtained is equal to the variance of the population divided by the sample size. This is because as the sample size increases, sample means cluster more closely around the population mean.

Therefore, the relationship between the standard error and the standard deviation is such that, for a given sample size, the standard error equals the standard deviation divided by the square root of the sample size. In other words, the standard error of the mean is a measure of the dispersion of sample means around the population mean.

When the standard deviation of the population is known, the standard of mean can be obtained by the equation $\dfrac{\sigma_p}{\sqrt{N}}$

$$\text{Standard error of Mean} = SE_{\bar{X}} = \dfrac{\sigma_p}{\sqrt{N}}$$

Here σ_p = Standard deviation of the population

N = Number of items in the sample

When the standard deviation of the population is not known, the standard of mean can be obtained by the equation $\dfrac{\sigma_s}{\sqrt{N}}$

Standard error of Mean $= SE_{\bar{X}} = \dfrac{\sigma_s}{\sqrt{N}}$

Here σ_s = Standard deviation of the sample

N = Number of items in the sample

The range of deviation of mean for 95% probable limits mean would lie can be obtained using Mean $\pm$ 1.96 $SE_{\bar{X}}$.

That is $\qquad\qquad\qquad \bar{X} \pm 1.96\ SE_{\bar{X}}$.

Example 1: If the average systolic blood pressure of population is 120 mmHg and a sample of size 200 is selected from the same population for clinical study with average BP 118 mmHg and Standard deviation is 15, find the range of BP of the population within which the means of the infinite number large sample of population mean would lie.

Solution:

The population mean μ = 120 and the sample mean $\bar{X}$ = 118,

Then the standard error of mean $SE_{\bar{X}} = \dfrac{\sigma_s}{\sqrt{N}} = 0.35$

The Range is $\bar{X} \pm 1.96\ SE_{\bar{X}}$. $= 118 \pm 0.35 = 119.06$ ----116.94

Example 2: The percentage saturation of bile in 15 female patient is as recorded below. Find the range of mean bile saturation of the population within which the means of the infinite number large sample of population mean would lie.

SLNO	percent Saturation of bile	d=(X-Mean(X)	d^2
1	40	-43.47	1889.641
2	86	2.53	6.4009
3	111	27.53	757.9009
4	86	2.53	6.4009
5	66	-17.47	305.2009
6	123	39.53	1562.621
7	90	6.53	42.6409
8	112	28.53	813.9609
9	52	-31.47	990.3609
10	88	4.53	20.5209
11	65	-18.47	341.1409
12	78	-5.47	29.9209
13	89	5.53	30.5809
14	56	-27.47	754.6009
15	110	26.53	703.8409
	$\sum X = 1252$		$\sum d^2 = 8255.734$

Mean $= \sum X/N = 1252/15 = 83.47$

Standard Deviation of sample $= S = \sqrt{\dfrac{\sum d^2}{n}} = \sqrt{\dfrac{8255.734}{23.46}} = 23.46$

Standard Error $= SE = S/\sqrt{N} = S/\sqrt{15} = 5.96$

Then the 95% confidence interval for the population within which the mean of infinite number of sample would lie is Mean $\pm 1.96(SE) = 83.47 \pm 1.96(5.96) = 71.78\text{-----}95.15$

Standard Error of the difference between the Means of two Samples

When two independent random samples chosen from same population with size N_1 and N_2 respectively. There may be some difference between the means of those two samples. The difference may be either due to some chance or due to some other factors. To find out this, the standard error of the difference between the means of two samples is calculated.

The standard error of the difference between two sample means can be calculated using the equation of formulae as listed below

1. When the standard deviation of the population is known (σ_p), then

$$S.E.(\overline{X1} - \overline{X2}) = \sigma p \sqrt{\dfrac{1}{N1} + \dfrac{1}{N2}}$$

   N1 and N2 sizes of the sample1 and sample2

2. When the standard deviation of the population is not known and samples are chosen from two different populations, then the standard error of the difference between their means would be

$$S.E.(\overline{X1} - \overline{X2}) = \sqrt{\dfrac{\sigma 1^2}{N1} + \dfrac{\sigma 2^2}{N2}}$$

   where σ_1 and σ_2 are standard deviations of the two samples.

Tests of Significance for a Single Mean

If $x_1, x_2, \ldots\ldots x_n$ are the n-observations of the sample or n-subjects who have been taken for study, these subjects are selected in a random way from the population whose mean is μ and standard deviation is σ

then

$$|Z| = \dfrac{|\bar{x} - \mu|}{\sigma/\sqrt{n}}$$

$\bar{x}$ is the mean or average of the sample chosen from / drawn from large population.

Note:

1. If the standard deviation of population is not known then $\sigma = s$, s – standard deviation of sample

2. Confidence limits for μ

For 95 and 99% confidence limits can be obtained for population mean μ using the equations

For 95% Confidence limits: $\bar{x} \pm 1.96 \ \sigma/n$ or $\bar{x} \pm 1.96 \ s/\sqrt{n}$

For 99% Confidence limits: $\bar{x} \pm 2.58 \ \sigma/n$ or $\bar{x} \pm 2.58 \ s/\sqrt{n}$

Example: It is claimed that the average life span of population is reduced to 75 years. A random sample of size 200 taken from the same large population and average life span is 73-years and standard deviation s is 5.2 years. Is there any significance difference between the means of population and sample.

Solution: The given values are Sample mean $\bar{x} = 73$ and sample size n = 200, standard deviation of sample s is 5.2 and population mean $\mu = 75$, then

$$|Z| = \frac{|\bar{x} - \mu|}{s/\sqrt{n}} = \frac{|73 - 75|}{5.2/\sqrt{200}} = \frac{2}{0.3676} = 8.158924$$

The calculated value of Z is greater than 1.96 at 95% confidence level. Hence the difference between the sample and population mean is significant. Hence the Null hypothesis H_0 is rejected and the alternative hypothesis H_1 is accepted and sample is not coming from the same population.

Tests of Significance for Difference of Means

The tests of significance between the means of two large samples can be obtained by the equation $Z = \dfrac{\overline{x1} - \overline{x2}}{\sqrt{\sigma\left(\frac{1}{n1} + \frac{1}{n2}\right)}}$ where $\overline{x1}$ is the mean sample$_1$ chosen from population1 and $\overline{x2}$ is the mean sample$_1$ chosen from population2. Here both the samples are taken from very large populations.

$$s = \sqrt{\frac{n1 s1^2 + n2 s2^2}{n1 + n2}}$$

s is combined standard deviation of two samples which are chosen from two large populations. If σ - standard deviation of the population is not known, then $s = \sigma$

Tests of Significance based on t-Distribution

To analyze the data of small sample, William S-Gosset developed statistical technique in the beginning of 20th – century and was later extended by Professor R. A. Fisher. The statistic which was given by Gosset known as student's t-test in the 1908.

The significance of the test based on the fundamental assumptions in all the exact sample test are:

(i) The parent population(s) from which the samples (s) is (are) drawn is (are) normally distributed.

(ii) The samples (s) is (are) random and independent of each other.

Students 'T' Distribution

The proportion of estimating population parameter from a small sample tackled with success by W. S. Gosset, under the name 'Student'. He referred to the ratio called 't' or Student's 't' and its sampling distribution is named as t-distribution. The t-distribution is obtained by the equation $t = \frac{|\bar{x}-\mu|}{s}\sqrt{n}$.

In this case, standard deviation of the population will be not known, but the standard deviation of the sample will be obtained by equation $s = \sqrt{\frac{\Sigma(x-\bar{x})^2}{n-1}}$.

Student's 'T'

Definition

If $x_1, x_2 \dots x_n$ is a random sample of size n chosen from a normal population with mean μ and standard deviation s, then student's t-statistic is defined as

$$t = \frac{|\bar{x}-\mu|}{s}\sqrt{n}$$

where $\bar{x}$ is the mean of sample and standard deviation of the sample. $s = \sqrt{\frac{\Sigma(x-\bar{x})^2}{n-1}}$.

Since size of the random sample taken for study is small and bias will be there in choosing sample, to reduce bias in random selection of sample, size n is reduced by (n–1), that is also called as degree of freedom and that is denoted as $\lambda = (n-1)$.

Critical Value of T

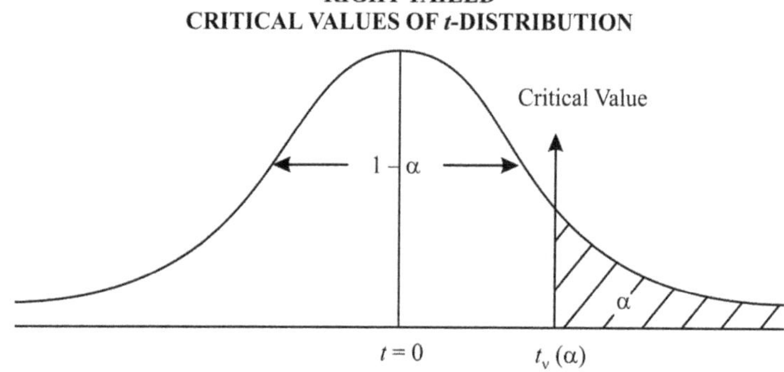

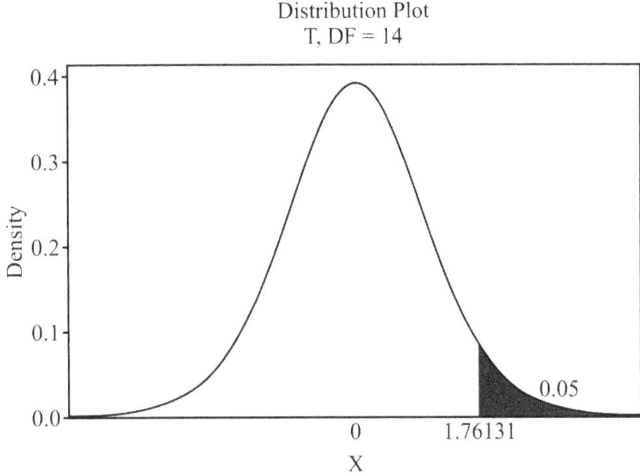

Here we define $P[t > t_\lambda(\alpha)] = \alpha$

The value of $t_\lambda(\alpha)$ is called as the upper (right tailed) – critical (or significant) value of t for ($t\,\lambda = df$) and the corresponding confidence coefficient ($1-\alpha$)

Two Tailed Test

TWO TAILED
CRITICAL VALUES OF *t*-DISTRIBUTION

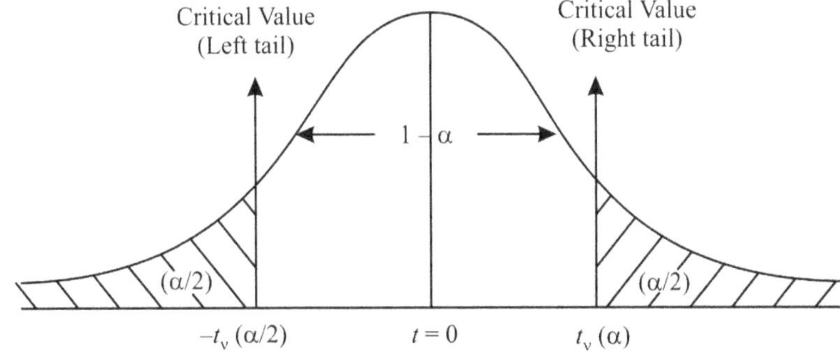

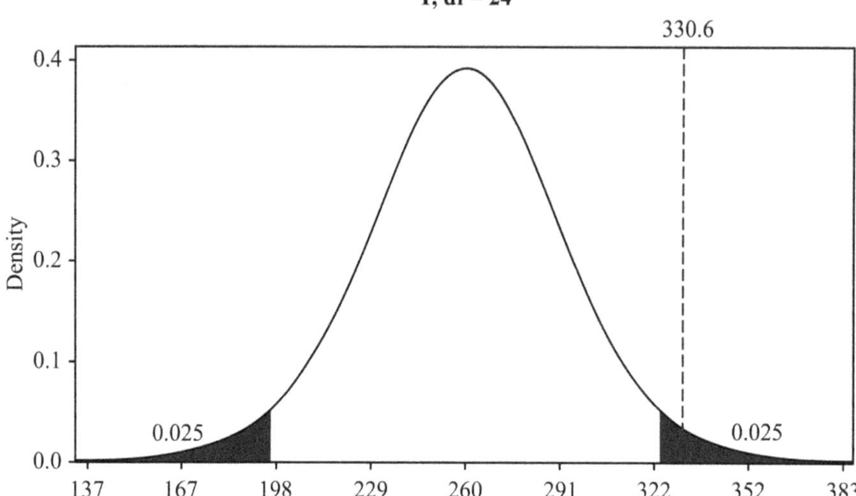

The two tailed critical values of t for degree of freedom λ with equal tails , each of area $(\alpha/2)$ are given by t_λ $(\alpha/2)$: +ve critical value and $- t_\lambda$ $(\alpha/2)$: -ve critical value. These critical values are tabulated in a t-distribution for different values α and λ.

T-test can be classified into three types, they are:

1. **Sample t-test:** This will be used to know the level of significance between population mean and sample or to know that the sample is coming from same population or from different population.

2. **Independent or Pooled sample t-test:** This t-test is most useful to know the level of significant difference between two independent samples which are taken from two different populations.

3. **Comparison or Difference or Paired or Student's t-test:** This test is applied to know the level of significance between the control and treatment, before and after treatment or Treatment and Placebo group.

Test for Single Mean: (Sample T-test)

The mathematical equation which is used calculate sample t-test is

$$t = \frac{|\bar{x}-\mu|}{s}\sqrt{n}$$

where $\bar{x}$ is the mean of sample, s is standard deviation of the sample. S is obtained by the equation $S = \sqrt{\dfrac{\Sigma(x-\bar{x})^2}{n-1}}$

To perform sample t-test, we have to set up null hypothesis.

Step 1. Set $H_0: \mu = \mu_0$. Here the investigator assume the population will be equal to sample μ_0.

Step 2: There is no significance difference between the means of sample and Population

Step 3: H_0: The sample which has been chosen for study has been drawn from the normal population with mean μ_0.

Step 4. Under the assumption H_0 the test statistics is performed by using the equations

$$t = \frac{|\bar{x}-\mu|}{s}\sqrt{n}, \quad \mu = \mu_0, \quad \bar{x} = \frac{\Sigma x}{n} \quad S = \sqrt{\frac{\Sigma(x-\bar{x})^2}{n-1}} \quad \text{where } \bar{x} \text{ is mean of the sample S is Standard}$$

deviation of the sample.

Step 5: The corresponding degree of freedom $\lambda = (n\text{-}1)$ for the sample size chosen for the study is computed

Step 6: To computed value of test statistics (t) under the assumption H_0 is compared with the standard table of 't' for the corresponding degree of freedom $\lambda = (n\text{-}1)$ at 5% or 1% level of significance.

Step 7: The inference is drawn, that the difference is significant, when the calculated value of t is greater than the table value or standard value and H_0 is rejected. If the calculated value of t is less than the standard or tabulated value of t, H_0 may be accepted at the level of significance.

Confidence or Fiducial Limits for Population Mean

The confidence limit can be obtained by the equation $\bar{x} \pm t_{(n\text{-}1)}(\alpha/2)\,\dfrac{s}{\sqrt{n}}$. The $t_{(n\text{-}1)}(\alpha/2)$ is the t-value which will be selected from the t-distribution table for the corresponding the degree of freedom $\lambda = (n\text{-}1)$. The t-value can be chosen for 95% or 99% confidence level of significance.

Example 1: A random sample of 16 patients have been selected for a clinical trial study, their average weight found to 66 kg. The sum of squares of deviation from mean is 150. Can this be regarded as taken from the population having mean weight 70 Kg? Also obtain 95% confidence limit for the sample mean.

Solution: The sample size $n = 16$ and $S^2 = 150$.

The average of Sample is $\bar{x}$ 66 and Population mean $= 70\,\text{kg} = 66$

Then the standard deviation $S = \sqrt{S^2}$

Then $S = \sqrt{150} = 12.25$

Then $t = \dfrac{|\bar{x}-\mu|}{s}\sqrt{n} = \dfrac{|66-70|}{12.25}\sqrt{10}$

$\qquad = \dfrac{4}{12.25}\,3.16$

$\qquad = 1.031837$

The Degree of freedom $\lambda = (n-1) = 10 - 1 = 9$

For DOF $= 9$ at 5% level of significance the t-value is 2.263.

The calculated value of t is less than the standard value. Hence the difference is not significant at 5% level of significance and H_0 is accepted. The sample is coming from the same population.

The confidence limit at 5% is $\bar{x} \pm t_{(n\text{-}1)}(\alpha/2)\,\dfrac{s}{\sqrt{n}}$

$$= 66 \pm t_{(10\text{-}1)}(\alpha/2)\,\dfrac{s}{\sqrt{n}}$$

$$= 66 \pm \quad 2.263 \,(12.25)/\sqrt{10}$$

$$= 66 \pm 8.77$$

$$= 57.23,\ 74.77$$

Exercises

1. A random sample of size 10 tablets chosen from a normal population and petencise of those 10 tablets are found to be as listed below.

Tablet number	1	2	3	4	5	6	7	8	9	10
Potency	199	196	198	199	201	196	198	202	200	201

   The average potency of population is 200 mg. Can this random sample be regarded as taken from the population whose mean is 200 mg? Also construct 95% confidence interval of mean for the corresponding degree of freedom.

2. A new drug manufacturer wants to market a new drug only, if he could be quite sure that the mean temperature of a healthy person after taking the new drug could not rise above 98.6^0 F, otherwise he will withhold the drug.

   The drug is administered to a random of 17 healthy persons. The mean temperature was found to 98.4^0 F, with a standard deviation of 0.6 F. Assuming that the distribution of the temperature is normal and $\alpha = 0.01$, what should the manufacturer do?

3. A random sample of 15 subjects were selected from the population where the average B.P. of the population is 130. The B.P of 15 subjects who have chosen from that population are as listed below.

Patient Number	1	2	3	4	5	6	7	8	9	10	11	12	13	14	14
Blood pressure	125	120	135	140	135	130	130	135	125	120	135	140	135	140	140

   Can this random sample regarded as taken from the population, whose mean is 130. Also construct 95% confidence limit for the population mean for the corresponding degree of freedom.

4. The following data gives Body mass index (BMI) and Forced vital capacity (FVC) of 12 patients. Can we conclude that mean FVC in those BMI < 25 kg/m^2 is different form those with BMI ≥ 25 kg/m^2? Carry out an appropriate statistical test and verify the level of significance at 95% level of confidence

Patient No.	1	2	3	4	5	6	7	8	9	10	11	12
BMI	21	18	25	27	22	21	24	20	19	24	25	20
FVC	3.5	2.7	4.2	3.9	3.1	2.8	3.7	4.1	3.0	3.8	3.1	3.7

Ans: $t = 1.03$ and DOF $= 10$, $T_{cal} = 1.03 < 2.228 = T_{ble}$ at 5% level of significant. Difference is not significant

T-test for the difference of Means (Unpaired T-test)

When an investigators wants to test two independent samples, which are chosen or drawn from two normal populations, where the means of those two populations are same and variance are also equal., then to verify the level of significance difference between the means of those two samples, pooled t-test is used.

The t-value is computed using the equation

$$t = \frac{|\bar{x_1} - \bar{x}_2|}{s} \sqrt{\frac{n_1 * n_2}{n_1 + n_2}}$$

where $\bar{x_1} = \frac{\Sigma x1}{n1}$ and $\bar{x_2} = \frac{\Sigma \bar{x}_2}{n_2}$ and standard deviation

$$s = \sqrt{\frac{\Sigma d_1{}^2 + \Sigma d_2{}^2}{n_1 + n_2 - 2}}$$

$\Sigma d_1{}^2 = \Sigma(x_1 - \bar{x}_1)^2$ and $\Sigma d_2{}^2 = \Sigma(x_2 - \bar{x}_2)^2$ and $(n_1 + n_2 - 2)$ is degree of freedom.

After obtaining the t-value, the computed value will be compared with the table or standard value for the corresponding degree of freedom $\lambda = (n_1 + n_2 - 2)$ at 5% or 1% level of significance to accept or to reject null hypothesis H_0.

Assumption for Pooled T-test

1. The parent populations from which samples are chosen or drawn are normally distributed

2. Both the samples which are drawn for study are independent

3. Here the investigator assumes that the standard deviations of both the populations are equal.

   i.e., $\sigma_1 = \sigma_2 = \sigma$

This is the most important test because, this is commonly used in clinical studies (a parallel-group design). This test can be applied for the comparison of an active drug and a placebo where each treatment is treated to test on different groups of patients.

To perform pooled t-test, steps to be followed are:

Step 1. Set H_0: $\mu1 = \mu_2$. Here the investigator assume the population of two samples equal

Step 2: There is no significance difference between the means two Population

Step 3: H_0 : The samples which are chosen for study has been drawn from the normal population

Step 4: Under the assumption H_0 the test statistics is performed by using the equations equation

$$t = \frac{|\bar{x_1} - \bar{x}_2|}{s} \sqrt{\frac{n_1 * n_2}{n_1 + n_2}}$$

where $\qquad \bar{x_1} = \frac{\Sigma x1}{n1}$ and $\bar{x_2} = \frac{\Sigma \bar{x}_2}{n_2}$

and standard deviation $\quad s = \sqrt{\dfrac{\Sigma d_1^2 + \Sigma d_2^2}{n_1 + n_2 - 2}}$

Step 5: The corresponding degree of freedom $\lambda = (n-1)$ for the sample size chosen for the study is computed

Step 6: To computed value of test statistics (t) under the assumption H_0 is compared with the standard table of 't' for the corresponding degree of freedom $\lambda = (n_1 + n_2 - 2)$ at 5% or 1% level of significance.

Step 7: The inference is drawn , that the difference is significant, when the calculated value of t is greater than the table value or standard value and H_0 is rejected. If the calculated value of t is less than the standard or tabulated value of t, H_0 may be accepted at the level of significance.

Example: The nicotine content in milligrams of two samples of tobacco were found to be as listed below:

Sample X1	24	27	26	21	25	
Sample X2	27	30	28	31	22	36

Can we conclude that both the samples come from normal population having same mean?

X1	d1 = (X1-mean(x1))	X2	d_2 = (X2-mean(x2))	$d1^2$	$d2^2$
24	-0.6	27	-2	0.36	4
27	2.4	30	1	5.76	1
26	1.4	28	-1	1.96	1
21	-3.6	31	2	12.96	4
25	0.4	22	-7	0.16	49
123		36	7	21.2	49
		174			108
Mean(x1)	24.6				
Mean(x2)	29				
$S = \sqrt{\dfrac{\Sigma d_1^2 + \Sigma d_2^2}{n_1 + n_2 - 2}}$	3.79				
t	1.917816095				

Exercise

A batch of 5 patients were advised to perform an exercise and that will raise systolic level of blood pressure (sys BP) for at least one hour.

Do these data acceptably support the hypothesis that the exercise raises average sys BP for at least one hour?

Sys before exercise (mmHg)	118	120	140	128	130
Sys after exercise (mmHg)	127	128	132	136	130

Confidence Interval for difference of Means ($\mu 1 - \mu 2$)

(Small Samples)

The confidence interval for the difference of mean ($\mu 1 - \mu 2$) is constructed by using the equation $\left[\overline{x1} - \overline{x2} \mp t_{(n1+n2-2)}(\alpha/2)s \sqrt{\left(\frac{1}{n1} + \frac{1}{n2}\right)} \right]$. The $(n_1 + n_2 - 2)$ is degree of freedom, S is combined standard deviation and $t(\alpha/2)$ is the critical value of t for the corresponding degree of freedom at 5% and 1% level of significance.

Exercise

1. A certain drug administered to 10 patients showed the following additional hours of sleep.

SLNO	1	2	3	4	5	6	7	8	9	10
Additional hours of sleep	-1.0	0.5	2.7	-0.6	1.2	1.8	1.6	3.5	0.2	-1.7

   Can it concluded that the drug does produce additional hours of sleep?

2. In a sample of 10 patients, the mean percentage of obese adults was 28.3 and standard deviation of that sample is 3.5. The standard deviation of the population is not known. Construct 95% confidence interval for population mean.

Ans: Confidence interval is 25.6 and 30.6

3. The coronary health improvement project (CHIP) there were 337 volunteers aged 43 to 85. Here participants are divided into two groups, named as intervention and control groups. The total number of volunteers in interventional group is 167 and in control group is 170. The average age of intervention group is 50.39 and the control group is 50.39, combined standard deviation is 11.05. Test whether the mean age differs significantly between the participants of intervention and control group.

Ans: t = 0.37

Paired T-test for the Difference of Means

This paired t-test is also named as comparison, difference and student's t-test. In general this test will be applied to know the level of significance difference between before and after treatment.

Suppose an investigators wants to find the whether the drug is really effective in curing the disease or not. Let x1, x2,.....xn be the disease status of patients before treatment and y1, y2,.......yn be the condition of the disease or disease status of the patients after treatment. In order to test level of significance difference between before and after treatment, we apply paired t-test.

Let di= xi – yi (i= 1, 2, ... n) denote the difference in the observations of subjects or items.

The test – value can be computed using the equation

$$t = \frac{\overline{d}}{s}\sqrt{n} \quad \text{where } d = x - y \text{ and } \overline{d} = \frac{\Sigma d}{n} \text{ and } s = \sqrt{\frac{\Sigma d^2 - (\overline{d})^2 * n}{n-1}}$$

In such cases, the degree of freedom $\lambda = (n-1)$

Example 1: The systolic blood pressure of 12 patients between the ages of 20 and 35 were measured before and after administration of a newly developed oral contraceptive and data is recorded as listed below. Is there any significance difference before and after treatment.

SL No (Subjects)	Systolic Blood Pressure		Difference $d=(A-B)$	d^2
	Before treatment(B)	After treatment(A)		
1	122	127	5	25
2	126	128	2	04
3	132	140	8	64
4	120	119	-1	01
5	142	145	3	09
6	130	130	0	00
7	142	148	6	36
8	137	135	-2	04
9	128	129	1	01
10	132	137	5	25
11	128	128	0	00
12	129	133	4	16
			$\sum d = 31$	$\sum d^2 = 185$

Here n = 12 subjects and $\bar{d}$ = average of the difference and $\bar{d} = \dfrac{\sum d}{n}$ = 31/12 = 2.58. Then the standard deviation is calculated using the equation s $= \sqrt{\dfrac{\sum d^2 - (\bar{d})^2 \times n}{n-1}}$.

$$S = \sqrt{\frac{185 - (2.58)^2 * 12}{12 - 1}} = 3.09$$

Then $\qquad t = \dfrac{\bar{d}}{s}\sqrt{n} = \dfrac{2.58}{3.09}\sqrt{12} = 2.90$

Then the degree of freedom $\lambda = (n-1) = (12-1) = 11$

At 5% level of significance the standard value of t for $\lambda = 11$ is 2.201. Calculated value of t = 2.90 > 2.201. Hence H_0 is rejected. Difference is significant and H_1 is accepted.

Exercises: In a certain experiment to compare the effects of two types of food A and B were advised for 8-subjects in each group (8+8). The subjects who have been drawn from two independent samples and increase /gain in weight due to consumption of food A and B for one month is as listed below(lb).

Subjects		1	2	3	4	5	6	7	8
Increase in Weight	A	49	51	52	47	50	52	53	53
	B	52	55	52	53	50	54	54	53

Assume subjects selected from two samples are independent, can we conclude that food B is better than food A in promoting weight gain?

1. Two laboratories carryout independent estimates of particular chemical in a medicine produced by a certain firm. A sample is taken from each batch, halved and separate halves are sent to the two laboratories. The following data is obtained.

No. of samples $\qquad$: 10

Mean Value of difference : 0.6

Of estimates

Sum of squares of the : 20

Differences (from Mean)

Is the difference is significant?

T-test for significance of an observed Sample from Correlation Coefficient

When a random sample (x_i, y_i), $i = 1, 2, 3, ..., n$ of size 'n' has been drawn from a bivariate normal distribution and r be the coefficient of correlation between the bivariate (x_i, y_i). Here we are computing 't' value to verify the whether correlation coefficient is significant or not. t is computed using the equation $t = \dfrac{r}{\sqrt{1-r^2}} \sqrt{n-2}$

i.e., t follows student's t – distribution with degree of freedom (n-2), n is taken as sample size.

95% and 99% Confidence limit for ρ where ρ - population coefficient of correlation

$r \pm t_{(n-2)}*S.E(r)$

$r \pm t_{(n-2)}* \dfrac{1-r^2}{\sqrt{n}}$

Example 1: A random sample of 27 pairs of observations from a normal population gives correlation coefficient of 0.42. Is it likely that the variables in the populations are uncorrelated?

Solution: Under null hypothesis $H_0: \rho = 0$ i.e., the value of r = 0.42 is not significant.

$$t = \dfrac{r}{\sqrt{1-r^2}} \sqrt{n-2}$$

$$t = \dfrac{0.42}{\sqrt{1-0.42^2}} \sqrt{27-2}$$

$$t = \dfrac{0.42}{0.9075} * 5 = 2.313$$

Degree of Freedom = $n - 2 = 27 - 2 = 25$, for DOF 25 the standard value of t at 5% level of significance is 2.060. Here the calculated value of t is greater than the table value, hence difference is significant at 5% level of significance. Null hypothesis is rejected.

Example 2: A coefficient of correlation of 0.2 is derived from a random sample of 625 pairs of observations.

(i)　Is the value significant

(ii) What are the 95% and 99% confidence limits for the correlation coefficient in the population?

Under null hypothesis H_0: $\rho = 0$ i.e., the value of $r = 0.2$ is not significant.

$$t = \frac{r}{\sqrt{1-r^2}} \sqrt{n-2}$$

$$t = \frac{0.40}{\sqrt{1-0.2^2}} \sqrt{625-2}$$

$$t = \frac{0.2}{0.9797} \times 24.9599 = 5.09$$

Degree of Freedom $= n - 2 = 625 - 2 = 623$, for DOF 623 the standard value of t at 5% level of significance is 1.95 and 2.58 for large sample at 5% and 1% level of significance. Here the calculated value of t is greater than the table value, hence difference is significant at 5% and 1% level of significance. Null hypothesis is rejected.

(ii) 95% confidence limits for ρ (population correlation coefficient)

$$r \pm 1.96 \times \frac{1-r^2}{\sqrt{n}}$$

$$0.2 \pm 1.96 \times \frac{1-0.2^2}{\sqrt{625}}$$

$$0.125 \quad - \quad 0.275$$

99% confidence limits for ρ (population correlation coefficient)

$$r \pm 2.58 \times \frac{1-r^2}{\sqrt{n}}$$

$$0.2 \pm 2.58 \times \frac{1-0.2^2}{\sqrt{625}}$$

$$(0.101 - 0.299)$$

Variance – Ratio Test F-test

To test to whether two samples differs significantly, which are chosen or drawn from normal population having the same variance. Such tests are carried out with the help of F-ratio, the formula used to analyze the data of two samples is

$$F = \frac{S_1^2}{S_2^2}, \text{ when } S_1^2 > S_2^2 \text{ then } \quad F = \frac{S_1^2}{S_2^2}$$

Else

$$F = \frac{S_2^2}{S_1^2} \text{ when } S_2^2 > S_1^2 \text{ then } \quad F = \frac{S_2^2}{S_1^2}$$

In general the F is obtained by the equation

$$F = \frac{Larger\ estimate\ of\ Variance}{Smaller\ estimat\ of\ Variance}$$

$$S_1^2 = \frac{\Sigma(X1-\overline{X1})^2}{N1-1}, S_2^2 = \frac{\Sigma(X2-2)^2}{N2-1}$$

λ_1 = degree of freedom of the sample having larger variance

λ_2 = degree of freedom of the sample having smaller variance

The value of F at 5% and 1% level of significance will be compared with F-distribution table for the corresponding degree freedom of $\lambda 1$ and $\lambda 2$.

If the calculated value of F found greater than table, then the ratio is considered significant at 5% or 1%. Else it is not significant, then the samples are considered to be taken from the populations having same variance.

Example: A random sample of 10 patients were fed on diet A , the increase in weight in terms of pound over a period of time found to be 10 6 16 17 13 12 8 14 15 9

And another group of patients were fed on diet B, the increase in weight were found to be 7 13 22 15 12 14 18 8 21 23 10 17

Apply F-test and verify whether both group of diets come from different populations or same from population

X1	X2	d1=(X1 $-\overline{X1}$	d2=(X2- $\overline{X2}$)	d1^2	d2^2
10	7	-2	-8	4	64
6	13	-6	-2	36	4
16	22	4	7	16	49
17	15	5	0	25	0
13	12	1	-3	1	9
12	14	0	-1	0	1
8	18	-4	3	16	9
14	8	2	-7	4	49
15	21	3	6	9	36
9	23	-3	8	9	64
	10		-5		25
	17		2		4
$\sum$X1 =120	$\sum$X2 =180			$\sum d_1^2$ 120	$\sum d_2^2$ 314

$$\overline{x_1} = \frac{\sum x1}{n1} = 120/10 = 12 \text{ and } \overline{x_2} = \frac{\sum X_2}{n_2} = 180/12 = 15$$

$$S_1^2 = \frac{\sum d1^2}{N1-1} = \frac{120}{10-1} = 13.3$$

$$S_2^2 = \frac{\sum d2^2}{N2-1} = \frac{314}{12-1} = 28.55$$

$$F = \frac{S_2^2}{S_1^2} = \frac{28.55}{13.3} = 2.14$$

F_{cal} = 2.14 < 3.112 = F_{ble} at 5% level of significance. Hence there is no significant difference between population variance of two samples.

Larger Sample Test

Here the investigator shall develop the tests of significance for large samples. For the practical purpose, sample size which is greater than 30 considered as large sample.

Here biostatistician use the equation $Z = \dfrac{t - E(t)}{SE(t)}$ to compute test value and to verify the level of significance at 5% and 1% level.

As per the normal distribution $P(1\text{-}1.96 \leq Z \leq 1.96)$ at 5% level of significance and $P(2.58 \leq Z \leq 2.58)$ at 1% level of significance.

The significance of Z for both two-tailed and one-tailed test is given in the standard Z-distribution table.

The working principle for numerical problems in tests of hypothesis for large samples has been explained in the steps listed below.

Steps:

1. Set up Null hypothesis H_0
2. Set up alternative hypothesis H_1
3. Set up levels of significance (α)
4. Obtain the test statistics Z using the equation $Z = \dfrac{t - E(t)}{SE(t)}$ where $n \rightarrow \infty$, t -Statistics value and E(t) – expected value. These are the values due to the fluctuations of sampling.
5. Obtain the critical values of Z and critical region (under H_1) at the desired level of significance (α).
6. Conclusion: Compare the computed values with the critical values
    (a) If $|Z| > 3$, then the result is significant and null hypothesis is rejected, at the level of significance.
    (b) If $|Z| \leq 3$, then we discuss the significance of Z at the desired level of significance, in general 5% or 1% level.

Two-Tailed Test

If $|Z| > 1.96$, then the investigator concludes that the difference is significant at 5%, hence H_0 is rejected. That is the difference between t and E(t) cannot be due to fluctuation of sampling.

If $|Z| \leq 1.96$, here we conclude that difference is not significant at 5% level of significance.

The Conclusion given here is that data do not provide any evidence for the investigator against the null hypothesis H_0. Hence H_0 is not rejected.

Similarly comparison of $|Z|$ with 2.58 at 1% for rejecting or accepting H0 can be done.

Single Tailed Test

When $|Z| > 1.645$ or $|Z| > 2.33$, then H_0 will be rejected at 5% and 1% of significance.

Test for Single Proportion

If X is number of individuals or units or items having attribute (it can be called as success) for a random sample of size n, which is chosen from a large population then,

$p = \dfrac{X}{n}$, p = observed proportion of sample or

p = Proportion of success for n-trial, where X- is number of success.

$E(p) = P$ is the proportion of success for population and $SE(p) = \sqrt{\dfrac{PQ}{n}}$, where $Q = 1 - P$

Q – is the probability of failure or proportion of failure. Then

$$Z = \frac{p - E(p)}{SE(p)} = \frac{p - P}{\sqrt{\dfrac{PQ}{n}}}$$

The limits of P at the level of significance are given by $p \pm Z_{\alpha/2} \sqrt{\dfrac{pq}{n}}$

Example: In a random sample of 400 subjects from a large population, 120 are females. Can it be said that males and females are in the ratio 5:3 in the population? Use 1% level of significance.

Solution: Given that n = 400 and

X = number of females in the sample is 120

P = observed proportion of females in the sample $= \dfrac{120}{400} = 0.30$

Null Hypothesis: The males and females in the population are in the ratio 5:3 i.e., H_0: P = Proportion of females in the population is = 3/8 = 0.375

Alternate Hypothesis H1: P# 0.375 (Two tailed)

The level of significance $\alpha = 0.01$.

Test statistics under H_0 , $Z = \dfrac{p - E(p)}{SE(p)} = \dfrac{p - P}{\sqrt{\dfrac{PQ}{n}}} = \dfrac{0.3000 - 0.375}{\sqrt{\dfrac{0.375 * 0.625}{400}}}$

$$= \frac{-0.075}{0.024} = \text{-3.125}$$

$$|Z| = 3.125$$

The significance value of Z at 1% level of significance for two tailed test is 2.58. Since the calculated value of $|Z|$ is greater than 2.58, hence it is significant at 1% level of significance. Hence the null hypothesis H_0 is rejected and we conclude that the males and females in the population are not in the ratio 5:3.

Example 2: In a sample 400 drugs produced by a machine, 30 were found to be discolored. But pharmaceutical industry claimed at most 5% of their tablets are discolored. Is the claim tenable?

Solution:

Given that n = 400 and X = number of discoloured tablets in the sample = 30.

The proportion of discoloured tablets in the sample $= \dfrac{X}{n} = \dfrac{30}{400} = 0.075$

Null Hypothesis Says : $H_0 : P \le 0.05$

Alternative Hypothesis : $H_1 : P > 0.05$

H : 0.05 implies P = 0.05 and Q = 0.95

Level of significance $\alpha = 0.05$

Then $\qquad Z = \dfrac{p-P}{\sqrt{\dfrac{PQ}{n}}} = \dfrac{0.075 - 0.050}{\sqrt{\dfrac{0.075 \times 0.050}{400}}} = 8.16$

For two tailed test Z = 1.96 at 5% level of significance.

Here Z = 8.16 > 1.96

Hence the result is significant at 5% level of significance.

Hence H_0 is rejected.

Hence the Pharmaceutical industry claim P = 0.05 is not acceptable.

Tests of Significance between the Proportions

Let A and B be the prevalence of certain attributes of two large populations among the subjects considered from those two large populations.

If we take two independent samples of large sizes say, n_1 and n_2 from two large samples.

Let X1 and X2 be the observed number of success (Number of Patients or subjects possessing the given attribute) in these samples respectively.

p_1 = Observed proportion of success in the sample from first population

$$p_1 = \dfrac{X1}{n1}$$

Similarly p_2 = Observed proportion of success in the sample from second population

$q_1 = 1 - p_1$

$q_2 = 1 - p_2$

If $E(p_1) = P_1$ and $E(p_2) = P_2$, then $Q_1 = 1 - P_1$ and $Q_2 = 1 - P_2$

Then $\qquad \text{S.E}_{(p1\text{-}p2)} = \sqrt{\dfrac{P1\,Q1}{n1} + \dfrac{P2\,Q2}{n2}}$

Then $\qquad Z = \dfrac{(p1-p2) - (P1-P2)}{\sqrt{\dfrac{P1\,Q1}{n1} + \dfrac{P2\,Q2}{n2}}}$

If $\qquad \hat{P} = \dfrac{n1P1 + n2P2}{n1+n2}$, then $\hat{Q} = 1 - \hat{P}$ then

$|Z| = \dfrac{(P1-P2)}{\sqrt{PQ\left(\dfrac{1}{n1} + \dfrac{1}{n2}\right)}}$ when P1 = P2 = P, this implies that Q1 = Q2 = Q

Then the 95% limits for P is

$$\hat{P} \pm 1.96 \sqrt{\frac{\hat{P}\hat{Q}}{n}}$$

Example: Before educating about the food habits, about in group 400 subjects in the sample$_1$, 300 subjects were suffering due to particular disease A, after educating a group of 300 subjects in sample$_2$ 200 were suffering due to a particular disease A. Both the samples were taken from two large populations. Using standard error of proportion, state is there any significance difference in decrease of disease.

Solution:

We have n1 = 400 and n2 = 300

P1 = Proportion of the persons were suffering due to disease A, before educating about food habit.

$$P1 = \frac{X1}{n1} = \frac{300}{400} = 0.75$$

P2 = Proportion of second sample

$$P2 = \frac{X2}{n2} = \frac{200}{300} = 0.66$$

Set null Hypothesis H_0 : P1 = P2. There is significance difference in disease before and after education.

Alternative Hypothesis H_1 : P1 > P2 or (P2 < P1)

Level of significance is $\alpha = 0.05$

$$|Z| = \frac{(P1-P2)}{S.E\,(P1-P2)}$$

$$|Z| = \frac{(P1-P2)}{\sqrt{PQ\left(\frac{1}{n1}+\frac{1}{n2}\right)}} = \frac{(0.75-0.66)}{\sqrt{PQ\left(\frac{1}{n1}+\frac{1}{n2}\right)}}$$

$$P = \frac{n1*p1+n2*p2}{n1+n2}$$

$$P = \frac{400*0.75+300*0.66}{400+300} = 0.711$$

then   Q = 1 - P

then   Q = 1 -0.711 = 0 289

then   Z = 2.599 > 1.96

Hence the difference is significant

9 Analysis of Variance (ANOVA)

The analysis of variance is a powerful statistical tool for tests of significance. Analysis of variance is a general method of analyzing data from designed experiments, whose objective is to compare two or more than groups means.

The term analysis of variance, was introduced by Prof. R. A. Fisher in 1920. In the short form Analysis of variance can be written as ANOVA.

Definition

Analysis of variance (ANOVA) is "Separation of variance ascribable to one group causes from the variance ascribable to the other group".

In general if the investigator has a goal in research project is to discover, where there are differences in the means of several independent groups. In this situation ANOVA is most suitable method to verify the level of significance difference between more than two samples.

Assumption for ANOVA Test

ANOVA test is based on the test statistics F (Variance ratio). To verify the validity of F-test in ANOVA, there are three important assumptions, which we have consider, they are:

(i)   The observations made are independent

(ii)   Parent populations are normal, from which the observation or subjects or items are drawn randomly.

(iii)   The different treatments chosen and environmental effects are additive in nature.

Classification of ANOVA

ANOVA is classified into two methods, they are named as:

1. ONE WAY ANOVA
2. TWO WAY ANOVA

One Way ANOVA

One way ANOVA is used , when an investigator wish to test the equality of treatment means in experiments, where two or more than two treatments are randomly assigned to different, independent experimental units.

The null hypothesis is written as H_0: $\mu_1 = : \mu_2 =: \mu_3 = \mu_k$, where $\mu_1 =$ the mean of treatmant1, $\mu_2 =$ The mean the treatment2 and so on.

Suppose there are 15 – tables are available for the comparison of three assay methods, 5-tablets are assigned for each assay. Here one way ANOVA design would result from a random assignment of the tablets to three groups.

Hypothesis Testing between more than Two Means (ANOVA)

The investigator can carry out the test for the equality of several Population (k) means by the rejection region method. The various steps involved in testing hypothesis are as listed below.

Step 1: Compute $G=\sum_i \sum_j x_{ij} =$ Grand total of all the observations

Step 2: Compute correction factor (CF) $= \dfrac{G^2}{N}$ where $N = n_1 + n_2 + \ldots n_K$

    $N =$ total number of observation chosen for study.

Step 3: Computation of raw Sum squares (RSS)

$$RSS = \sum_i \sum_j x_{ij}^2 = \text{Sum of the squares of all the observations or experimental results}$$

Step 4: Total sum squares $=$ SST $=$ RSS $-$ CF

Step 5: Computation of $T_i = \sum_{j=1}^{nj} x_{ij}$

    $T_i =$ The sum of all the observations in the ith class, $i=1, 2, 3 \ldots k$

Step 6: Computations of sum of squares between treatments (Columns)

$$SCC = \frac{T1^2}{n1} + \frac{T2^2}{n2} + \ldots + \frac{Tk^2}{nk} - CF$$

Step 7: Sum of the squares due to error. This is denoted as SSE

    SSE $=$ SST $-$ SCC

        $=$ Total sum squares $-$ Sum of squares between the treatments.

Step 8: Mean squares between columns or treatment is computed as MSC $= \dfrac{SSC}{k-1}$

    K$=$ Number of samples.

Step 9: Mean squares due to error. It is denoted as MSE

    MSE $= \dfrac{SSE}{N-k}$

Step 10: Computation of test statistics under H_0:

$$F = \frac{Mean\ squares\ between\ samples\ or\ columns}{Means\ squares\ due\ to\ err\ or}$$

$$F = \frac{MSC}{MSE}$$

Step 11: The computation of degrees of freedom of numerator and denominator value of F -Distribution.

$$\lambda_1 = k - 1 = \text{DOF of numerator}$$

$$\lambda_2 = N - k = \text{DOF of denominator}$$

If the computed value of F for the corresponding DOF λ_1 and λ_2 is greater than the table value or critical value of F at a particular level of significance (5% or 1%), then H_0 is rejected at that level of significance, otherwise it may regarded as true.

Step 12: Critical difference between the samples

After the computation of frequency distribution value, result shows the difference is significant between the samples or treatments, then investigator has to verify which sample is more significant among the samples, which are selected randomly for studies.

To perform this, Least Significance difference (LSD) has to be obtained and that has to be compared with the absolute difference between the means of samples. LSD is computed using the equation

LSD = [The critical value of t at the level of significance for DOF (N – K) of mean square due to error] × S.E(xi – xj)

$$LSD = t_{(\alpha/2)(N-k)}\sqrt{MSE\left(\frac{1}{n1} + \frac{1}{n2}\right)}$$

t($\alpha/2$ – t-value for the corresponding degree of freedom N-k, taken from t-distribution table

MSE - Mean sum square due to error

OR

$$LSD = t_{(\alpha/2)(N-k)}\sqrt{MSE\left(\frac{2}{n_i}\right)}, \quad \text{if } n_i = n_j$$

If the difference $|x_i - x_j|$ between the means of any two treatments is greater than LSD, it is said to be significant, otherwise it is not significant.

Example 1: Test the hypothesis, that the average number of days a patient was kept in the three local hospitals say A, B and C is same, a random check on the number of days that seven patients stayed in each hospital reveals the following.

Hospital 1 X1	Hospital 2 X2	Hospital 3 X3
8	4	1
5	3	4
9	8	9
2	7	8
7	7	7
8	1	2
2	5	3

Test the hypothesis at $\alpha = 0.05$

Solution:

Hospital 1 X1	$X1^2$	Hospital 2 X2	$X2^2$	Hospital 3 X3	$X3^2$
8	64	4	16	1	1
5	25	3	9	4	16
9	81	8	64	9	81
2	4	7	49	8	64
7	49	7	49	7	49
8	64	1	1	2	4
2	4	5	25	3	9
41	291	35	213	34	224
$\sum X1$	$\sum X1^2$	$\sum X2$	$\sum X2^2$	$\sum X3$	$\sum X3^2$

1. Grand Total =

$$G = \sum X1 + \sum X2 + \sum X3$$
$$= 41 + 35 + 34 = 110$$

2. Correction Factor = $CF = \dfrac{G^2}{N} = \dfrac{110^2}{21}$
$$= 576.1905$$

$$N = n1 + n2 = n3 = 7 + 7 + 7 = 21$$

3. Raw sum squares = $RSS = \sum X1^2 + \sum X2^2 + \sum X3^2$
$$= 291 + 213 + 224 = 728$$

4. Total sum Squares = $SST = RSS - CF = 728 - 576.1905$
$$= 151.8095$$

5. Sum of squares between columns or samples = SSC

$$SSC = \left(\left(\frac{\sum(X1)^2}{n1} \right) + \left(\frac{\sum(X2)^2}{n2} \right) + \left(\frac{\sum(X3)^2}{n3} \right) \right) - CF$$

$$= \left(\left(\frac{(41)^2}{7} \right) + \left(\frac{(35)^2}{7} \right) + \left(\frac{(34)^2}{7} \right) \right) - 576.1905$$

$$SSC = 4.095238$$

6. Sum of squares due to error = SSE

    SSE = SST − SSC = 151.8095 − 4.095238 = 147.7143

7. Mean Squares between columns or treatment = MSC $= \dfrac{SSC}{K-1}$

    K = number of samples taken for study = 3

    $$MSC = \frac{4.095238}{3-1} = 2.048$$

8. Mean square due to error = MSE $= \dfrac{SSE}{N-K} = \dfrac{147.7143}{21-3}$

    MSE = 8.206

9. Computation of Test value , F − distribution
    $$F = \frac{MSC}{MSE} = \frac{2.048}{8.206}$$

    F = 0.250

10. Computation of degree of freedom of numerator (MSC) and denominator (MSE) of F-distribution

    $\lambda 1 = K - 1 = 3 - 1 = 2$
    $\lambda 2 = N - k = 21 - 3 = 18$

11. Computed value of F-distribution should be compared with standard table value of F-distribution at 5% or 1% level of significance.

    Here the table value the degree of freedom 2 and 18 is $F_{ble} = 3.08$

    $F = 0.250 < F_{ble} = 3.08$,

Hence the difference is not significant between the means of different samples. Null hypothesis is true.

When the difference is not significant, there is no need to compute LSD to verify which sample is more significant.

Example 2: Students were given different drug treatments before revising for their exams. Some were given a memory drug, some a placebo and some no treatment. The examination scores obtained in Percentage (%) given below for three different groups. Apply one-way ANOVA to verify the level of significance between these three treatments.

	Memory Drug	Placebo	No treatment
1	70	37	3
2	77	43	10
3	83	50	17
4	90	57	23
5	97	63	30

Solution:

Memory Drug X1	$X1^2$	Placebo X2	$X2^2$	No treatment X3	$X3^2$
70	4900	37	1369	3	9
77	5929	43	1849	10	100
83	6889	50	2500	17	289
90	8100	57	3249	23	529
97	9409	63	3969	30	900
	0		0		0
	0		0		0
417	35227	250	12936	83	1827
$\sum X1$	$\sum X1^2$	$\sum X2$	$\sum X2^2$	$\sum X3$	$\sum X3^2$

1. Grand Total $= G = \sum X1 + \sum X2 + \sum X3$

$$= 250 + 83 = 750$$

2. Correction Factor $= CF = \dfrac{G^2}{N} = \dfrac{750^2}{15}$

$$= 37500$$

$$N = n1 + n2 = n3 = 5 + 5 + 5 = 15$$

3. Raw sum squares $= RSS = \sum X1^2 + \sum X2^2 + \sum X3^2$

$$= 35227 + 12936 + 1827 = 49990$$

4. Total sum Squares $= SST = RSS - CF = 499990 - 37500$

$$SST = 12490$$

5. Sum of squares between columns or samples $= SSC$

$$SSC = \left(\left(\frac{\sum (X1)^2}{n1} \right) + \left(\frac{\sum (X2)^2}{n2} \right) + \left(\frac{\sum (X3)^2}{n3} \right) \right) - CF$$

$$= \left(\left(\frac{(417)^2}{5} \right) + \left(\frac{(250)^2}{5} \right) + \left(\frac{(83)^2}{5} \right) \right) - 37500$$

$$SSC = 11155.6$$

6. Sum of squares due to error $= SSE$

$$SSE = SST - SSC = 12490 - 11155.6 = 1334.4$$

7. Mean Squares between columns or treatment $= MSC = \dfrac{SSC}{K-1}$

$$K = \text{number of samples taken for study} = 3$$

$$MSC = \frac{11155.6}{3-1} = 5577.800$$

8. Mean square due to error $= MSE = \dfrac{SSE}{N-K} = \dfrac{1334.4}{15-3}$

   $MSE = 111.200$

9. Computation of Test value , F – distribution

   $$F = \dfrac{MSC}{MSE} = \dfrac{5577.8}{111.200}$$

   $F = 50.160$

10. Computation of degree of freedom of numerator (MSC) and denominator (MSE) of F-distribution

    $\lambda 1 = K - 1 = 3 - 1 = 2$

    $\lambda 2 = N - k = 15 - 3 = 12$

11. Computed value of F-distribution should be compared with standard table value of F-distribution at 5% or 1% level of significance.

    Here the table value the degree of freedom for degree of freedom 2 and 18 is $F_{ble} = 3.08$

    $F_{cal} = 50.160 < F_{ble} = 3.69,$

Hence the difference is significant between the means of different samples or treatments.

Null hypothesis is not true.

When the difference is significant, we need to compute LSD to verify which sample is more significant.

$$LSD = t_{(\alpha/2)(N-k)}\sqrt{MSE\left(\dfrac{2}{n_i}\right)}, \quad \text{if} \quad n_i = n_j$$

$$LSD = 1.7823 \times \sqrt{111.20\left(\dfrac{2}{5}\right)} = 11.88$$

Mean	Absolute difference between means of any samples	Comparison with LSD	Remark
Mean1 $= \overline{X1} =$ **83.4**	$Abs(\overline{X1} - \overline{X2})$ $= 83.4 - 50 = 33.4$ $Abs(\overline{X1} - \overline{X3})$ $= 83.4 - 16.6 = 66.8$	$33.4 > 11.88 = LSD$ $66.8 > 11.88 = LSD$	Difference is significant
Mean2 $= \overline{X2} = 50$	$Abs(\overline{X2} - \overline{X3})$ $= 50 - 16.6 = 33.4$	$33.4 > 11.88 = LSD$	Difference is significant
Mean3 $= \overline{X3} =$ 16.6			
The average value of X1 is more than the remaining two samples, hence X1 is more significant than remaining two samples			

ANOVA TABLE

	Sum of squares	DOF	Mean Squares	F	Significant
Between samples	11155.6	2	5577.800	50.160	P< 0.0001
Within samples	1334.4	12	111.200		
Total	12490.0	14			

Example

Calcium is an essential mineral that regulates the heart, is important for blood clotting and for building healthy bones. The National Osteoporosis Foundation recommends a daily calcium intake of 1000-1200 mg/day for adult men and women. While calcium is contained in some foods, most adults do not get enough calcium in their diets and take supplements. Unfortunately some of the supplements have side effects such as gastric distress, making them difficult for some patients to take on a regular basis.

A study is designed to test whether there is a difference in mean daily calcium intake in adults with normal bone density, adults with osteopenia (a low bone density which may lead to osteoporosis) and adults with osteoporosis. Adults 60 years of age with normal bone density, osteopenia and osteoporosis are selected at random from hospital records and invited to participate in the study. Each participant's daily calcium intake is measured based on reported food intake and supplements. The data are shown below.

Normal Bone Density	Osteopenia	Osteoporosis
1200	1000	890
1000	1100	650
980	700	1100
900	800	900
750	500	400
800	700	350

Is there a statistically significant difference in mean calcium intake in patients with normal bone density as compared to patients with osteopenia and osteoporosis?

We will run the ANOVA using the five-step approach.

1. Correction Factor = CF $= \dfrac{G^2}{N} = \dfrac{14720^2}{18} = 12037689$

    $N = n1 + n2 = n3 = 6 + 6 + 6 = 18$

2. Raw sum squares = RSS $= \sum X1^2 + \sum X2^2 + \sum X3^2$

    $= 5412900 + 4080000 + 3517100 = 13010000$

3. Total sum Squares = SST = RSS − CF = $13010000 - 12037689$

    SST = 972311

4. Sum of squares between columns or samples = SSC

$$SSC = \left(\left(\frac{\sum(X1)^2}{n1}\right) + \left(\frac{\sum(X2)^2}{n2}\right) + \left(\frac{\sum(X3)^2}{n3}\right) \right) - CF$$

$$= \left(\left(\frac{(5630)^2}{6} \right) + \left(\frac{(4800)^2}{6} \right) + \left(\frac{(4290)^2}{6} \right) \right) - 12037689$$

$$\text{SSC} = 152477.8$$

5.   Sum of squares due to error = SSE

SSE = SST – SSC = 972311.1 – 152477.8

$$= 819833.3$$

6   Mean Squares between columns or treatment = MSC $= \dfrac{SSC}{K-1}$

K = number of samples taken for study = 3

$$\text{MSC} = \frac{152477.8}{3-1} = 76238.889$$

7.   Mean square due to error $= \text{MSE} = \dfrac{SSE}{N-K} = \dfrac{819833.3}{18-3}$

MSE = 54655.556

7   Computation of Test value , F – distribution

$$F = \frac{MSC}{MSE} = \frac{76238.889}{54655.556}$$

F = 1.395

8.   Computation of degree of freedom of numerator (MSC) and denominator (MSE) of F-distribution

$\lambda 1 = K - 1 = 3 - 1 = 2$

$\lambda 2 = N - k = 18 - 3 = 15$

8   Computed value of F-distribution should be compared with standard table value of F-distribution at 5% or 1% level of significance.

Here the table value the degree of freedom 2 and 18 is $F_{ble} = 3.08$

F = 1.395 < F_{ble} = 3.68,

Hence the difference is significant between the means of different samples or treatments.

Null hypothesis is true.

ANOVA TABLE

	Sum of squares	DOF	Mean Squares	F	Not Significant
Between samples	152477.8	2	76238.889	1.395	P > 0.05
Within samples	819833.3	15	54655.556		
Total	972311.1	17			

Critical Values of the F Distribution with Alpha Level of .05

Upper 5% points

$n_2 \backslash n_1$	1	2	3	4	5	6	7	8	9	10	12	15	20	24	30	40	60	120	∞
1	161.4	199.5	215.7	224.6	230.2	234.0	236.8	238.9	240.5	241.9	243.9	245.9	248.0	249.1	250.1	251.1	252.2	253.3	254.3
2	18.51	19.00	19.16	19.25	19.30	19.33	19.35	19.37	19.38	19.40	19.41	19.43	19.45	19.45	19.46	19.47	19.48	19.49	19.50
3	10.13	9.55	9.28	9.12	9.01	8.94	8.89	8.85	8.81	8.79	8.74	8.70	8.66	8.64	8.62	8.59	8.57	8.55	8.53
4	7.71	6.94	6.59	6.39	6.26	6.16	6.09	6.04	6.00	5.96	5.91	5.86	5.80	5.77	5.75	5.72	5.69	5.66	5.63
5	6.61	5.79	5.41	5.19	5.05	4.95	4.88	4.82	4.77	4.74	4.68	4.62	4.56	4.53	4.50	4.46	4.43	4.40	4.36
6	5.99	5.14	4.76	4.53	4.39	4.28	4.21	4.15	4.10	4.06	4.00	3.94	3.87	3.84	3.81	3.77	3.74	3.70	3.67
7	5.59	4.74	4.35	4.12	3.97	3.87	3.79	3.73	3.68	3.64	3.57	3.51	3.44	3.41	3.38	3.34	3.30	3.27	3.23
8	5.32	4.46	4.07	3.84	3.69	3.58	3.50	3.44	3.39	3.35	3.28	3.22	3.15	3.12	3.08	3.04	3.01	2.97	2.93
9	5.12	4.26	3.86	3.63	3.48	3.37	3.29	3.23	3.18	3.14	3.07	3.01	2.94	2.90	2.86	2.83	2.79	2.75	2.71
10	4.96	4.10	3.71	3.48	3.33	3.22	3.14	3.07	3.02	2.98	2.91	2.85	2.77	2.74	2.70	2.66	2.62	2.58	2.54
11	4.84	3.98	3.59	3.36	3.20	3.09	3.01	2.95	2.90	2.85	2.79	2.72	2.65	2.61	2.57	2.53	2.49	2.45	2.40
12	4.75	3.89	3.49	3.26	3.11	3.00	2.91	2.85	2.80	2.75	2.69	2.62	2.54	2.51	2.47	2.43	2.38	2.34	2.30
13	4.67	3.81	3.41	3.18	3.03	2.92	2.83	2.77	2.71	2.67	2.60	2.53	2.46	2.42	2.38	2.34	2.30	2.25	2.21
14	4.60	3.74	3.34	3.11	2.96	2.85	2.76	2.70	2.65	2.60	2.53	2.46	2.39	2.35	2.31	2.27	2.22	2.18	2.13
15	4.54	3.68	3.29	3.06	2.90	2.79	2.71	2.64	2.59	2.54	2.48	2.40	2.33	2.29	2.25	2.20	2.16	2.11	2.07
16	4.49	3.63	3.24	3.01	2.85	2.74	2.66	2.59	2.54	2.49	2.42	2.35	2.28	2.24	2.19	2.15	2.11	2.06	2.01
17	4.45	3.59	3.20	2.96	2.81	2.70	2.61	2.55	2.49	2.45	2.38	2.31	2.23	2.19	2.15	2.10	2.06	2.01	1.96
18	4.41	3.55	3.16	2.93	2.77	2.66	2.58	2.51	2.46	2.41	2.34	2.27	2.19	2.15	2.11	2.06	2.02	1.97	1.92
19	4.38	3.52	3.13	2.90	2.74	2.63	2.54	2.48	2.42	2.38	2.31	2.23	2.16	2.11	2.07	2.03	1.98	1.93	1.88
20	4.35	3.49	3.10	2.87	2.71	2.60	2.51	2.45	2.39	2.35	2.28	2.20	2.12	2.08	2.04	1.99	1.95	1.90	1.84
21	4.32	3.47	3.07	2.84	2.68	2.57	2.49	2.42	2.37	2.32	2.25	2.18	2.10	2.05	2.01	1.96	1.92	1.87	1.81
22	4.30	3.44	3.05	2.82	2.66	2.55	2.46	2.40	2.34	2.30	2.23	2.15	2.07	2.03	1.98	1.94	1.89	1.84	1.78
23	4.28	3.42	3.03	2.80	2.64	2.53	2.44	2.37	2.32	2.27	2.20	2.13	2.05	2.01	1.96	1.91	1.86	1.81	1.76
24	4.26	3.40	3.01	2.78	2.62	2.51	2.42	2.36	2.30	2.25	2.18	2.11	2.03	1.98	1.94	1.89	1.84	1.79	1.73
25	4.24	3.39	2.99	2.76	2.60	2.49	2.40	2.34	2.28	2.24	2.16	2.09	2.01	1.96	1.92	1.87	1.82	1.77	1.71
26	4.23	3.37	2.98	2.74	2.59	2.47	2.39	2.32	2.27	2.22	2.15	2.07	1.99	1.95	1.90	1.85	1.80	1.75	1.69
27	4.21	3.35	2.96	2.73	2.57	2.46	2.37	2.31	2.25	2.20	2.13	2.06	1.97	1.93	1.88	1.84	1.79	1.73	1.67
28	4.20	3.34	2.95	2.71	2.56	2.45	2.36	2.29	2.24	2.19	2.12	2.04	1.96	1.91	1.87	1.82	1.77	1.71	1.65
29	4.18	3.33	2.93	2.70	2.55	2.43	2.35	2.28	2.22	2.18	2.10	2.03	1.94	1.90	1.85	1.81	1.75	1.70	1.64
30	4.17	3.32	2.92	2.69	2.53	2.42	2.33	2.27	2.21	2.16	2.09	2.01	1.93	1.89	1.84	1.79	1.74	1.68	1.62
40	4.08	3.23	2.84	2.61	2.45	2.34	2.25	2.18	2.12	2.08	2.00	1.92	1.84	1.79	1.74	1.69	1.64	1.58	1.51
60	4.00	3.15	2.76	2.53	2.37	2.25	2.17	2.10	2.04	1.99	1.92	1.84	1.75	1.70	1.65	1.59	1.53	1.47	1.39
120	3.92	3.07	2.68	2.45	2.29	2.17	2.09	2.02	1.96	1.91	1.83	1.75	1.66	1.61	1.55	1.50	1.43	1.35	1.25

Critical Values of the F Distribution with Alpha Level of .001

Upper 0·1% points

$v_2 \backslash v_1$	1	2	3	4	5	6	7	8	9	10	12	15	20	24	30	40	60	120	∞
1	4053*	5000*	5404*	5625*	5764*	5859*	5929*	5981*	6023*	6056*	6107*	6158*	6209*	6235*	6261*	6287*	6313*	6340*	6366*
2	998.5	999.0	999.2	999.2	999.3	999.3	999.4	999.4	999.4	999.4	999.4	999.4	999.4	999.5	999.5	999.5	999.5	999.5	999.5
3	167.0	148.5	141.1	137.1	134.6	132.8	131.6	130.6	129.9	129.2	128.3	127.4	126.4	125.9	125.4	125.0	124.5	124.0	123.5
4	74.14	61.25	56.18	53.44	51.71	50.53	49.66	49.00	48.47	48.05	47.41	46.76	46.10	45.77	45.43	45.09	44.75	44.40	44.05
5	47.18	37.12	33.20	31.09	29.75	28.84	28.16	27.64	27.24	26.92	26.42	25.91	25.39	25.14	24.87	24.60	24.33	24.06	23.79
6	35.51	27.00	23.70	21.92	20.81	20.03	19.46	19.03	18.69	18.41	17.99	17.56	17.12	16.89	16.67	16.44	16.21	15.99	15.75
7	29.25	21.69	18.77	17.19	16.21	15.52	15.02	14.63	14.33	14.08	13.71	13.32	12.93	12.73	12.53	12.33	12.12	11.91	11.70
8	25.42	18.49	15.83	14.39	13.49	12.86	12.40	12.04	11.77	11.54	11.19	10.84	10.48	10.30	10.11	9.92	9.73	9.53	9.33
9	22.86	16.39	13.90	12.56	11.71	11.13	10.70	10.37	10.11	9.89	9.57	9.24	8.90	8.72	8.55	8.37	8.19	8.00	7.81
10	21.04	14.91	12.55	11.28	10.48	9.92	9.52	9.20	8.96	8.75	8.45	8.13	7.80	7.64	7.47	7.30	7.12	6.94	6.76
11	19.69	13.81	11.56	10.35	9.58	9.05	8.66	8.35	8.12	7.92	7.63	7.32	7.01	6.85	6.68	6.52	6.35	6.17	6.00
12	18.64	12.97	10.80	9.63	8.89	8.38	8.00	7.71	7.48	7.29	7.00	6.71	6.40	6.25	6.09	5.93	5.76	5.59	5.42
13	17.81	12.31	10.21	9.07	8.35	7.86	7.49	7.21	6.98	6.80	6.52	6.23	5.93	5.78	5.63	5.47	5.30	5.14	4.97
14	17.14	11.78	9.73	8.62	7.92	7.43	7.08	6.80	6.58	6.40	6.13	5.85	5.56	5.41	5.25	5.10	4.94	4.77	4.60
15	16.59	11.34	9.34	8.25	7.57	7.09	6.74	6.47	6.26	6.08	5.81	5.54	5.25	5.10	4.95	4.80	4.64	4.47	4.31
16	16.12	10.97	9.00	7.94	7.27	6.81	6.46	6.19	5.98	5.81	5.55	5.27	4.99	4.85	4.70	4.54	4.39	4.23	4.06
17	15.72	10.66	8.73	7.68	7.02	6.56	6.22	5.96	5.75	5.58	5.32	5.05	4.78	4.63	4.48	4.33	4.18	4.02	3.85
18	15.38	10.39	8.49	7.46	6.81	6.35	6.02	5.76	5.56	5.39	5.13	4.87	4.59	4.45	4.30	4.15	4.00	3.84	3.67
19	15.08	10.16	8.28	7.26	6.62	6.18	5.85	5.59	5.39	5.22	4.97	4.70	4.43	4.29	4.14	3.99	3.84	3.68	3.51
20	14.82	9.95	8.10	7.10	6.46	6.02	5.69	5.44	5.24	5.08	4.82	4.56	4.29	4.15	4.00	3.86	3.70	3.54	3.38
21	14.59	9.77	7.94	6.95	6.32	5.88	5.56	5.31	5.11	4.95	4.70	4.44	4.17	4.03	3.88	3.74	3.58	3.42	3.26
22	14.38	9.61	7.80	6.81	6.19	5.76	5.44	5.19	4.99	4.83	4.58	4.33	4.06	3.92	3.78	3.63	3.48	3.32	3.15
23	14.19	9.47	7.67	6.69	6.08	5.65	5.33	5.09	4.89	4.73	4.48	4.23	3.96	3.82	3.68	3.53	3.38	3.22	3.05
24	14.03	9.34	7.55	6.59	5.98	5.55	5.23	4.99	4.80	4.64	4.39	4.14	3.87	3.74	3.59	3.45	3.29	3.14	2.97
25	13.88	9.22	7.45	6.49	5.88	5.46	5.15	4.91	4.71	4.56	4.31	4.06	3.79	3.66	3.52	3.37	3.22	3.06	2.89
26	13.74	9.12	7.36	6.41	5.80	5.38	5.07	4.83	4.64	4.48	4.24	3.99	3.72	3.59	3.44	3.30	3.15	2.99	2.82
27	13.61	9.02	7.27	6.33	5.73	5.31	5.00	4.76	4.57	4.41	4.17	3.92	3.66	3.52	3.38	3.23	3.08	2.92	2.75
28	13.50	8.93	7.19	6.25	5.66	5.24	4.93	4.69	4.50	4.35	4.11	3.86	3.60	3.46	3.32	3.18	3.02	2.86	2.69
29	13.39	8.85	7.12	6.19	5.59	5.18	4.87	4.64	4.45	4.29	4.05	3.80	3.54	3.41	3.27	3.12	2.97	2.81	2.64
30	13.29	8.77	7.05	6.12	5.53	5.12	4.82	4.58	4.39	4.24	4.00	3.75	3.49	3.36	3.22	3.07	2.92	2.76	2.59
40	12.61	8.25	6.60	5.70	5.13	4.73	4.44	4.21	4.02	3.87	3.64	3.40	3.15	3.01	2.87	2.73	2.57	2.41	2.23
60	11.97	7.76	6.17	5.31	4.76	4.37	4.09	3.87	3.69	3.54	3.31	3.08	2.83	2.69	2.55	2.41	2.25	2.08	1.89
120	11.38	7.32	5.79	4.95	4.42	4.04	3.77	3.55	3.38	3.24	3.02	2.78	2.53	2.40	2.26	2.11	1.95	1.76	1.54
∞	10.83	6.91	5.42	4.62	4.10	3.74	3.47	3.27	3.10	2.96	2.74	2.51	2.27	2.13	1.99	1.84	1.66	1.45	1.00

Two - Way ANOVA

Suppose the n-observations are classified into k-categories (or classes) say A1, A2,- - - - Ak according to some criterion A and into h-categories say B1, B2- - - - - -Bh according to some criterion B, having kh combinations.

(Ai, Bj) i = 1, 2, 3 ... k, j = 1, 2, 3 ... h often they are called as cells.

This type of classification, according to two factor or criteria is called as two way classification and its analysis is called as two way analysis of variance.

In the two way classification, the response variables are affected by two factors. In two – way classification, the total variation in the observation x_{ij} can split into the following three components.

1. The variation between the classes due to the other factor represented along the k-rows of the table.
2. The variation between the classes due to the other factor represented along the columns of the table.
3. The inherent variation within the observation of each class due to a combination of a large number of uncontrolled or extraneous factors of random nature, termed as chance variation

Statistical Analysis of Two Way ANOVA

Step 1: Here we are considering two factors of variation say A and B.

Step 2: Set null hypothesis: The factors A and B are homogeneous

H_{oA}: $\mu_1 = \mu_2 = \mu_3 \dots \mu_k$, i.e., there is no significant difference between the factors B

Step 3: Alternate Hypothesis:

H_{1A}: At least two of $\mu_1, \mu_2, \mu_3 \dots \mu_k$ are different

H_{1B} : At least two of $\mu_1, \mu_2, \mu_3 \dots \mu_h$ are different

k = number of classes represented along the rows

h = Number of classes represented along the columns

Ri = Total or sum of the observations in the ith – rows

Cj = Total number of observations in the jth – Column

Step 4 : Computation of raw sum squares

$$RSS = \sum_i \sum_j x_{ij}^2 = \text{Sum of the squares of all the observations or experimental results}$$

Step 5: Computation of Grand total

$$G = \sum_{i=1}^{k} \sum_{j=1}^{h} x_{ij} = \sum Ri \;\; = \;\; \sum Cj$$

N = total number of observations

Step 6: Compute correction factor (CF) $= \dfrac{G^2}{N}$ where N = $n_1 + n_2 + \text{-------} n_K$

Step 7: Sum of squares due to factor A (Row)

$$SSA = \left(\frac{R_1^2}{h} + \frac{R_2^2}{h} + \frac{R_3^2}{h} ... + \frac{R_k^2}{h}\right) - CF$$

$$SSA = \left(\frac{R_1^2 + R_2^2 + ... + R_k^2}{h}\right) - CF$$

Step 8 : Sum of squares due to factor B (Column)

$$SSB = \left(\frac{C_1^2}{k} + \frac{C_2^2}{k} + \frac{C_3^2}{k} ... + \frac{C_h^2}{k}\right) - CF$$

$$SSB = \left(\frac{C_1^2 + c_2^2 + ... + c_h^2}{k}\right) - CF$$

Step 9: Total sum squares = SST

$$SST = RSS - CF$$

Step 10 : Sum of squares due to error = SSE

$$SSE = SST - SSA - SSB$$

Step 11: Mean squares due to factor A

$$MSA = \left(\frac{SSA}{k-1}\right)$$

Step 12: Mean squares due to factor B

$$MSB = \left(\frac{SSB}{h-1}\right)$$

Step 13: Mean squares due to Error

$$MSE = \left(\frac{SSE}{(k-1)(h-1)}\right)$$

Step 14: Computation of F - distribution for A and B

$$F_A = \frac{MSA}{MSE}, \qquad F_B = \frac{MSB}{MSE}$$

Step 15: Degree of freedom for F_A

Degree of freedom for numerator value is $\lambda_{nr} = (k - 1)$

Degree of freedom for denominator value $\lambda_{dr} = (k - 1)(h - 1)$

Step 15: Degree of freedom for F_B

Degree of freedom for numerator value is $\lambda_{nr} = (h - 1)$

Degree of freedom for denominator value $\lambda_{dr} = (k - 1)(h - 1)$

Step 16: TEST STATISTICS

Under null hypothesis H_{0A} and H_{0B}

The test values are compared with standard or tabulated value of F at 5% or 1% level of significance.

$F_A > F_{ble}$ – Difference is significant between different factors of A . Then the alternative hypothesis is true and null hypothesis is rejected.

Similarly

$F_B > F_{ble}$ – Difference is significant between different factors of B . Then the alternative hypothesis is true and null hypothesis is rejected.

Step 17: Next Least Significant difference (LSD) between the factors of A and Between the factors of B should be computed to verify which pairs of data are significant.

$$LSD = t_{(N-h-k+1)(\alpha/2)} \sqrt{\frac{2MSE}{k}}$$

Step 18: Significant difference can be verified by comparing absolute difference of any two means with LSD.

Example 1: Five doctors take five treatment or drugs to treat certain disease and teach doctors were assigned five patients to treat with five different drugs. The numbers day taken by each patients to recover from the diseases is as listed in the table

Doctors	Treatments / Drugs					
	1	2	3	4	5	
1	10	14	23	18	20	
2	11	15	24	17	21	
3	9	12	20	16	19	
4	8	13	17	17	20	
5	12	15	19	15	22	

Discuss the difference between

a. The doctors and

b. The treatments at 5% level of significance($\alpha = 0.05$)

If the difference between doctors and between treatments is significant, find which pair of means differ significantly.

Solution:

Doctors	Treatments / Drugs					
	1-C1	2-C2	3-C3	4-C4	5-C5	
1(R1)	10	14	23	18	20	R1=
2(R2)	11	15	24	17	21	R2=
3(R3)	9	12	20	16	19	R3=
4(R4)	8	13	17	17	20	R4=
5(R5)	12	15	19	15	22	R5=
Column Totals(C)	C1=	C2=	C3=	C4=	C5=	

Solution:

Drug1 X1	$X1^2$	Drug2 X2	$X2^2$	Drug 3 X3	$X3^2$	Drug 4 X4	$X4^2$	Drug 5 X5	$X5^2$	Total
10	100	14	196	23	529	18	324	20	400	R1=85
11	121	15	225	24	576	17	289	21	441	R2=88
9	81	12	144	20	400	16	256	19	361	R3=76
8	64	13	169	17	289	17	289	20	400	R4=75
12	144	15	225	19	361	15	225	22	484	R5=83
C1=50	510	C2=69	959	C3=103	2155	C4=83	1383	C5=102	2086	G=407

Step1 : Here we are considering two factors of variation say A and B.

Step 2 : Set null hypothesis : The factors A and B are homogeneous

H_{oA}: $\mu_1 = \mu_2 = \mu_3 \ldots \mu_k$, ie., there is no significant difference between the factors B

Step3 : Alternate Hypothesis :

H_{1A}: At least two of $\mu_1, \mu_2, \mu_3 \ldots \mu_k$ are different

H_{1B} : At least two of $\mu_1, \mu_2, \mu_3 \ldots \mu_h$ are different

k = number of classes represented along the rows

h = Number of classes represented along the columns

Ri = Total or sum of the observations in the ith – rows

Cj = Total number of observations in the jth – Column

Step 4 : Computation of raw sum squares

$$\text{RSS} = \sum_i \sum_j x_{ij}^2 = 510 + 959 + 2155 + 1383 + 2086 = 7093$$

Step 5 : Computation of Grand total

$$G = \sum_{i=1}^{k} \sum_{j=1}^{h} x_{ij} = \sum Ri = \sum Cj = 50 + 69 + 103 + 83 + 102 = 407$$

N = total number of observations = 25

Step 6 : Compute correction factor (CF) $= \dfrac{G^2}{N} = \dfrac{407^2}{25} = 6625.96$

where N = $n_1 + n_2 + \ldots n_K$ = 5 + 5 + 5 + 5 + 5 = 25

Step 7 : Sum of squares due to factor A (Row)

$$\text{SSA} = \left(\frac{R_1^2}{h} + \frac{R_2^2}{h} + \frac{R_3^2}{h} \ldots + \frac{R_k^2}{h} \right) - \text{CF}$$

$$\text{SSA} = \left(\frac{R_1^2 + R_2^2 + \ldots + R_k^2}{h} \right) - \text{CF}$$

$$= \left(\frac{85^2 + 88^2 + 76^2 + 75^2 + 83^2}{5} \right) - 6625.96 = 25.84$$

Step 8 : Sum of squares due to factor B (Column)

$$SSB = \left(\frac{C_1^2}{k} + \frac{C_2^2}{k} + \frac{C_3^2}{k} - - - - + \frac{C_h^2}{k}\right) - CF$$

$$SSB = \left(\frac{50^2 + 69^2 + 103^2 + 83^2 + 102^2}{5}\right) - 6625.96 = 406.64$$

Step 9: Total sum squares = SST

$$SST = RSS - CF = 7093 - 6625.96 = 467.04$$

Step 10 : Sum of squares due to error = SSE

$$SSE = SST - SSA - SSB = 467.04 - 406.64 - 25.84 = 34.56$$

Step 11: Mean squares due to factor A

$$MSA = \left(\frac{SSA}{k-1}\right) = \times \left(\frac{25.84}{5-1}\right) = 6.460$$

Step 12: Mean squares due to factor B

$$MSB = \left(\frac{SSB}{h-1}\right) = \left(\frac{406.64}{5-1}\right) = 101.660$$

Step 13: Mean squares due to Error

$$MSE = \left(\frac{SSE}{(k-1)(h-1)}\right) = \left(\frac{34.56}{(5-1)(5-1)}\right) = 2.160$$

Step 14: Computation of F - distribution for A and B

$$F_A = \frac{MSA}{MSE} = = \frac{6.460}{2.160} = 2.991,$$

$$F_B = \frac{MSB}{MSE} = = \frac{101.660}{2.160} = 47.06481$$

Step 15: Degree of freedom for F_A

Degree of freedom for numerator value is $\lambda_{nr} = (k - 1) = (5 - 1) = 4$

Degree of freedom for denominator value $\lambda_{dr} = (k - 1)(h - 1) = (5 - 1)(5 - 1)$

$$= 4 \times 4 = 16$$

Step 15: Degree of freedom for F_B

Degree of freedom for numerator value is $\lambda_{nr} = (h - 1) = (5 - 1) = 4$

Degree of freedom for denominator value $\lambda_{dr} = (k - 1)(h - 1) = (5 - 1)(5 - 1)$

$$= 4 \times 4 = 16$$

Step 16: TEST STATISTICS

Under null hypothesis is H_{0A} and H_{0B}

The test values are compared with standard or tabulated value of F at 5% or 1% level of significance.

FA <F_{ble} – Difference is significant between different doctors (factors A) . Then the alternative hypothesis is not true and null hypothesis is Accepted.

$FB > F_{ble}$ – Difference is significant between different drugs (factors B). Then the alternative hypothesis is   true and null hypothesis is rejected.

Step 17: Next Least Significant difference (LSD) between the factors of A and Between the factors of B should be computed to verify which pairs of data are significant.

$$LSD = t_{(N-h-k+1)(\alpha/2)} \sqrt{\frac{2MSE}{k}}$$

$$LSD = t_{(25-5-5+1)(\alpha/2)} \sqrt{\frac{2MSE}{k}}$$

$$LSD = t_{(16)(\alpha/2)} \sqrt{\frac{2*21160}{5}} = 2.12 \sqrt{\frac{2*2.16}{5}} = 1.97$$

Step 18: Significant difference can be verified by comparing absolute difference of any two means with LSD.

Mean	Absolute difference between means of any samples		Comparison with LSD		Remark
Mean(X1) =10	x1-x2	=3.8	3.8	> LSD	Significant
	x1-x3	= 10.6	10.6	> LSD	Significant
	x1-x4	=6.6	6.6	> LSD	Significant
	x1-x5	= 10.4	10.4	> LSD	Significant
Mean(X2) =13.8	x2-x3	=6.8	6.8	> LSD	
	x2-x4	=2.8	2.8	> LSD	Significant
	x2-x5	=6.6	6.6	> LSD	Significant
Mean(X3) =20.6					Significant
Mean(X4) =16.6	x3-x4	=4	4	> LSD	Significant
	x3-x5	=0.2	0.2	< LSD	Not Significant
Mean(X5) =20.4	X4 - x5	=3.8	3.8	> LSD	Significant
The average value of X_1 is more than the remaining two samples, hence X_1 is more significant than remaining two samples					

Example 2: The tablet dissolutions after 30 minutes for three products (Percent dissolution) is summarized in the following.

Generic

Lab	A	B	Standard
1	90	83	94
2	94	75	78
3	86	76	89
4	81	78	85
5	83	80	84
6	85	82	87

Perform two way ANOVA and verify the level of significance between them , if the difference is significant, which sample is more significant.

Solution:

Apply SPSS–Software and Analyze the data

Tests of Between-Subjects Effects						
Dependent Variable: Drug						
Source		Type III Sum of Squares	df	Mean Square	F	Sig.
Intercept	Hypothesis	126672.222	1	126672.222	5534.223	0.000
	Error	114.444	5	22.889[a]		
Group	Hypothesis	215.444	2	107.722	5.556	0.024
	Error	193.889	10	19.389[b]		
Laboratories	Hypothesis	114.444	5	22.889	1.181	0.384
	Error	193.889	10	19.389[b]		
Group * Laboratories	Hypothesis	193.889	10	19.389[c]	.	.
	Error	0.000	0			
a. MS(Laboratories)						
b. MS(Group * Laboratories)						
c. MS(Error)						

Tukey's Multiple Comparison Test

Tukey's Test

Tukey's multiple comparison test is one of several tests that can be used to determine which means amongst a set of means differ from the rest. Tukey's multiple comparison test is also called Tukey's honestly significant difference test or Tukey's LSD. Hence this Tukey's multiple comparison test is used verify the level of significance between more than two samples.

Tukey multiple comparison test, like both the t-test and ANOVA, assumes that the data from the different groups come from populations where the observations have a normal distribution and the standard deviation is the same for each group.

This test is more conservative than LSD. This means that a larger difference between treatments is needed for significance in the Tukey test than in the LSD test,

In the multiple range test, treatments can be compared without the need for a prior significant F test. However, the ANOVA should always be carried out. The error term for the treatment comparisons comes from the ANOVA and within mean square in the one-way ANOVA. Here also a least significance difference will be calculated, that will be similar to LSD Procedure.

If any of the difference of treatment means exceeding $Q\sqrt{\dfrac{s^2}{N}}$, then that will be considered as significant. S^2 is the error variance from ANOVA (within mean square for the one-way ANOVA) and N is the sample size. This test is based on equal sample sizes in each groups. When two groups to be compared are unequal in size , then N is replaced by $\dfrac{2\,N1N2}{(N1+N2)}$ and Q is the value of the "Studentized range" that can be chosen from the standard Studentized table.

Exercise

The sleeping medicine A was prescribed for 12 male and 12 female, with different doses like 10 mg, 40 mg and 70 mg. For each 4 male and 4 female patients are assigned and additional time taken by patients in minutes is as recorded below.

Sex	Factor (A –Dose)				
	10 mg	40 mg	70 mg		
Male	12	9	19		A1B1 = 48
	17	12	32	B1 =197	A1B2 =128
	11	12	28		A2B1 =42
	18	9	18		A2B2 =97
Female	18	37	38		A3B1 = 97
	48	15	39	B2 = 382	A3B2 = 157
	19	20	34		k=4
	43	25	46		N = 24
					a = 3
					b =2
	A1= 186	139	254	G = 579	

Compute F-distribution between dose and also between male and female patients using two-way ANOVA and also verify the level of significance between dose and sex.

Example 3: The Assessment of knowledge, attitude and practice of parents on vaccination was conducted having one child, 2 children's and 3 children's and scores obtained after the assessment is as listed below. Is there significance difference between the patients having 1, 2 and 3 children's.

10	13	5
6	18	9
19	23	5
17	20	4
12	23	5
18	22	10
21	19	11
13	21	14
13	22	19
25	21	5
11	25	9
13	22	5
18	3	5
14	4	6
10	19	5
10	19	9
11	21	16
16	8	5
17	19	4
26	18	5
29	16	5
18	20	10
11	16	5
15	6	10
14	18	4
10	19	10
19	22	
9	19	
	18	

Answer:

ANOVA

VAR00001

	Sum of Squares	df	Mean Square	F	Sig.
Between Groups	1469.188	2	734.594	27.912	0.000
Within Groups	2105.439	80	26.318		
Total	3574.627	82			

Multiple Comparisons

Dependent Variable: LSD

Variables	Groups	Mean Difference	Std. Error	Sig.	95% Confidence Interval	
					Lower Bound	Upper Bound
1.00	2.00	-2.54557	1.35921	.065	-5.2505	.1593
	3.00	7.48626*	1.39720	.000	4.7058	10.2668
2.00	1.00	2.54557	1.35921	.065	-.1593	5.2505
	3.00	10.03183*	1.38555	.000	7.2745	12.7892
3.00	1.00	-7.48626*	1.39720	.000	-10.2668	-4.7058
	2.00	-10.03183*	1.38555	.000	-12.7892	-7.2745
*. The mean difference is significant at the 0.05 level.						

Example 4: The Assessment of knowledge, attitude and practice of parents on vaccination was conducted on the basis of socio economic status like Lower middle, upper middle, upper lower and Upper middle. The scores obtained after the assessment is as listed below. Is there significance difference between the parents of having different economic status.

Lower Middle	Upper Middle	Upper lower	Upper Middle
10	19	5	13
6	17	9	18
19	25	5	23
21	29	4	20
22	18	5	23
21	19	12	22
22	10	18	21
3	19	19	25
4	10	19	18
13	19	21	16
13	23	8	20
11	19	19	13
14	19	10	18

Lower Middle	Upper Middle	Upper lower	Upper Middle
11	17	16	10
16	17	6	17
19	25	26	18
11	25	10	22
11	20	11	18

Answer:

Descriptive

VAR00003

	N	Mean	Std. Deviation	Std. Error	95% Confidence Interval for Mean		Minimum	Maximum
					Lower Bound	Upper Bound		
1.00	18	13.7222	6.02744	1.42068	10.7248	16.7196	3.00	22.00
2.00	18	19.4444	4.82911	1.13823	17.0430	21.8459	10.00	29.00
3.00	18	12.3889	6.66103	1.57002	9.0764	15.7013	4.00	26.00
4.00	18	18.6111	3.91286	.92227	16.6653	20.5569	10.00	25.00
Total	72	16.0417	6.15856	.72579	14.5945	17.4889	3.00	29.00

ANOVA

VAR00003

	Sum of Squares	df	Mean Square	F	Sig.
Between Groups	664.264	3	221.421	7.422	.000
Within Groups	2028.611	68	29.833		
Total	2692.875	71			

Multiple Comparisons

Dependent Variable: VAR00003

LSD

(I) Group	(J) Groups	Mean Difference (I-J)	Std. Error	Sig.	95% Confidence Interval	
					Lower Bound	Upper Bound
1.00	2.00	-5.72222[*]	1.82064	.002	-9.3552	-2.0892
	3.00	1.33333	1.82064	.466	-2.2997	4.9664
	4.00	-4.88889[*]	1.82064	.009	-8.5219	-1.2559
2.00	1.00	5.72222[*]	1.82064	.002	2.0892	9.3552
	3.00	7.05556[*]	1.82064	.000	3.4225	10.6886
	4.00	.83333	1.82064	.649	-2.7997	4.4664

(I) Group	(J) Groups	Mean Difference (I-J)	Std. Error	Sig.	95% Confidence Interval	
					Lower Bound	Upper Bound
3.00	1.00	-1.33333	1.82064	.466	-4.9664	2.2997
	2.00	-7.05556*	1.82064	.000	-10.6886	-3.4225
	4.00	-6.22222*	1.82064	.001	-9.8552	-2.5892
4.00	1.00	4.88889*	1.82064	.009	1.2559	8.5219
	2.00	-.83333	1.82064	.649	-4.4664	2.7997
	3.00	6.22222*	1.82064	.001	2.5892	9.8552

*. The mean difference is significant at the 0.05 level.

Example 5

Experiment was conducted in replicate by 8 laboratories for testing the dissolution rate of three formulations or products and the dissolution rate recorded as listed below. Perform two-way ANOVA and verify the level of significance between these three products

Solution:

APPLY SPSS Statistical Software

Laboratory	Generic										Standard					Row Total
	A					B										
1	88	90	2	7744	8100	80	84	8	6400	7056	92	95	4.5	8464	9025	529
2	92	96	8	8464	9216	75	76	0.5	5625	5776	73	82	40.5	5329	6724	494
3	81	91	50	6561	8281	72	76	8	5184	5776	84	94	50	7056	8836	498
4	76	85	40.5	5776	7225	74	79	12.5	5476	6241	81	89	32	6561	7921	484
5	76	82	18	5776	6724	75	78	4.5	5625	6084	82	88	18	6724	7744	481
6	84	89	12.5	7056	7921	70	76	18	4900	5776	79	88	40.5	6241	7744	486
7	79	85	18	6241	7225	74	87	84.5	5476	7569	71	79	32	5041	6241	475
8	66	72	18	4356	5184	72	81	40.5	5184	6561	70	81	60.5	4900	6561	442
	642	690	167	51974	59876	592	637	176.5	43870	50839	632	696	278	50316	60796	3889
	1332					1229					1328					
	83.25					76.8125					83					

Sum	3889
cf	315090.02
TSS	2580.98
Product SS	425.5
Laboratory SS	690.5
Within -cell SS	621.5
CXR	843.46

Source	DF	SS	Mean Squares	F	
Drug Product	2	425.5	212.77	3.53	2,14
Lab SS	7	690.5	98.64	3.81	4,24
CXR (Residuals)	14	843.46	60.25	2.33	14, 24
Within Cell	24	621.5	25.89583333		

Example 6: Experiment was conducted in replicate by 8 laboratories for testing the dissolution rate of three formulations or products and the dissolution rate recorded as listed below. Perform two-way ANOVA and verify the level of significance between these three products

Solution:

APPLY SPSS Statistical Software

Laboratory	Generic										Standard					Row Total
	A					B										
1	88	90	2	7744	8100	80	84	8	6400	7056	92	95	4.5	8464	9025	529
2	92	96	8	8464	9216	75	76	0.5	5625	5776	73	82	40.5	5329	6724	494
3	81	91	50	6561	8281	72	76	8	5184	5776	84	94	50	7056	8836	498
4	76	85	40.5	5776	7225	74	79	12.5	5476	6241	81	89	32	6561	7921	484
5	76	82	18	5776	6724	75	78	4.5	5625	6084	82	88	18	6724	7744	481
6	84	89	12.5	7056	7921	70	76	18	4900	5776	79	88	40.5	6241	7744	486
7	79	85	18	6241	7225	74	87	84.5	5476	7569	71	79	32	5041	6241	475
8	66	72	18	4356	5184	72	81	40.5	5184	6561	70	81	60.5	4900	6561	442
	642	690	167	51974	59876	592	637	176.5	43870	50839	632	696	278	50316	60796	3889
	1332					1229					1328					
	83.25					76.8125					83					

Sum	3889
cf	315090.02
TSS	2580.98
Product SS	425.5
Laboratory SS	690.5
Within -cell SS	621.5
CXR	843.46

Source	DF	SS	Mean Squares	F	
Drug Product	2	425.5	212.77	3.53	2,14
Lab SS	7	690.5	98.64	3.81	4,24
CXR (Residuals)	14	843.46	60.25	2.33	14, 24
Within Cell	24	621.5	25.89583333		

10 Chi-Square Test

The Chi-Square test (λ^2) is an extremely useful type of test instrument and is used to provide a probability basis for testing the variation between sample values and values obtained from a frequency (Probability) model.

There are many situations in which it is not possible for the statistician to make rigid assumptions about the shape of population from which samples are being drawn. The limitation has led to the development of a group of alternative techniques known as non-parametric or distribution-free methods. A non-parametric method may be defined as a statistical test in which no hypothesis that does not depend on assumptions concerning the form of the underlying distribution.

Chi-Square (λ^2) Distribution

The square of a standard normal variable is called as a Chi-square variate with 1 degree of freedom (DOF). If X is a random variable following normal distribution with mean μ and standard deviation σ, then $\left(\dfrac{X-\mu}{\sigma}\right)$ is a standard normal variate $\left(\dfrac{X-\mu}{\sigma}\right)^2$ is called as Chi-Square variate with DOF 1.

If we take $x_1, x_2, x_3, \ldots\ldots\ldots x_n$ are n-independent variables, having normal distribution with average (Mean) $\mu_1, \mu_2, \mu_3 \text{-------} \mu_n$ and standard deviations $\sigma_1, \sigma_2, \sigma_3, \text{-------} \sigma_n$ are standard deviations. Then the variate $\lambda^2 = \left(\dfrac{X1-\mu1}{\sigma1}\right)^2 + \left(\dfrac{X2-\mu2}{\sigma2}\right)^2 \text{-------------+} \left(\dfrac{Xn-\mu n}{\sigma n}\right)^2 = \sum_{i=1}^{n}\left(\dfrac{Xi-\mu i}{\sigma i}\right)^2$ which is the sum of the squares of n-independent standard normal variates, this follows Chi-square distribution with n-DOF.

Chi-Square test: This is one the most useful test which was introduced in the year 1900 by Karl Pearson. This is one of the simplest and most widely used non-parametric test in standard analysis. Chi-Square test is used for measuring the significance of the difference between an observed statistical distribution and theoretical distribution. This test is also known as λ^2 . test of goodness of fit. This will be used to test, if the deviation between observation (experiment) and theory may be attributed to chance (fluctuations of sampling).

Under null hypothesis, that there is no significant difference between the observed (experimental) and the theoretical or hypothetical value, ie there is good compatibility between theory and experiment, Karl Pearson proved that the statistic $\chi^2 = \sum_{i=1}^{n} \frac{(Oi-Ei)^2}{Ei} = \frac{(O1-E1)^2}{E1} + \frac{(O2-E2)^2}{E2} + ... + \frac{(On-En)^2}{En}$ follows χ^2 distribution with $v = n-1$ DOF, where $O_1, O_2 ... O_n$ are the observed frequencies and E1, E2, ... En are corresponding expected or theoretical frequencies obtained under some theory or hypothesis.

Steps for computation of χ^2 and drawing conclusions:

(i) Compute the expected frequencies E1, E2, ..., En corresponding to the observed frequencies O1, O2, ... On under some theory or hypothesis.

(ii) Compute the deviations (O-E) for each frequency and then square them to obtain $(O-E)^2$.

(iii) Compute the deviations $(O-E)$ for each frequency and then square them to obtain $(O-E)^2$

(iv) Divide the square of the deviations $(O-E)^2$ by the corresponding expected frequency to find $(O-E)^2/E$.

(v) Obtain $\chi^2 = \sum \left[\frac{(O-E)^2}{E} \right]$

(vi) Assume Null Hypothesis (H_0). The theory fits the data well, and follows χ^2 distribution with degree of freedom under the null hypothesis of independence. The DOF $= (r-1)(c-1)$. $r =$ row numbers and c=Columns numbers.

1. The data listed in the table gives the list of people who are doing their service in military and they were having sleep problem due to possible exposure of some chemical. Is there any significance difference between chemical exposure and sleep between working in military and non-working.

Sleeping Problem	Service in Military		
	YES	NO	Total
Yes	173	160	333
NO	599	851	1450
Total	772	1011	1783

$$E_{11} = \frac{(333)(772)}{1783} = 144.18,$$

$$E_{12} = \frac{(333)(1011)}{1783} = 188.82,$$

$$E_{21} = \frac{(772)(1450)}{1783} = 627.82,$$

$$E_{22} = \frac{(1011)(1450)}{1783} = 822.18.18,$$

O	E	(O-E)	$(O-E)^2$	$(O-E)^2/E$
173	144.18	28.82	830.5924	5.76
160	188.82	-28.82	830.5924	4.40
599	627.82	-28.82	830.5924	1.32
851	822.18	28.82	830.5924	1.01
				$\sum \left[\frac{(O-E)^2}{E} \right] = 12.49$

DOF = (r -1) (C-1) = (2 – 1) (2 -1) = 1

$$\lambda^2_{cal} = 12.49$$

$$\lambda^2_{tle} = 3.84$$

$$\lambda^2_{cal} > \lambda^2_{tle}$$

This indicates that difference is significant and soldier are getting sleep problem due to the exposure of chemicals.

2. Doctors performed a study to examine two types of preoperative skin preparation before performing open heart surgery. Doctors used aqueous iodine and insoluble Iodine and result obtained is as listed below.

Preparations	Comparison of two Preparations		
	Infected	Not Infected	Total
Aqueous Iodine	14	94	108
Insoluble Iodine	04	97	101
Total	18	191	209

Is there any significance difference between Aqueous Iodine and Insoluble Iodine preparations

Solution:

E1 (18*108)/209

    9.30

E2 (18*101)/209

    8.70

E3 (191*108)/208

    99.17

E4 (191*101)/208

    92.75

O	E.	O-E	$(O-E)^2$	$(O-E)^2/E$
14	9.30	4.7	22.09	2.38
4	8.70	-4.7	22.09	2.54
94	99.17	-5.17	26.7289	0.27
97	92.75	4.25	18.0625	0.19
				$\sum \left[\dfrac{(O-E)^2}{E}\right] = 5.38$

$$DOF = (r-1)\,(C-1) = (2-1)\,(2-1) = 1$$

$$\lambda^2_{cal} = 5.34$$

$$\lambda^2_{tble} = 3.84$$

$$\lambda^2_{cal} > \lambda^2_{tble}$$

This indicates that difference is significant between Aqueous Iodine and Insoluble Iodine preparations

3.   The effect of new treatment of a particular disease is summarized in the following table

	Old treatment	New Treatment	Total
Cured	20	30	50
Not Cured	40	70	110
Total	60	100	160

Apply Chi-square test and verify the effect of new treatment

Solution:

Status * TREATMENT * Ttotal Cross tabulation

Ttotal				TREATMENT		Total
				N	O	
Total	Status	C	Count	30	20	50
			Expected Count	31.3	18.8	50.0
		NC	Count	70	40	110
			Expected Count	68.8	41.3	110.0
	Total		Count	100	60	160
			Expected Count	100.0	60.0	160.0

Total		Value	df	Asymp. Sig. (2-sided)
Total	Pearson Chi-Square	.194[a]	1	.660
	Continuity Correction	.070	1	.792
	Likelihood Ratio	.193	1	.660

P>0.05, therefore the difference is not significant.

4. A New drug was used to for anaesthetizing patients. The degree of consciousness of patients 10 minutes after operation was observed and compared with the results which were obtained by using standard drug and gases. The result obtained is as listed below.

	Unconscious	Semi Conscious	Conscious	Total
New Drug	30	25	15	70
Standard Drug	35	40	25	10
Total	65	65	40	170

Apply Chi-Square test and determine, whether the new drug has any on the degree of consciousness.

Solution:

Total		Value	df	Asymp. Sig. (2-sided)
Total	Pearson Chi-square	8.871[a]	2	.012
	N of Valid Cases	170		

P < 0.05 , therefore the difference is significant.

5. A survey was made by health department to verify the effect due to the exposure to a chemical in a pharmaceutical industry on sleep and data collected after interviewing is as listed below in the table.

Data collected from workers after conducting interview

(Exposed and Non-Exposed group)

Sleep Problem	Yes	No	Total
Yes	150	120	270
No	400	680	1080
Total	60	100	1350

Apply chi-square test and verify whether the sleep is affected due to the exposure of chemical in pharmaceutical industry or not

Solution:

Sleep hours* Workers exposed and Not exposed group * total Cross tabulation						
		1	Count	150	120	270
			Expected Count	110.0	160.0	270.0
		2	Count	400	680	1080
			Expected Count	440.0	640.0	1080.0
	Total		Count	550	800	1350
			Expected Count	550.0	800.0	1350.0

Chi-Square Tests

	Total	Value	df	Asymp. Sig. (2-sided)	Exact Sig. (2-sided)	Exact Sig. (1-sided)
Total	Pearson Chi-Square	30.682[a]	1	.000	.000	.000
	N of Valid Cases	1350				

$P < 0.05$, therefore the difference is significant. Sleep is affected due to the chemical exposure.

6. A carcinogenicity study was conducted on animals using drug and placebo. The summary of the data is as listed below.

	Drug	Placebo	Total
Animal with Carcinoma	10	7	17
Animal without Carcinoma	60	73	133
Total	70	80	150

Apply Chi-square test verify the effect of drug in carcinogenicity study.

Solution:

Row * Column * Total Cross tabulation							
	Total				Column		Total
					1	2	
Total	Row	1	Count		10	7	17
			Expected Count		7.9	9.1	17.0
		2	Count		60	73	133
			Expected Count		62.1	70.9	133.0
	Total		Count		70	80	150
			Expected Count		70.0	80.0	150.0

Total		Value	df	Asymp. Sig. (2-sided)	Exact Sig. (2-sided)	Exact Sig. (1-sided)
Total	Pearson Chi-Square	3.795[a]	1	.051	.056	.037
	N of Valid Cases	230				

$P > 0.05$, therefore the difference is not significant. Drug is not effective.

7. Number of people who were affected by measles among vaccinated and unvaccinated as listed below in the table. Apply chi-square test to observe protective value of vaccination.

	Attacked	Not attacked	Total
Control (Placebo)	15	35	50
Experiment (On Drug)	10	70	80
Total	25	105	130

Apply chi-square test to observe protective value of vaccination.

Solution:

Row * Column * Total Cross tabulation					Column		Total
Total					1	2	
Total	Row	1	Count		20	100	120
			Expected Count		26.1	93.9	120.0
		2	Count		30	80	110
			Expected Count		23.9	86.1	110.0
	Total		Count		50	180	230
			Expected Count		50.0	180.0	230.0

Chi-Square Tests

Total		Value	df	Asymp. Sig. (2-sided)	Exact Sig. (2-sided)	Exact Sig. (1-sided)
Total	Pearson Chi-Square	3.795[a]	1	.051	.056	.037
	N of Valid Cases	230				

$P > 0.05$, therefore the difference is not significant. Drug is not effective.

8. A cancer screening test was conducted by a group of oncologist and a total of 500 people were screened to know that how many are suffering from oral cancer due to the consumption and not consumption of tobacco. The information collected by oncologist is as listed below.

	Tobacco Consumer	Not Consuming tobacco	Total
Oral Cancer	30	90	120
No Oral Cancer	120	100	220
Total	150	190	340

Apply Chi-square test and verify, whether the tobacco consumption is the main cause for getting oral cancer or not.

Solution:

Row * Column * Total Cross tabulation					Column		Total
					1	2	
Total	Row	1	Count		30	90	120
			Expected Count		52.9	67.1	120.0
		2	Count		120	100	220
			Expected Count		97.1	122.9	220.0
	Total		Count		150	190	340
			Expected Count		150.0	190.0	340.0

Chi-Square Tests

Total		Value	df	Asymp. Sig. (2-sided)	Exact Sig. (2-sided)	Exact Sig. (1-sided)
Total	Pearson Chi-Square	27.493[a]	1	.000	.000	.000
	N of Valid Cases	340				

$P < 0.05$, therefore the difference is significant. Tobacco consumption is effective in causing the oral cancer.

9. A clinical trial study which was sponsored by a pharmaceutical was jointly conducted by Medicine and Pharmacology departments to measure out the efficiency of neomycin in preventing infection during first two weeks of burns. The data recorded after performing the clinical trials, as listed below.

Infection

Dressing	Tobacco Consumer	Not Consuming tobacco	Total
Penicillin	30	10	40
Penicillin + Neomycin	15	35	50
Total	45	45	90

Apply Chi-square test and what conclusion will you draw about the data listed above.

Solution:

Row * Column * Total Cross tabulation					
Total				Column	Total
				1	2	
Total	Row	1	Count	30	10	40
			Expected Count	20.0	20.0	40.0
		2	Count	15	35	50
			Expected Count	25.0	25.0	50.0
	Total		Count	45	45	90
			Expected Count	45.0	45.0	90.0

Chi-Square Tests

Total			Value	df	Asymp. Sig. (2-sided)	Exact Sig. (2-sided)	Exact Sig. (1-sided)
Total	Pearson Chi-Square		18.000[a]	1	.000	.000	.000
	N of Valid Cases		90				

$P < 0.05$, therefore the difference is significant and neomycin is more effective in preventing the infection.

10. A sample of 200 college students participated in a study, which was designed to evaluate or to assess the level of student knowledge about a particular group of diseases. The following table gives the list of students classified on a major field of study and level of knowledge on a particular group of diseases.

Major field of study

Knowledge about disease	Premedical	Others	Total
Good	35	15	50
Poor	90	360	450
Total	125	375	500

Apply Chi-square test and assess whether there is any relationship between the knowledge about disease and major field of study of the college students from which the sample was (drawn) taken for study.

Solution:

Apply Chi-square test and assess whether there is any relationship between the knowledge about disease and major field of study of the college students from which the sample was (drawn) taken for study.

Solution:

<table>
<tr><th colspan="8">Row * Column * Total Cross tabulation</th></tr>
<tr><td colspan="4">Total</td><td colspan="2">Column</td><td>Total</td></tr>
<tr><td colspan="4"></td><td>1</td><td>2</td><td></td></tr>
<tr><td>Total</td><td>Row</td><td>1</td><td>Count</td><td>35</td><td>15</td><td>50</td></tr>
<tr><td></td><td></td><td></td><td>Expected Count</td><td>12.5</td><td>37.5</td><td>50.0</td></tr>
<tr><td></td><td></td><td>2</td><td>Count</td><td>90</td><td>360</td><td>450</td></tr>
<tr><td></td><td></td><td></td><td>Expected Count</td><td>112.5</td><td>337.5</td><td>450.0</td></tr>
<tr><td></td><td>Total</td><td></td><td>Count</td><td>125</td><td>375</td><td>500</td></tr>
<tr><td></td><td></td><td></td><td>Expected Count</td><td>125.0</td><td>375.0</td><td>500.0</td></tr>
</table>

Chi-Square Tests

Total		Value	df	Asymp. Sig. (2-sided)	Exact Sig. (2-sided)	Exact Sig. (1-sided)
Total	Pearson Chi-Square	60.000[a]	1	.000	.000	.000
	N of Valid Cases	500				

$P < 0.05$, therefore the difference is significant between the knowledge and major field of study

Total		Value	df	Asymp. Sig. (2-sided)	Exact Sig. (2-sided)	Exact Sig. (1-sided)
Total	Pearson Chi-Square	60.000[a]	1	.000	.000	.000
	N of Valid Cases	500				

$P < 0.05$, therefore the difference is significant between the knowledge and major field of study.

11. A clinical trial study which was jointly conducted by clinical trial centre and Pharmaceutical industry by selecting 320 cases of Typhoid in a hospital. The purpose of study was to verify the effect of ciprofloxacin over chloramphenicol. The data obtained after treatment as listed below.

Drug	Cured	Not Cured	Total
Ciprofloxacin	150	15	165
Chloramphenicol	130	25	155
Total	280	40	320

Verify the level of significance difference between these two drugs by applying Chi-square test.

Solution:

Row * Column * Total Cross tabulation					
Total				Column		Total
				1	2	
Total	Row	1	Count	150	15	165
			Expected Count	144.4	20.6	165.0
		2	Count	130	25	155
			Expected Count	135.6	19.4	155.0
	Total		Count	280	40	320
			Expected Count	280.0	40.0	320.0

Chi-Square Tests

Total		Value	df	Asymp. Sig. (2-sided)	Exact Sig. (2-sided)	Exact Sig. (1-sided)
Total	Pearson Chi-Square	3.620[a]	1	.057	.064	.041
	N of Valid Cases	320				

$P > 0.05$, therefore the difference is not significant between the drugs.

11 Design of Experiment

11.1 INTRODUCTION TO DESIGNED EXPERIMENT

STRATEGY OF EXPERIMENT

When an investigator perform any experiment, to discover something about a particular process. In general experiment can be called as test. When we perform experiment on human being to verify the effectiveness of a drug is a test.

In general, experiment can be defined as a test or series of tests in which purposeful changes are made due to some input variables of a process or system. After getting output or response or result, we can know the reason for changes or for getting result.

Here we mainly focus about planning and conducting experiments and also about the resulting data, so that valid and objective conclusion can be obtained.

Experimentation plays an important role in how commercialization of the technology and product realization activities, that may be a new product design, and formulation of a pharmaceutical product along with manufacturing process development.

In many experiment designs develop robust process, that is a process affected minimally by external sources of variability.

Example: To study the hardness of a tablet, here we are interested to know which ingredient produces maximum hardness and what is the quantity that we have considered to increase the hardness of a tablet.

Generally experiments are designed to study the performance of process and system. Here process includes operations, machine, methods, people and other ingredients or resources that are used to transforms some input into an output, that may be one or two observable response variable.

In an experimental design some of the process variables and properties of some materials of $x_1, x_2 \ldots\ldots x_p$ are controllable variables. In addition to these variables, there are some uncontrollable variables they are written as $z_1, z_2 \ldots z_q$.

The objectives of designing an experiment includes

1. To determine which variables are most effective or influential for getting good response's'

2. To determine where to set the values of x, which is more influential, so that desired value of y-(response) can be obtained.

3. To determine where to set the influential 'x's so that variability in 'y' can be minimized.

4. To determine how to set the variables x, which are more influential, so that the effects of uncontrollable variables can be minimized.

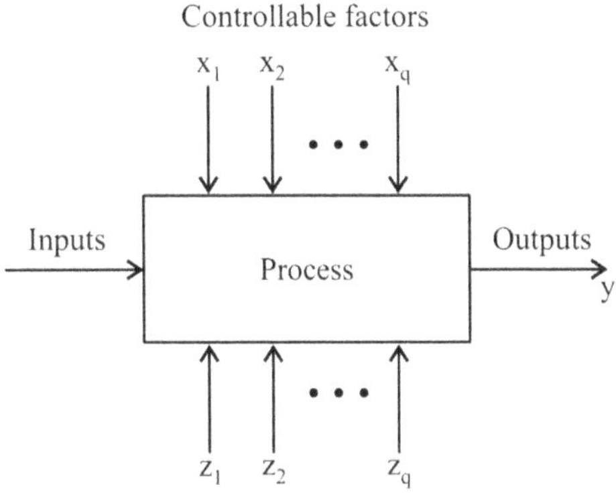

The general approach to planning and conducting the experiments is called the strategy of experiments.

GUIDANCE FOR DESIGNING EXPERIMENTS

For any investigator when he is going for the statistical approach in designing, analyzing the result or response of an experiment, it is very important for all the investigators, who are involved in research activity, should have a clear idea in advance, exactly what is to be studied, how one has to collect data and how data's to be analyzed. This includes seven important steps as listed below:

1. Recognition and defining the problems

2. Selection of response or output variable

3. choice of factors or variables to be selected and the levels of each variable and ranges

4. Choice of experimental design

5. Performing the experiment

6. Statistical analysis of data

7. Conclusion and recommendations.

Recognitions and Defining the Problem

It is necessary to develop all ideas about the objectives of the experiment to solicit input from all concerned parties like quality assurance, manufacturing, customer, R and D section and operating personnel (who usually have much insight and who are too often ignored). In general we can say that team approach is most important in designing experiment.

It is more important to prepare a list of specific problems or questions that are to be addressed by the experiment. A clear statement of the problem often contributes substantially to better understandings of the phenomenon being studies and the final solution of the problem.

Selection of the Responsible or Output Variable

While selecting the responsible variable investigator must be certain about variable chosen really provides useful information about the process order study. Most often the average or standard deviation (or both) of the measured characteristic will be the response variables. After getting the response, if we gauge the change capability is inadequate, only relatively large factor or variable effects will be detected by the experiment or by repeating the same experiment

Choice of Factors Levels or Range

When an investigator going to select factors, which are going to influence performance of process he classifies them as:

1. Potential design factors
2. Nuisance factors

The potential design factors are those factors, where the investigator can vary in the experiment.

Nuisance factors on the other hand may have large effects that must be accounted, where we may not be interested in them in the context of the present experiment. Nuisance factors are often classified as controllable factor, uncontrollable or noise factors.

A controllable nuisance factor is one, whose levels may be set by the investigator or experimenter.

The uncontrollable nuisance factor can be measured by a method called analysis of covariance to compensate its effect.

Example: Humidity is a variable it can be uncontrollable variable or factor but is can be measured and treated as a covariate.

When a variable or factor varies naturally and uncontrollably in the process can be controlled for the purpose of experiment can be called as noise factor.

Choice of Experimental Design

Choice of design requires consideration of sample size (number of replicates) or selection of a suitable run order for the experimental trials.

Design also involves what type empirical model to describe result. The model can be defined as a quantitative relationship (equation) between the output or response and important factor which are selected as inputs, these are design factors. We can choose first order model when two input variables are chosen as $y = a_0 + b_1 x_1 + b_2 x_2 + e$

Where y is the response and x_1 and x_2 are the design factors and b_1 or b_2 are unknown parameters can be obtained from the data which are obtained from experiment. If there is an interaction between the factor, the first order can be extended to $Y = a + b_1 x_1 + b_2 x_2 + b_{12} x_1 x_2 + e$

It the investigator wants include higher order interactions then the second order model like

$$Y = a_0 + b_1x_1 + b_2x_2 + b_{12}x_1x_2 + b_{11}x_1^2 + b_{22}x^2 + e$$

This model is often used in the optimization of the experiments

Performing the Experiment

When we are performing an experiment it is very important to monitor the process carefully to ensure that everything we are doing according plan which has been designed. Some time someone should be assigned to check factor setting before each trial or run.

Coleman and Montgomery suggests that prior to conducting experiment a few trial or pilot runs are required, which will give the information about the consistency of experimental material, a check on the measurement system, a rough idea about experimental error and a chance to practice the overall experimental technique.

Statistical Analysis of the Data

After the collection complete experimental results to analyze the data statistical methods should be applied to get conclusion about the result. This can be done using different types of statistical software

But the investigator must remember that statistical method cannot prove that the factor (factors) have a particular effect. They only can produce guidelines about the reliability and the validity of the result

Conclusion and Recommendation

After the complete analysis of data, the investigator must draw conclusion about the results and recommends a course of action.

Data should be presented graphically at the conclusion stage, when we are presenting results to others.

Follow-up runs and confirmation testing should also be performed to validate the conclusions from the experiment.

Finally investigator should recommend which factors should be considered to get an optimized result. It is a major mistake to design a single large, comprehensive experiment at the start of the study. In this regard investigator should recommend for pilot study. This will help the investigator to understand problems and difficulties. Finally it is important to recognize that all experience they are designed in experiments, but important thing here is whether they are well designed are not.

A well designed experiment will usually lead to a good, successful experiment and reduce your time, money and save other recourses.

DOE is an **essential** piece of the reliability program. It plays an **important** role in **Design** for Reliability (DFR) programs, allowing the simultaneous investigation of the effects of various factors and thereby facilitating **design** optimization. DOE also helps to identifying relationships between cause and effect in a mathematical equation. Those equations may linear, polynomial, quadratic and cubic etc. The selection of equation depends on the type of reaction which is taking place between the factors or variables which are chosen to prepare a formulation. Those points will be discussed with suitable formulation experimental results as examples.

The basic principles of experimental design are

(i)   Randomization,

(ii) Replication and

(iii) Local Control.

Randomization: Randomization is the corner stone underlying the use of statistical methods in experimental designs.

Replication: By replication we means that repetition of the basic experiments.

Local Control: The variables which are around the experimental area and experimenter has to control those variables to optimize the experimental result or response

Introduction

Need for Research: The growing global competition makes companies and service organizations to perform with utmost efficiency, mainly to have edge over competitors.

The goal of improving the efficiency of any organization leads to usage of different statistical operation research tools for better decision making. Within Pharmacy the potential areas of research are wide and varied surveying patients, weight management patent's owed medicines and targeted medicines use reviews. It is striking just how closely the research projects matches the needs of pharmacy business,

Pharmacist may follow career tracks that provide opportunities beyond dispensing prescription drugs in a drug store. Pharmacies in academia delve into the research behind the discovery and testing of new medicines. In pharmaceutical companies pharmacists often are employed to oversee research project.

The project pharmacists are hand on pharmacist involved directly with the research. Most of the time they study in different stages of clinical research. The Pharmacist who are doing research will be the investigator in different stages as basis, in clinical and translation research. The study also focus some issues relating to the cost of R&D, the performance of the pharmaceutical industry in developing innovative drugs and the role of expected profile in private firms decisions about investing in R & D.

The efficiency will lead the improvement of industry, which is a main key for the success of any industry or organization.

The productivity of a business system can be defined as the ratio between the output and input, where the output means to the annual total income of an industry or business system and input refers to total amount spent on different resources and services utilized in their business system and the annual production and services rendered,

There is an avenue for pharmacist in pharmaceutical industry to carryout their research in the development of new compounds and drugs. In private industry pharmacist are involved in the actual production of drugs once clinical trials have been completed. Their research continues as they monitor usage of drugs and oversee quality control and continues research. Pharmacists are also hired to monitor the chemical plants that produce the drugs and supervise the processes. Now a day's pharmaceutical industry using Design of experiment statical software which will be assisting to design the experiment and analyze the experimental result.

Research

To get a better result in the practical situation, the investigator should visualize the fact that a detailed study which is required. The research is the only way to achieve a better result. Research is an well defined and organized set of activities to study and develop a model or Procedure/Technique to find the results of a realistic problem supported by the literature and data such that its objectives are optimized and further makes recommendations and interferences for implementations.

In the pharmaceutical field (industry, academic institutions) different statistical tools which are used to analyze data are

1. Methods to find measures of central tendency viz mean, median and mode
2. Methods to find measures of dispersion viz variance, coefficient of variance, standard deviation etc.
3. Forecasting methods.
4. Design of experiments.
5. Testing of hypothesis.

In most of the pharmaceutical research, design of experiments aims to design the experiments with one or more factors or variables, where the investigator suspects these factors have effect on one or more response(output) variable and analyze, what is the effect of these factor on the response variable(s).

If the research is the design and analysis experimental result includes, there focus will be on systems, procedure, processes, machine, materials, employees and other resources which are used to produce drugs or items.

To design an experiment and to analyze the result most often in industry the (DOE) design of experiment software will be used.

The use of DOE with different methods is explained in details in different chapters. Technology, Definitions (vocabulary)

Factor

A factor is an assigned variable, which are taken as ingredient to prepare a formulation.

Ex: concentration, temperature, lubricant agent etc.

A factor which we are chosen to perform an experiment may be quantitative and qualitative. The choice of factors to be selected to perform experiment depends on the objectives and is pre determined by the experimenter.

QUANTITATIVE FACTOR

A quantitative factor has a numerical value assigned to it.

Ex: When we choose ingredient or factor with 2%, 3%, 4% they are quantitative factors.

Qualitative Factor

The Qualitative factor is one where numerical value is not involved in the factor

Ex: Diet, Drug (used to perform clinical trial experiment)etc.

In addition to these two factors there are two more factors; named as fixed factor and random factor.

Fixed Factor: In an experiment, if a specific set of variable or factors selected with certainty, and then those factors are termed as fixed factors

Ex: If four doctors choose a drug to treat patients, each doctor treats 5 patients using same drug.

n is total number of patients treated.

(n-1)) Degree of freedom of the factor - drug.

Effect of fixed factor A (drug)= $\sum_{i=0}^{n} A^2$ / (n-1)

Random factor: In an experiment, if a set of treatments of a factor (drug – factor – any factor can be chosen) is selected randomly with the available treatments, then it is termed as random factor.

Ex: If four drugs are chosen randomly to verify the level of significance, then these four drugs are random factors.

Levels: The levels of variable or factor are the values or designations assigned to the factor

OR

Setting of the factors at a particular values or categories.

Ex: 20^0 and 40^0 are the levels of temperature, which is one factor in the preparation of formulation and 0.1 moles and 0.3 moles are levels for the factor concentration.

Replication: When an investigator designs any experiment to prepare a formulation, there will be some error due to some uncontrollable factors, to estimate effect of those factors, the same experiment has to be repeated under the same condition(s), such repetition of an experiment is called as replication.

Effect: The change in response variable or output variable is due to the change in the levels of factors is called or termed as effect.

When two factors or variables A and B chosen to perform experiment and levels are low and high, then the different combinations are

Runs	A	B	Combination	AB(interaction)
1	-	-	Low-low	+
a	+	-	High-low	-
b	-	+	Low -high	-
ab	+	+	High-high	+

The main effect $A = \frac{1}{2n}\{[(ab-b)]+[a-1]\}$

The main effect $B = \dfrac{1}{2n}\{[(ab-a)]+[b-1]\}$

Then the interaction effect $AB = \dfrac{1}{2n}\{[ab-b]-[a-1]\}$

OR

The formulas to obtain the effects of A, B and AB may be desired by another method

The formulas used are to find effect A is

$$A = \bar{Y}_A^+ - \bar{Y}_A^-$$

$$= [\dfrac{(ab+a)}{2n} - \dfrac{(b+1)}{2n}]$$

and effect of B is obtained by

$$B = \bar{Y}_B^+ - \bar{Y}_B^-$$

$$B = [\dfrac{(ab+b)}{2n} - \dfrac{(a+1)}{2n}]$$

Then the interaction effect of AB is obtained by equation

$$AB = [\dfrac{(ab+1)}{2n} - \dfrac{(a+b)}{2n}]$$

Need for Design of Experiments in Pharmacy

Design of experiment (DOE) in Pharmaceutical experiments, mainly in formulation development required to:

1. To identify the relation in between cause and effect of the reality
2. To know the interactions between or among the factors or different variables which are used in the experiment.
3. To find what level should be fixed in order to obtain optimized result and enhance the performance of the experiment
4. Is it possible to use technique to minimize the error
5. To improve the robustness of the design or process to variation. To derive the knowledge about the product and processes in the formulation development in pharmaceutical industry mainly they have to focus on experimentation. Any experiment can be defined as a series conducted in a systematic manners to understand the existing process or to explore new product or process. In the present situation the design of experiments (DOE) is a tool for developing an experimentation strategy, which helps investigator to maximize their learning by using minimum recourses. This also helps in the manufacturing process to increase yield of the process and decrease the variability and errors.

The methodology of DOE ensures the investigators, that all the factors or variables and interaction of these variable are systematically investigated. The information what the investigator gets from a DOE analysis is more reliable and complete

Methods of designing experiments in formulation developments

In the design and analysis of experiments there are different methods as listed below

1. Factorial design
2. Regression approach
3. Response surface methodology

1. Factorial design : 2^n factorial experiment

In a factorial design experiment the base 2 stands for number of levels (low or high). In this case only two levels are selected. The power indicates the number of ingredient or variable which are selected for the formulation development by an investigator. In this section the concept 2^2 and 2^3 factorial designs are discussed.

In the design of 2^n- factorial design experiments, the investigator assume that

(a)   The factor are fixed

(b)   The design is completely randomized

(c)   The distribution is normal

The 2^n design is particularly useful in early stages of experimental work, when the investigator wants do experiments with many factors. This method provides the limited number of runs within which n-factor can be studied in a complete factorial design. Here in formulation development designs are used in factor screening experiments

Concept of 2^2 Factorial Experiments

The 2^2 factorial design is the first design in 2^k - series two factors with two levels say low and high. These two factors can be named as A and B. Each factors are represented by 0 and 1 respectively. The graphical view of 2^2 design is as represented below.

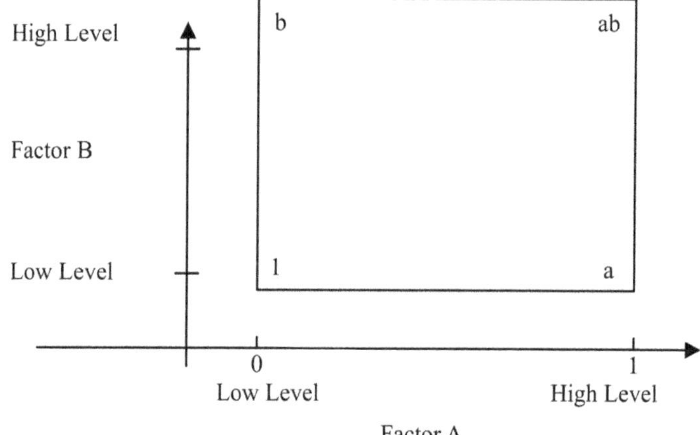

The 2^2 – factorial design is a completely randomized experiment the factors levels and treatment combination are as shown in the table

Runs	A	B	Treatment Combination
1	-	-	Low-low
a	+	-	High-low
b	-	+	Low -high
ab	+	+	High-high

The treatment combinations in the 2^2 factorial design are represented as 1, a, b and ab. In 2^2 design we measure the effect of factor which are used in the formulation development.

Effect of Factor

The average effect of the factor is the average of changes of the response due to the change in that factor under the levels of all other factors which are considered in the experimental design.

Here in 2^2 design experiment, Investigator obtains the main effect or average effect of A and B and the interaction effect of AB.

The main or average effect of A is obtained by using the equation

$$A=\frac{1}{2k}\{[(ab-b)]+[a-1]\}$$

$$A=\frac{1}{2k}\{[ab+a-b-1]\}$$

where k – is named as number of replicates taken at the treatment combinations.

The average or main effect of B is computed as

$$B=\frac{1}{2k}\{[ab-b)]+[b-1]\}$$

$$B=\frac{1}{2k}[ab+b-a-1]$$

Then the interaction effect of AB is obtained by the equation

$$AB=\frac{1}{2k}\{[ab-b]-[a-1]\}$$

$$=\frac{1}{2k}[ab+b-a-1]$$

Main effect of A:

Now the effect of A at low level of B is $\left[\frac{[a-1]}{n}\right]$ and the effect of A at high level of B is $\left[\frac{[ab-b]}{n}\right]$. The average of these quantities is called as main effect of A.

MAIN EFFECT OF B:

Main effect of B is found from the effect of B at the low levels of A is $\left[\frac{[b-1]}{n}\right]$, at the high level of A is $\left[\frac{[ab-a]}{n}\right]$. The average of these quantities is called as main effect of B.

Interaction effect of AB: The interaction effect of AB is defined as the average differences between the effect of A at the High level of B and the effect of A at low level of B.

The effect of A is positive, indicates that increasing A from the low level to high level will increase the yield. Similarly if the effect of B is Negative, Indicates that the increase of B from low to high level, suggest increase of quantity B, decrease the yield.

The interaction effect always appears to be small, when compared with two main effects.

In 2^k factorial, it is always important to examine the magnitude and direction of the factor effects to verify which variables plays very important role in preparing formulation. The ANOVA can be used to draw the interpretation about result or data which we have obtained by performing an experiments.

To perform ANOVA, investigator should determine the sum of squares of A, B and AB.

The sum of the squares can be obtained by taking contrast of main effect of A, B and AB.

The contrast of A is

$$\text{Contrast}_A = ab+a-b-1$$

This also can be called total effect of A.

Similarly the contrast B and AB can be obtained using equations.

$$\text{Contrast}_B = [ab+b-a-1]$$

$$\text{Contrast}_{AB} = [ab+1-a-b]$$

Then sum of squares A, B and AB are obtained using equations as listed below.

$$SS_A = \frac{[ab+a-b-1]^2}{4K}$$

$$SS_B = \frac{[ab+b-a-1]^2}{4K}$$

$$SS_{AB} = \frac{[ab+1-b-a]^2}{4K}$$

K is number of replication of the formulation experiments.

The total sum of squares is obtained in the usual way, but that is

$$SST = \sum_{i=1}^{2}\sum_{j=1}^{2}\sum_{k=1}^{n}Y^2{}_{ijk} - \frac{y^2}{4n}$$

Y = Grand sum of the results which are obtained.

In general SST has 4n -1 degrees of freedom.

The sum of squares due to error with 4(n-1) degree of freedom is obtained by the equation.

$$SSE = SS_T - SS_A - SS_B - SS_{AB}$$

All these values can be summarised in a ANOVA table as shown below.

Sources of variations	Sum of Squares	Degree of Freedom	Mean Squares	Fisher distribution value 'F'	P-Values
A	SS_A	(a-1)	$MS_A = \dfrac{SS_A}{a-1}$	$F = \dfrac{MS_A}{MS_E}$	-
B	SS_B	(b-1)	$MS_B = \dfrac{SS_B}{b-1}$	$F = \dfrac{MS_B}{MS_E}$	-
AB	SS_{AB}	(a-1) (b-1)	$MS_{AB} = \dfrac{SS_{AB}}{(a-1)(b-1)}$	$F = \dfrac{MS_{AB}}{MS_E}$	-
Error	SS_E	4(k-1) or ab(k-1)	$MSE = \dfrac{SS_E}{4(k-1)}$	-	-

n= 2   k = 3

a = 2   b = 2   (a-1) (b-1)

a-1 = 2-1 = 1   b -1 =2-1 = 1   1×1 = **1**

ab(K -1) = 2*2(3-1) = **8**

Example:

Factor			Replication			Total
A	B	AB	I	II	III	
–	–	+	28	25	27	80
+	–	–	36	32	32	100
–	+	–	18	19	23	60
+	+	+1	31	30	29	90

This data can be represented in the form of graph

$$SS_A = \frac{[ab+a-b-1]^2}{4K}$$

$$SS_A = \frac{[90+100-60-80]^2}{4 \times 3}$$

$$= 208.33$$

$$SS_B = \frac{[90+60-100-80]^2}{4 \times 3}$$

$$= 75$$

$$SS_{AB} = \frac{[ab+1-a-b]^2}{4K}$$

$$SS_{AB} = \frac{[90+80-100-60]^2}{4 \times 3}$$

$$= 8.33$$

$$\text{Sum of squares} = 28^2 + 36^2 + 18^2 + 31^2 + \text{-------} + 23^2 + 29^2$$

$$= 9398.06$$

Y = Grand total

Y = 80 + 100 + 60 + 90 = 330

$$SST = \text{Sum of squares} - \frac{Y^2}{4K}$$

$$= 9398 - \frac{(330)^2}{12}$$

SST = 323.00

$$SSE = SST - SS_A - SS_B - SS_{AB}$$

$$= 323.00 + 208.33 + 75.00 - 8.33$$

$$= 31.34$$

Sources of variations	Sum of Squares	Degree of Freedom	Mean Squares	Fisher distribution value 'F'	P-Values
A	208-33	(2-1) =1	$MS_A = \frac{208.33}{2-1}$ 208.33	$F = \frac{MS_A}{MS_E} = \frac{208.33}{31.34}$	-
B	$SS_B = 75$	(2-1) =	$MS_B = \frac{75}{2-1}$ $= 75$	$F = \frac{MS_B}{MS_E}$ $= \frac{75}{31.34}$	-
AB	$SS_{AB} = 8.33$	(2-1) (2-1) = 1	$MS_{AB} = \frac{8.33}{(2-1)(2-1)}$ $= 8.33$	$F = \frac{MS_{AB}}{MS_E}$ $= \frac{8.33}{31.34}$	-
Error	$SS_E = 31.34$	4(k-1) or ab(k-1)	$MSE = \frac{SS_E}{4(k-1)}$	-	-

Blocking a Replicated 2^k Factorial Design

When it is not possible to perform all the runs or experiments in 2^k factorial design experiment with a homogeneous condition, then the investigator can deliberately vary the experimental conditions to ensure that the treatments are equally effective across many situations that are likely to be encountered in practice. For example while preparing formulation experiment with several batches of raw material or chemicals will be used to know the effect of those materials in preparing formulation.

In the statistical theory of the **design of experiments, blocking** is the arranging of **experimental** units in groups (**blocks**) that are similar to one another. Typically, a

blocking factor is a source of variability that is not of primary interest to the investigator or experimenter. The runs in block (replicate) would be made in random order.

Blocking increases the sample size, which in turn reduces variability; individuals within blocks should be as different as possible to create a more heterogeneous experiment. Blocking reduces bias in **experiments**; individuals should be randomly divided into their blocks.

Example: In general to prepare and optimize a formulation by applying 2^2 – factorial design, only four experimental trials can be made from a single batch of ingredients. Therefore to perform three replicates, three different batches of ingredients will be required in this design. The results obtained after performing in three different blocks as listed below.

BOLCK-1	BOLCK-2	BOLCK-3
1 = 28	1 = 25	1 = 27
a = 36	a = 32	a = 32
b = 18	b = 19	b = 23
ab = 31	ab = 30	ab = 29

Total B1 = 113   Block2 = 106   Block3 = 111

$$SS_{Block} = \sum_{i=1}^{3} \frac{Bi^2}{4} - \frac{G^2}{12} = \frac{(113)^2 + (106)^2 + (111)^2}{4} - \frac{(330)^2}{12}$$

$SS_{Block} = 6.50$

Analysis of variance for the formulation process experiment performed in three blocks

Confounding in the 2^k Factorial Design Experiment

In many of the pharmaceutical formulation problems, it is not possible to conduct or perform complete replicate of a factorial design in one block. In order to overcome this problem, Confounding technique will be applied to prepare or perform formulation experiments. Confounding is a design technique for arranging a complete factorial experiment in blocks and in this method the block size will be smaller than the number of treatment combinations in one replicate. The confounding technique gives complete information about certain treatment effects (that is high order interactions) to be indistinguishable from, or confounded with, blocks. Even though the designs presented are incomplete block designs, because each block does not contain all the treatments or treatment combinations.

Definition: Confounding is a design technique for arranging a complete factorial experiment in blocks, where block size is smaller than the number of treatment combinations in one replicate. Cause information about certain treatment effects to be indistinguishable from (confounded with) blocks.

Confounding in the 2^k Factorial Design in Two Blocks

If an experimenter wish to run a single replicate of the 2^2 design, then each of $2^2 = 4$ treatment combinations requires a quantity of ingredients and here each batch of ingredient/raw materials is large enough for two treatment combinations which are to be tested. To perform experiment to prepare a formulation, two batches of ingredients or raw materials are required. When we consider the ingredients or raw materials as blocks, then the investigator or experimenter must assign two of the four treatment combinations for each block.

The combination of 2^2–factorial design are assigned to two different blocks and block1 contains the treatment combinations of (1) and (ab) and Block2 contains (a) and (b). The order in which the treatment combinations are run within a block is randomly determined. Here the experimenter or the investigator must decide which block to run first.

Combinations	I	A	B	AB	BOLCK-1
1	+	-	-	+	2
a	+	+	-	-	1
b	+	-	+	-	1
ab	+	+	+	+	2

BOLCK-1	BOLCK-2
1	a
ab	b

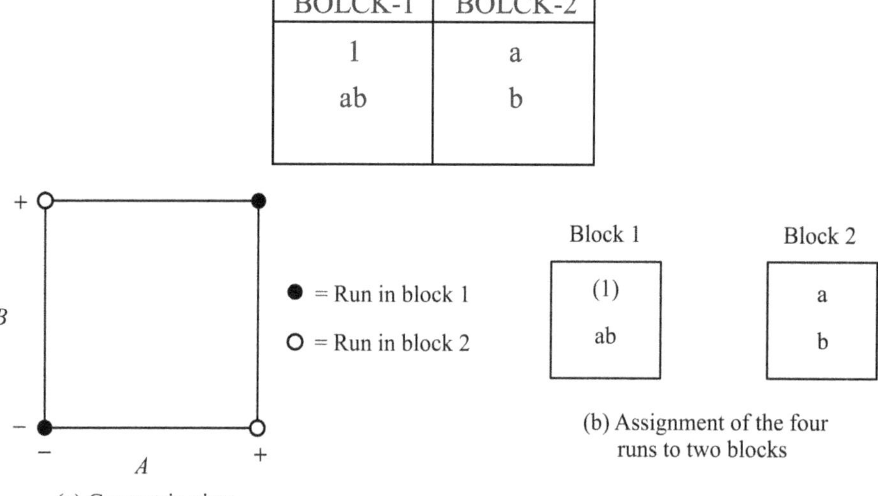

(a) Geometric view

(b) Assignment of the four runs to two blocks

Here both the main effects A and B are unaffected by blocking, because each estimate there is one plus and one minus treatment combination from each block. Then any difference between block1 and block2 will be canceled out.

Because of two treatment combinations with plus sing in block1 and minus sign in block2, the block effect and the AB interaction are identical. We can say that AB is confounded with blocks.

Confounding with 2^3–Factorial Design

This confounding can be extended for 2^3–factorial design. When 2^3–factorial design is considered, the investigator can perform formulation experiments in 8 –runs and they will divided into 2–blocks. If the investigator wish to confound the three-factor interaction ABC with blocks, there the investigator assign the treatment combinations with minus sign on ABC to block1 and those that are with plus sign are assigned to block 2. Here we emphasize that the treatment combinations within a block are run in a random order.

Combinations	I	A	B	AB	C	AC	BC	ABC	Block
1	+	-	-	+	-	+	+	-	1
a	+	+	-	-	-	-	+	+	2
b	+	-	+	-	-	+	-	+	2
ab	+	+	+	+	-	-	-	-	1
c	+	-	-	+	+	-	-	+	2
ac	+	+	-	-	+	+	-	-	1
bc	+	-	+	-	+	-	+	-	1
abc	+	+	+	+	+	+	+	+	2

In order to find the main effect of A , the difference between average of the four runs of A with high level (+) and average of the four runs of A with low level (-) and the equation used to calculate the main effect of A is

$$A = \bar{Y}_{A+} - \bar{Y}_{A^-} = \frac{a+ab+ac+abc}{4n} - \frac{1+b+c+bc}{4n} = \frac{a+ab+ac+abc-1-b-c-bc}{4n}$$

$$A = \frac{1}{4n}\{a + ab + ac + abc - 1 - b - c - bc\}$$

Similarly by applying the procedure the main effect of B can be obtained and the equation used is

$$B = \bar{Y}_{B+} - \bar{Y}_{B-} = \frac{b+ab+bc+abc}{4n} - \frac{1+a+c+ac}{4n} = \frac{b+ab+bc+abc-1-a-c-ac}{4n}$$

$$B = \frac{1}{4n}\{b + ab + bc + abc - 1 - a - c - ac\}$$

Similarly the effect of C can be obtained using the equation

$$C = \frac{1}{4n}\{c + ac + bc + abc - 1 - a - b - ab\}$$

The interaction effect of AB can obtained by the equation by the same procedure

$$AB = \bar{Y}_{AB+} - \bar{Y}_{AB^-}$$

$$AB = \frac{1}{4n}\{abc + ab + c + 1 - ac - bc - b - a\}$$

Similarly the effect of AC, BC and ABC can be obtained by choosing the +ve and –Ve sign values from the respective columns of the treatment combinations and respective equations are

$$AC = \frac{1}{4n}\{1 + b + ac + abc - a - c - ab - bc\}$$

$$B = \frac{1}{4n}\{1 + a + bc + abc - a - b - ab - c\}$$

$$ABC = \frac{1}{4n}\{abc + a + b + c - ab - ac - bc - 1\}$$

In case of 2^3 – design the sums of squares with n – replication can be obtained by the equation SS $= \dfrac{(Contrast)^2}{8n}$; the value 8 is taken as the number of runs in case of 2^3– factorial design.

ANOVA for selected factorial model

Analysis of variance table [Partial sum of squares - Type III]

Source Of variation	Sum of Squares	df	Mean Square	F Value	p-value Prob > F	Inference
A	SS_A	$(a\text{-}1)$	MS_A	MS_A/MS_E		
B	SS_B	$(b\text{-}1)$	MS_B	MS_B/MS_E		
C	SS_C	$(c\text{-}1)$	MS_C	MS_C/MS_E		
AB	SS_{AB}	$(a\text{-}1)(b\text{-}1)$	MS_{AB}	MS_{AB}/MS_E		
AC	SS_{AC}	$(a\text{-}1)(c\text{-}1)$	MS_{AC}	MS_{AC}/MS_E		
BC	SS_{BC}	$(b\text{-}1)(c\text{-}1)$	MS_{BC}	MS_{BC}/MS_E		
ABC	SS_{ABC}	$(a\text{-}1)(b\text{-}1)(c\text{-}1)$	MS_{ABC}	MS_{ABC}/MS_E		
Pure Error	SS_E	$abc(n\text{-}1)$	MS_E			
Total						

Example:

An experiment was performed by an investigator to measure the improve in the yield of a chemical process. The investigator selected three factors A, B, and C and each with 2-levels (low and High) and three replicates of a completely randomized experiments were performed. The results obtained after performing the experiments are as recorded in the table.

Combinations	A	B	C	Replicate1	Replicate2	Replicate3
1	-	-	-	20	30	26
a	+	-	-	32	42	28
b	-	+	-	35	35	51
ab	+	+	-	57	48	47
c	-	-	+	42	46	37
ac	+	-	+	40	38	35
bc	-	+	+	62	51	54
abc	+	+	+	41	42	46

Analyze the effect of each factors and verify which factor is most effective?

ANOVA for selected factorial model

Analysis of variance table [Partial sum of squares - Type III]

Source	Sum of Squares	df	Mean Square	F Value	p-value Prob > F	Inference
Model	1856.96	7	265.28	8.19	0.0003	significant
A-A	*2.04*	*1*	*2.04*	*0.063*	*0.8049*	
B-B	*975.38*	*1*	*975.38*	*30.13*	*< 0.0001*	
C-C	*287.04*	*1*	*287.04*	*8.87*	*0.0089*	
AB	*18.38*	*1*	*18.38*	*0.57*	*0.4622*	
AC	*477.04*	*1*	*477.04*	*14.73*	*0.0014*	
BC	*57.04*	*1*	*57.04*	*1.76*	*0.2030*	
ABC	*40.04*	*1*	*40.04*	*1.24*	*0.2825*	
Pure Error	518.00	16	32.37			
Cor Total	2374.96	23				

REGRESION MODEL

In a 2^n factorial design, the results obtained after performing an experiment, can be expressed in the form of regression model. The regression model approach is much more natural and infusive. In general for chemical process experiment the commonly used model is regression model

$$Y = \beta_0 + + \beta_1 x_1 + \beta_2 x_2 + e$$

Here x_1 and x_2 are two factors or variables which are chosen to perform experiment.

β_0 is intercept

β_1 and β_2 are slopes of the factors x_1 and x_2

When we consider only one factor the regression model is $Y = \beta_0 + \beta_1 x_1$.

This can be extended for multiple regressions like

$$Y = \beta_0 + \beta_1 x_1 + \beta_2 x_2 + \beta_3 x_3 + - - - - - - - - + \beta_k x_k$$

In the design of experiment to obtain the values of $\beta_0, \beta_1, \beta_2, - - - - \beta_k$, Matrix method will be used.

When we consider the regression model

$$Y = \beta_0 + \beta_1 x_1 + \beta_2 x_2 + \beta_3 x_3 + - - - - - - - - + \beta_k x_k$$

$$Y = \text{Dependent Variable}$$

$x_1 \; x_2 \text{....} x_k$ are independent variables

$$Y = \beta_0 + \beta_1 x_1 + \beta_2 x_2 + \beta_3 x_3 + \text{- - - - - - - -} + \beta_k x_k$$

$\beta_1, \; \beta_2, \; \beta_3 \; \text{.........} \beta_k$ are slopes of factors or variables $x_1, x_2, x_3 \text{......} x_k$

k is the number of independent variables.

The theoretical model of the regression equation can be represented as

Y	X_1	X_2	X_3	----------	X_5	-----------	-----------	X_k
y_1	X_{11}	X_{12}	X_{13}	----------	X_{15}	-----------	-----------	X_{1k}
y_2	X_{21}	X_{22}	X_{23}	----------	X_{25}	-----------	-----------	X_{2k}
y_3	X_{31}	X_{32}	X_{33}	----------	X_{35}	-----------	-----------	X_{3k}
y_n	X_{n1}	X_{n2}	X_{n3}	----------	X_{n5}	-----------	-----------	X_{nk}

The general form of matrix can be

$$X = \begin{bmatrix} x11 & x12 & - - - - - - - - & x1k \\ x21 & x22 & - - - - - - - - & x2k \\ & & - - - - - - - - - - - - & \\ & & - - - - - - - - - - - - & \\ xn1 & xn1 & - - - - - - - - & xnk \end{bmatrix}$$

$$Y = \begin{bmatrix} y1 \\ y2 \\ \\ \\ yn \end{bmatrix} \qquad \propto = \begin{bmatrix} \beta1 \\ \beta2 \\ \\ \\ \beta K \end{bmatrix}$$

The coefficients of regression model can be obtained by applying the following procedure

1. Find transpose of X (x^T)
2. Find the product of matrices $X^T X$
3. Obtain the co-factor matrix of $X^T X$
4. Obtain the value of the determine $1|X^T X|$
5. Obtained adjoint matrix of $X^T X$
6. Obtain inverse of $X^T X$ $\quad [X^T X]^{-1} = \dfrac{1}{|X^T X|} \text{adj}(X^T X)$
7. Obtain $X^T Y$

Then coefficient of regression model can be obtained by multiplying $[X^T X]^{-1}$ and $X^T Y$

$$\alpha = [X^T X]^{-1} [X^T X]$$

Then ß$_0$ ß$_1$ß$_2$ - - - - - - ß$_k$ can computed after obtaining the product of $[X^TX]^{-1}[X^TY]$

Example:

For the given data from the regression equation and obtain Predicted value and Perform one way ANOVA to verify the level of significance

X	Y
5	3
8	4
7	5
6	2
4	1

Solution: Matrix X = $\begin{bmatrix} 1 & 5 \\ 1 & 8 \\ 1 & 7 \\ 1 & 6 \\ 1 & 4 \end{bmatrix}$ D= $\begin{bmatrix} \alpha \\ \beta \end{bmatrix}$ and Y = $\begin{bmatrix} 3 \\ 4 \\ 5 \\ 2 \\ 1 \end{bmatrix}$

$$X^T = \begin{bmatrix} 1 & 1 & 1 & 1 & 1 \\ 5 & 8 & 7 & 6 & 4 \end{bmatrix}$$

Find the Product of $\quad$ X^T*X = $\begin{bmatrix} 1 & 1 & 1 & 1 & 1 \\ 5 & 8 & 7 & 6 & 4 \end{bmatrix}\begin{bmatrix} 1 & 5 \\ 1 & 8 \\ 1 & 7 \\ 1 & 6 \\ 1 & 4 \end{bmatrix}$

$$X^T*X = \begin{bmatrix} 5 & 30 \\ 30 & 190 \end{bmatrix}$$

Next co-factor of each element should be obtained and co-factor matrix should to written

C.F. of 5 = +(190) = 190

C.F. 30 = -(30) = -30

C.F. 30 = -(30) = -30

C.F. 190=+(5) $\quad$ = 5

Then the Cofactor matrix of X^T*X = $\begin{bmatrix} 190 & -30 \\ -30 & 5 \end{bmatrix}$

Adjoint(X^T*X) = Transpose of Cofactor Matrix of X^T*X

Adjoint(X^T*X) = = $\begin{bmatrix} 190 & -30 \\ -30 & 5 \end{bmatrix}$

The value of the determinant $| X^T * X | = \begin{vmatrix} 5 & 30 \\ 30 & 190 \end{vmatrix} = 950 - 900 = 50$

Then the Inverse of $| X^T * X |$ is written as $(X^T * X)^{-1} = \dfrac{1}{| X^T * X |}$ Adjoint($X^T * X$)

$$(X^T * X)^{-1} = \frac{1}{50} \begin{bmatrix} 190 & -30 \\ -30 & 5 \end{bmatrix}$$

Obtain $X^T * Y = \begin{bmatrix} 1 & 1 & 1 & 1 & 1 \\ 5 & 8 & 7 & 6 & 4 \end{bmatrix} \begin{bmatrix} 3 \\ 4 \\ 5 \\ 2 \\ 1 \end{bmatrix} = \begin{bmatrix} 15 \\ 98 \end{bmatrix}$

$$D = \begin{bmatrix} \alpha \\ \beta \end{bmatrix} = (X^T * X)^{-1} * (X^T * Y)$$

$$\begin{bmatrix} \alpha \\ \beta \end{bmatrix} = \frac{1}{50} \begin{bmatrix} 190 & -30 \\ -30 & 5 \end{bmatrix} \begin{bmatrix} 15 \\ 98 \end{bmatrix} = \frac{1}{50} \begin{bmatrix} -90 \\ 40 \end{bmatrix} = \begin{bmatrix} -1.8 \\ 0.8 \end{bmatrix}$$

$Y = \alpha + \beta X$

$Y = -.18 + 0.8X$

X	Y	$\hat{Y} = -.18 + 0.8X$	$(Y - Mean(Y))^2$	$(\hat{Y} - Mean(Y))^2$
5	3	2.2.	0	0.64
8	4	4.6	1	2.56
7	5	3.8	4	0.64
6	2	3	1	0
4	1	1.4	4	2.56
	$\sum Y = 15$		SST = 10	SSR = 6.4

$$Mean(Y) = \frac{15}{5} = 3$$

$$SSE = SST - SSR = 10 - 6.4 = 3.6$$

Sources of Variation	Sum of Squares	DOF	Mean Squares	F	p-value	
A-X	6.4	1	6.4	5.333	0.1040	not significant
Residual	3.6	3	1.2		0.1040	
Cor Total	10	4				

TESTING THE HYPOTHESIS ON THE SIGNIFICANCE OF REGRESION

After fitting regression model investigator should check the estimated result from regression model represent the real world data

Let $Y_n = n^{th}$ Observation of the dependent variable Y

$x_n = n^{th}$ value of the independent variable X

$\overline{Y}$ = Average of Y

$\widehat{Y}i$ = Predicted value of nth dependent variable Y

n = Total number values

a_0 = Intercept

a_i = Slope of the particular independent variable

e_n = Random error between $Y_n \propto \overline{Y}$ variables

Now model is $Y_n = a_0 + a_n x_n + e$

The sum of square of total

$$SS_T = \sum_1^n (yi - \bar{y})^2$$

The sum of Squares of regression is

$$SS_R = \sum_1^n (\widehat{y}i - y)^2$$

The sum of Squares due to error is SS_E

$$SS_E = \sum_{n=1}^n (yi - \widehat{y}i)^2$$

The degree of freedom for the total= SS_T = n-1

The degree of freedom due to regression is (for SS_R)=1

The degree of freedom for the error= SS_R = (n-2)

ANOVA Table to test the significance of regression

Source of variation	Sum of sequences	Degree of freedom	Means square	F-rates
Due to regression	SS_R	1	$MSS_R = \dfrac{SSE}{1}$	$F = \dfrac{MSSR}{MSE}$
Due to error	SS_E	n-2	$MSE = \dfrac{SSE}{n-2}$	

RESPONSE SURFACE METHODOLOGY

Response surface methodology (RSM) is used to analyze experimental results, when there are several variables or factors, influencing the output or response. The main purpose of this method is to optimize the response among the different results.

For example suppose that a pharmacist wishes to find which levels of factors should be fixed to get a maximum yield when he prepares a formulation.

IF x and x_2 are two factors, which are taken as inputs to yield the response or dependent or output variable Y.

The process yield of these two factor x_1 and x_2 with different levels is a function of the factors x_1 and x_2.

That function is written in mathematical equations as $Y=f(x_1, x_2)_{+}e$

Where e-represents the errors obtained in the response Y

If the expected response 'Y' is written as $E(y) = f(x_1, x_{2)} = \eta$, then surface is written as $\eta = f(x_1, x_2)$ is called response surface.

Generally the exact nature of response surface is unknown and the model the investigator decide to apply is an attempt at a reasonable approximation to it. The first order model which we prefer is

$$Y = \beta_0 + \beta_1 x_1 + \beta_2 x_2 + \beta_3 x_3 + \cdots \cdots + \beta_k x_k$$

$\beta_0 =$ intercept

$\beta n'^S =$ coefficient of respective factors which are chosen to perform experiment to prepare a formulation,

Where k is derived number of factor chosen or selected for that particular experiment.

X^S_i are different independent factors or variables chosen (Independent Variables)

Investigator can use the first order model when the response is a linear function of the independent variable.

If there is curve linear or curvature in the response or system, then a polynomial of higher degree must be selected, such as the second order model.

$$Y = \beta_0 + \sum_{i=1}^{k} \beta i x i + \Sigma$$

Example: $\beta_0 + \beta_1 X_1 + \beta_2 X_2 + \beta_{11} X^2_1 + \beta_{22} X^2 + \beta_{12} X_1 X_2 + \varepsilon$

RSM problems, very frequently apply one or both of these models to analyze the results. Of course, it is unlikely that a polynomial model will be a reasonable approximation of the time functional relationship over the entire space of the independent variables, but for a relatively small region they usually work quite well.

When an investigator use response surface method, investigator looks for the combination of the factors setting of selecting such that the response is optimised.

When the investigator says the optimum is maximizing type, then the result he/she is expecting is hill – climbing. Here we can take the path of steepest ascent in the direction of the maximum increase in the response or product or output.

If the optimum is a minimization type, then we are going down into the valley here we take the path of steepest descend in the direction of the maximum decrease in the response.

The overall objectives of RSM is to determine the optimum operating condition for the system or to determine a region of the factor space in which operating requirements are satisfied.

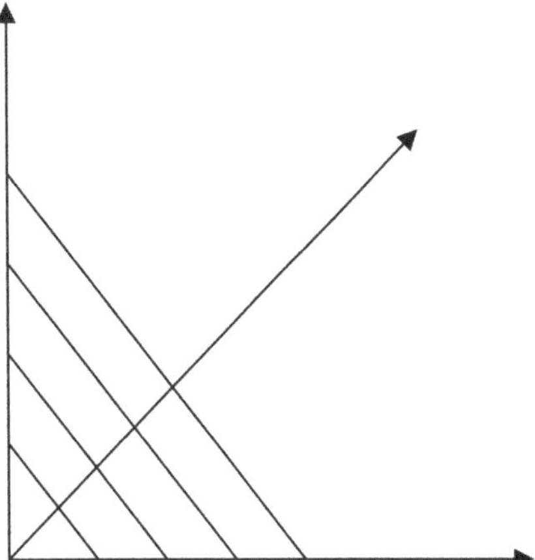

Path of steepest ascent of first order model.

3D surface of first circle model will be intersects.

TYPES OF DESIGNS IN RSM

1. CENTRAL COMPOSITE DESIGN

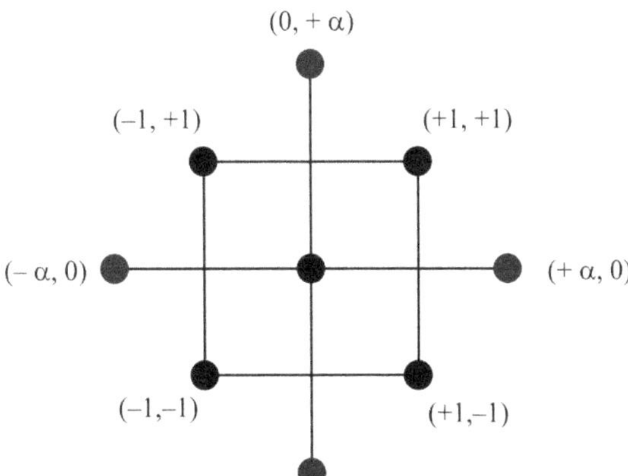

Two Factors Design

The most popular type of design for second order model is the central composite design in the short form, it is name as CCD.

This is a simple and highly effective in giving solution to augment the 2^k design with four axial runs as shown in the figure. In 2^k design, if k=2, this can used to fit the second order model.

when k = 3 factors, in this design there $14+n_c$ runs n_c usually lie between 3 and 5 $(3 \leq n_c \leq 5)$.

This design normally can be applied, when first order design provides an inadequate information for the data of result, in which the investigator has used to analyze the result.

In CCD there are two important parameters to be noted are.

1. $\alpha = n^{1/4}{}_f$ is the distance of the axial points from the design centre and n_f it is the number of factorial points in the design.

    n_c – the number of centre points runs, generally there will be 3 or 5 central point runs will be chosen for analysing the result.

The second order model for 2^2 – factorial design.

Runs	X_1	X_2
1	−1	−1
2	−1	+1
3	+1	−1
4	+1	+1
5	0	0
6	0	0
7	0	0
8	0	0
9	0	0
10	1.414	0
11	−1.414	0
12	0	1.414
13	0	−1.414

The graphical view of the points of CCD.

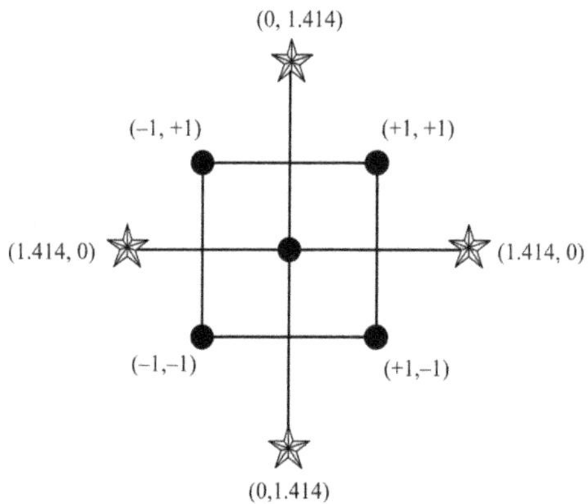

Central Composite Design (CCD)

The points or the values of ingredients on x-axis and Y-axis can be obtained by using the distance formulae between two points. If $A = (X_1, Y_1)$ and $B = (X_2, Y_2)$, then the distance between two point is obtained by the equation $d = \sqrt{(X2 - X1)^2 + (Y2 - Y1)^2}$

In the above table the first run consists of two low levels and those two levels are considered as B = (X2, Y2) = (-1, -1) in the third quadrant of XY- Plane and the centre point runs are as zero level (mid level) and coordinates are considered as A = (X1, Y1) = (0, 0) . Then the distance between these points

$$d=\sqrt{(X2-X1)^2+(Y2-Y1)^2}$$
$$=\sqrt{(-1-0)^2+(1-0)^2}$$
$$=\sqrt{1+1}$$
$$=\sqrt{2}=1.414$$

In the run number 10 of the above example, which is listed in the table, to the right side of the x-axis, x-coordinate is unknown and y-coordinate is 0, Then the coordinates of that point to the right side of x-axis is (x, 0). To find the value of x, we use distance formulae and we take the distance between two points as 1.414. Then the distance from origin O = (0, 0) and to the point lying on x-axis (x, 0) is $d=\sqrt{(X2-X1)^2+(Y2-Y1)^2}$ can be written as 1.414 $=\sqrt{(X-0)^2+(0-0)^2}$.

$$1.414=\sqrt{(X)^2}$$
$$1.414=x$$

Therefore the level of 10th run combination can be written as (1.414, 0).

Similarly the combination of 11th, 12th and 13th runs co-ordinates can be obtained by following above mentioned method and combinations obtained are written as (-1.414, 0), (0, 1.414) and (0, -1.414).

CONVERSION OF ACTUAL VALUES TO CODED VALUES

1. In an experiment to find the response variable spreadability, there are 3 ingredients which are random by chosen with two levels. The ingredients are water/(ml),PVP–k_{30}(in gms) and carbopol. The level of these three ingredients Are as listed below.

		Low	High
A	Water	25	30
B	PVP–k_{30}	0.1	6.2
C	Carbopol	0.4	6.6

The experimental design and response of spreadbility is listed below.

Std	RUN	Water	PVP–k_{30}	Carbopol	Spreaderbilty
1	1	25	0.1	0.4	4.2
7	2	25	0.2	0.6	5.9
2	3	30	0.1	0.4	6.1
6	4	30	0.1	0.6	7.2
8	5	30	0.2	0.6	7.8
3	6	25	0.2	0.4	4.8
4	7	30	0.2	0.4	6.4
5	8	25	0.1	0.6	5.4

(i)   Write the model of design

(ii)   Derive the expected means and compute F – Test value.

(iii)   Test the significance of each possible test at $\alpha = 0.05$.

2. An experiment is conducted to measure thickness of tablets in 2^3 – factorial experiment using three factors or variable of A-sterrate, B-drug and C– Starch with 2 levels as listed below. Convert the given values in coded form and write the combinations of different experiments.

Factor	Low level(mg)	High Level(mg)
A = Sterrate	1mg	2mg
B = Disease	50mg	100mg
C = Starch	25	50mg

Transforming the actual to coded.

The general formula is $\dfrac{X-(Average\ of\ two\ levels)}{\frac{1}{2}(difference\ of\ levels)}$

Low level A = $\dfrac{1-\left(\frac{1+2}{2}\right)}{\frac{1}{2}(2-1)} = \dfrac{1-(1.5)}{0.5} = -1$

High Level of A = $\dfrac{2-\left(\frac{1+2}{2}\right)}{\frac{1}{2}(2-1)} = \dfrac{2-(1.5)}{0.5} = 1$

Similarly Low Level of B = $\dfrac{50-\left(\frac{50+100}{2}\right)}{\frac{1}{2}(100-50)} = \dfrac{50-(75)}{25} = -1$

High Level of B = $\dfrac{100-\left(\frac{50+100}{2}\right)}{\frac{1}{2}(100-50)} = \dfrac{100-(75)}{25} = 1$

Similarly we can find the codes C, they also will be equal to -1 and 1.

Then the combination of the experiment can be written as.

Combination	Sterrate A	PMG B	Starch C	Response
1	−1	−1	−1	
a	+1	−1	−1	
b	−1	+1	−1	
ab	+1	+1	−1	
c	−1	−1	+1	
ac	+1	−1	+1	
bc	−1	+1	+1	
abc	+1	+1	+1	

Example 2: An experiment was designed to measure the response viscosity using two ingredient carbopol and badam, the level of these two ingredients are as listed below.

	Low	High
Carbopol	0.2	0.4
Badam	0.4	0.6

This experiment is using centre level(3 –level), the model is 3^2 – factorial design.

The design and response of the experiment is listed below.

Runs	Carbopol A	Badam B	Viscosity(Response)
1	0.2	0.6	0.581
2	0.2	0.5	0.718
3	0.4	0.6	2.85
4	0.4	0.4	2.33
5	0.2	0.4	1.15
6	0.4	0.5	2.88
7	0.3	0.5	1.69
8	0.3	0.6	2.19
9	0.3	0.4	2.31

1. Derive the expected mean squares and compute F – Test.

2. Test the significance of each possible test at $\alpha = 0.05$.

Example 3: An experiment was conducted to formulate NLC using oil phase and smix. The experiment is designed in two levels of factor and it was performed using central composite design of DOE and three responses EE, DL and PS are obtained as listed in the table. Analyse the result and verify the level of significance by computing F-distribution value using ONE – WAY ANOVA technique

Std	Run	Oil Phase	Smix	Response (Entrapment Efficiency) EE %	Response (Drug loading) DL %	Response (Particle size) PS (mn)
13	1	7.5	35	60.98	14.86	152.9
12	2	7.5	35	60.98	14.86	152.8
7	3	7.5	13.7868	52.48	11.85	183.2
9	4	7.5	35	60.98	14.86	152.9
2	5	10	20	77.49	18.64	220.6
3	6	5	50	49.85	10.58	99.7
1	7	5	20	40.82	7.89	98.7
8	8	7.5	56.2132	69.86	15.49	137.89

10	9	7.5	35	60.99	14.86	152.9
11	10	7.5	35	60.99	14.87	152.9
5	11	3.96447	35	35.84	4.94	102.6
4	12	10	50	81.67	20.36	169.7
6	13	11.0355	35	84.95	24.49	197.4

Solution:

The linear equation that is used to analyze the result of the response EE when coded values are used is

$$EE=+61.38+17.24* A+4.72* B$$

The linear equation that is used to analyze the result of the response EE when actual values are used is

$$EE=-1.37468 \quad +6.89710* Oil Phase+0.31491* Smix$$

These two linear equations are obtained by Matrix method

After performing One – Way ANOVA, result obtained is

Sources	Sum of Squares	df	Mean Square	F Value	p-value Prob > F	
Model	2557.00	2	1278.50	431.78	2.0E-10	significant
A-Oil Phase	2378.50	1	2378.50	803.28	7.0E-11	
B-Smix	178.50	1	178.50	60.28	1.5E-05	
Residual	29.61	10	2.96			
Lack of Fit	29.61	6	4.93	164498.06	9.9E-11	significant
Pure Error	0.00	4	0.00			
Cor Total	2586.61	12				

Descriptive Statistics

Factor	Coefficient Estimate	df	Standard Error	95% CI Low	95% CI High
Intercept	61.38	1	0.477	60.31	62.44
A-Oil Phase	17.24	1	0.608	15.89	18.60
B-Smix	4.72	1	0.608	3.37	6.08

Run Order	Actual Value	Predicted Value	Residual
1	60.98	61.38	-0.40
2	60.98	61.38	-0.40
3	52.48	54.70	-2.22
4	60.98	61.38	-0.40
5	77.49	73.89	3.60
6	49.85	48.86	0.99
7	40.82	39.41	1.41
8	69.86	68.06	1.80
9	60.99	61.38	-0.39
10	60.99	61.38	-0.39
11	35.84	36.99	-1.15
12	81.67	83.34	-1.67
13	84.95	85.76	-0.81

The graph between Predicted vs actual values.

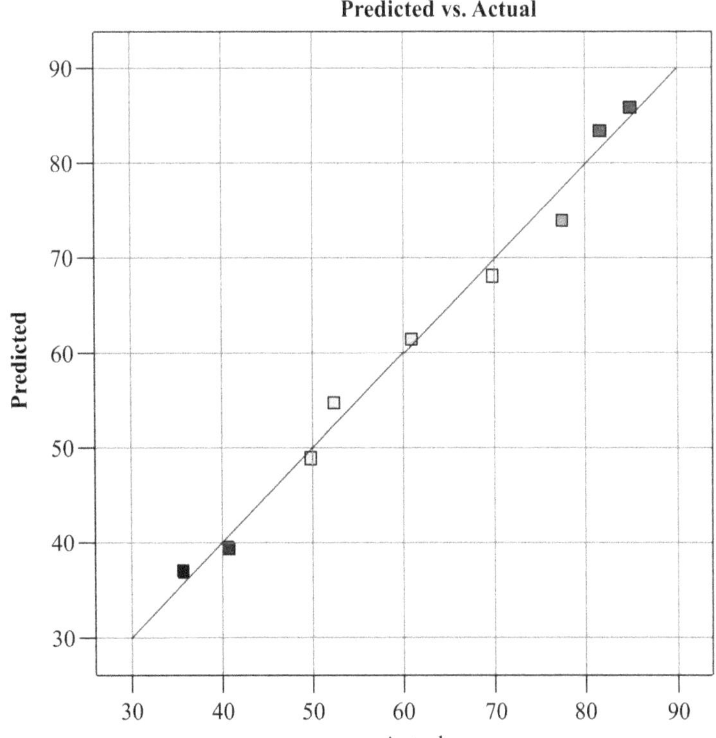

3D-Graph between input variables oil phase and smix and response Variable EE %

Oil Phase	Smix	Response EE %
7.5	35	60.98
7.5	35	60.98
7.5	13.7868	52.48
7.5	35	60.98
10	20	77.49
5	50	49.85
5	20	40.82
7.5	56.2132	69.86
7.5	35	60.99
7.5	35	60.99
3.96447	35	35.84
10	50	81.67
11.0355	35	84.95

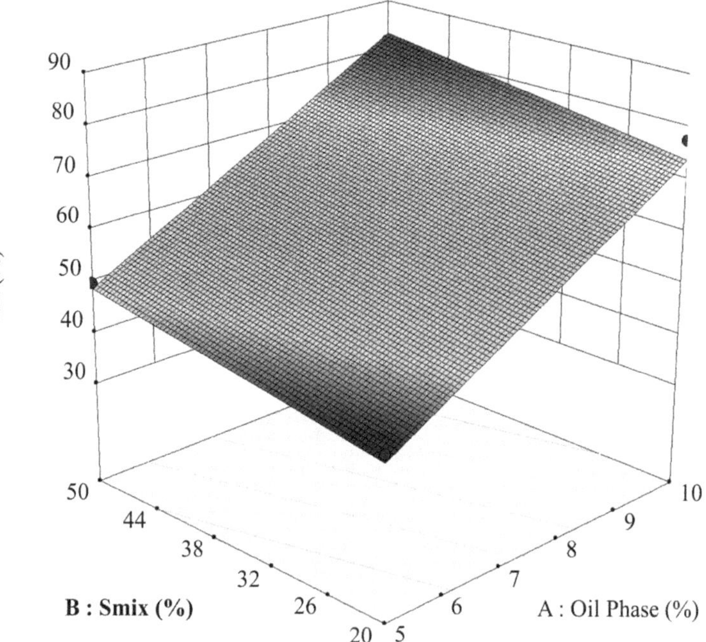

CANTOR-Graph between input variables oil phase and smix and response Variable EE %

Oil Phase	Smix	Response EE %
7.5	35	60.98
7.5	35	60.98
7.5	13.7868	52.48
7.5	35	60.98
10	20	77.49
5	50	49.85
5	20	40.82
7.5	56.2132	69.86
7.5	35	60.99
7.5	35	60.99
3.96447	35	35.84
10	50	81.67
11.0355	35	84.95

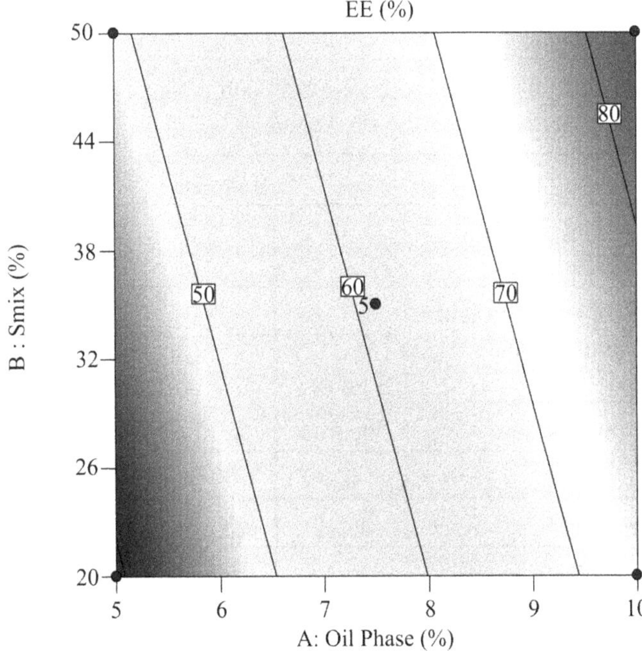

Historical Designing

Historical data design for importing data that already exists.

Here the investigator or the experimenter should specify the minimum and maximum level for equal numeric factor. Also should specify the level for categorical data. The level names are case sensitive and imported data must match exactly.

Here experimenter should set rows to equal numbers of historical data, which is already chosen, which shows how many runs are there in that experimental data. Here the investigator should copy and paste option to import data into the blank design layout.

Example 1: A formulation was to be prepared to optimize dissolution time. (The formulation with the dissolution time approximately 15 minutes is optimal) Stearic acid and mixing time were varied according to a historical design with the following results.

Runs	Formulation	Stearic Acid%	Mixing time (min)	Response
1	1	0.25	15	10
2	2	0.50	20	15
3	3	0.75	25	18
4	4	0.25	30	23
5	5	1	15	25
6	6	1	30	21

Construct a polynomial response equation. What concentration of stearic acid and mixing time would you choose for the final product?

Response						
ANOVA for Response Surface 2FI model						
Analysis of variance table [Partial sum of squares - Type III]	Sum of		Mean	F	p-	Remarks
Source of variation	Squares	df	Square	Value	value	
Model	142.89	3.00	47.63	9.12	0.10	not significant
A-Stearic Acid	43.12	1.00	43.12	8.26	0.10	
B-Mixing TIme	20.38	1.00	20.38	3.90	0.19	
AB	76.09	1.00	76.09	14.57	0.06	
Residual	10.45	2.00	5.22			
Cor Total	153.33	5.00				

Response = -14.48 +34.35*Stearic Acid +1.26*Mixing Time - 1.55*Stearic Acid * Mixing Time

Run Order	Actual Value	Predicted Value
1	10.00	9.08
2	15.00	16.54
3	18.00	20.14
4	23.00	22.18
5	25.00	24.18
6	21.00	19.88

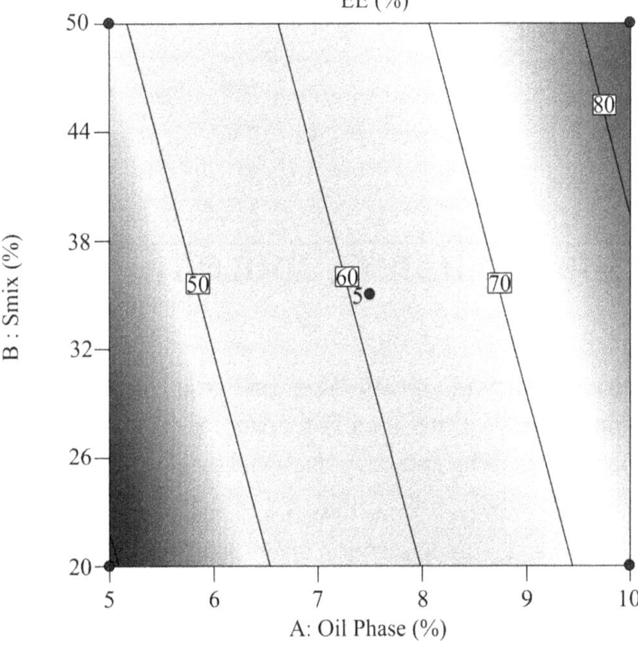

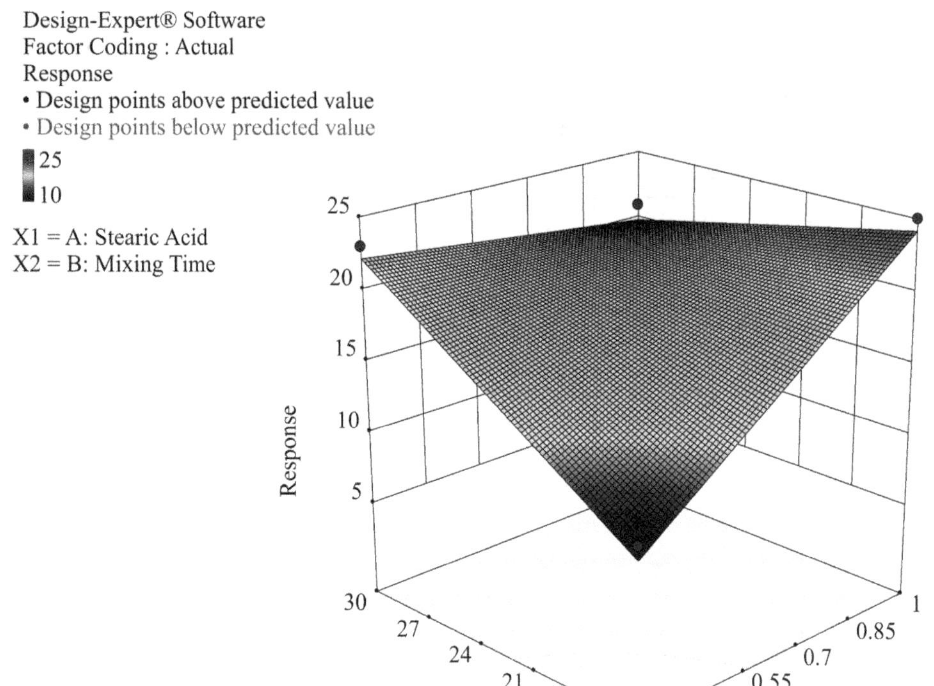

DESIGNING AND METHODOLOGY

DESIGN

Design consists of guide post to keep one going in right direction and sometime it may be a tentative not final. Working out of the plan consists of making certain decisions with respect to what, where, when, why and how much and by what means.

To design an experiment the investigator has to follow three important principles, and they are 1. Replication 2. Randomization and 3. Local control.

Replication: Replication will be useful to provide an estimate of experimental error when the same experiment is repeated more number of times.

Randomization: Randomization will ensure that this estimate is statistically valid.

Local control: Local control will reduce the experimental error by making the experiment more efficient.

STEPS IN METHODOLOGY AND DESIGNING

DEFINITION OF THE PROBLEM

The investigator has to define the problem that he intended to study. A problem statement is a concise description of an issue to be addressed or a condition to be improved upon. It identifies the gap between the current (problem) state and desired (goal) state of a process or product.

Ex: a. Pregnancy prevalence

    b   Rising trend in malaria

    d. Smoking and lung cancer

    e. Cholesterol and Coronary heart disease

AIM AND OBJECTIVE

AIM: The aim of the work, i.e., the overall purpose of the study, should be clearly and concisely defined. Aims are broad statements of desired outcomes, or the general intentions of the research, which is going to give a picture' of your research project. Emphasize what is to be accomplished (not how it is to be accomplished. Aims points out the general purpose of the study.

Ex: State whether nature of the problem has to be studied or solution has to be found out

OBJECTIVES: Objectives spell out exactly what one intends to do in the study. The goals of pharmacy practice research are to support the clinical and effective use of medicines, while ensuring that the risks of adverse drug reactions are minimized. It is undertaken by researchers, often based in universities, from a wide range of health care disciplines.

1. Objective to compare the efficiency of two lines of treatment to adopt better techniques in various method of heart surgery
2. Warn public against smoking if it is proved to be one of the causative factors in lung cancer

REVIEW THE LITERATURE ON THE PROBLEM UNDER STUDY

A literature review is a scholarly paper, which includes the current knowledge including substantive findings, as well as theoretical and methodological contributions to a particular topic. Literature reviews are secondary sources, and do not report new or original experimental work. The *process* of reviewing the literature is often ongoing and informs many aspects of the empirical research project.

Critically review the literature on the problem under study, because there is a possibility that the same or similar ideas had occurred to someone else, who has already carried out experiments and published the results a long time ago.

If so, clarify if you want to confirm the findings, challenge the conclusion, extend the work further and bridge some gaps in the existing knowledge

EX: Density of microfilaria Bancroft is higher at night, but you would like to know which part of the night

Hypothesis: State your Hypothesis

A hypothesis is a tentative statement about the relationship between two or more variables. It is a specific, testable prediction about what you expect to happen in a study. Let's take a closer look at how a hypothesis is used, formed, and tested in scientific research. You have to precisely start with an assumption Positive or Negative. A hypothesis helps to translate the research problem and objective into a clear explanation or prediction of the expected results or outcomes of the study

The hypothesis is what the researchers' predict the relationship between two or more variables, but it involves more than a guess. Most of the time, the hypothesis begins with a question which is then explored through background research. It is only at this point that researchers begin to develop a testable hypothesis.

In a study exploring the effects of a particular drug, the hypothesis might be that researchers expect the drug to have some type of effect on the symptoms of a specific illness. In psychology, the hypothesis might focus on how a certain aspect of the environment might influence a particular behaviour.

Unless you are creating a study that is exploratory in nature, your hypothesis should always explain what you *expect* to happen during the course of your experiment or research.

Investigator has to remember that defined hypothesis does not have to be correct. While the hypothesis predicts what the researchers expect to see, the goal of the research is to determine whether this guess or assumption is right or wrong. When conducting an experiment, researchers might explore a number of factors to determine which ones might contribute to the ultimate outcome.

In many cases, researchers may find that the results of an experiment *do not* support the original hypothesis. When writing up these results, the researchers might suggest other options that should be explored in future studies.

EX: There is no relationship between hypertension and Social status

As a whole cholera Vaccine is of no use in prevention of cholera and so on

PLAN OF ACTION

The plan of action is a document that lists what steps must one has to follow in order to achieve/reach a specific goal. The purpose of an action plan is to clarify what resources are required to reach the goal, formulate a timeline for when specific tasks need to be completed and determine what resources are required for completion of this research work in a stipulated time. Prepare overall plan of investigation for studying the problem and meeting the objective.

A work plan is a base to set the goals and processes by which a team and/or person can accomplish those goals, and offering the reader a better understanding of the scope of the project. Work plans, help you stay organized while working on projects.

DEFINITION OF POPULATION UNDER STUDY

It is from the accessible population that researchers selects sample from that population. It can defined as a subset of a population. The population, or target population, is the total population about which information is required. Ideally, this is a population at risk.

When an investigator selects the population for study, can take population from country, state, district, sub district, town, village, specified groups of population as per age, income, occupation etc. Investigator has to define clearly who are to be included and who are to be excluded.

SAMPLE SIZE

The term sample size denotes the number of subjects/animals to be used for study. The size has to be sufficiently large, so as to draw valid inferences about the population under study. Sample size determination is the act of choosing the number of observations or replicates to include in a statistical sample. The sample size is an important feature of any empirical study in which the goal is to make inferences about a population from a sample.

SPECIFYING THE NATURE OF STUDY:

Meta-Analysis

A way of combining data from many different research studies. A meta-analysis is a statistical process that combines the findings from individual studies.

Systematic Review

A summary of the clinical literature. A systematic review is a critical assessment and evaluation of all research studies that address a particular clinical issue. The researchers use an organized method of locating, assembling, and evaluating a body of literature on a particular topic using a set of specific criteria. A systematic review typically includes a description of the findings of the collection of research studies. The systematic review may also include a quantitative pooling of data, called a meta-analysis.

Randomized Controlled Trial

A controlled clinical trial that randomly (by chance) assigns participants to two or more groups. There are different methods to randomize study subjects into their groups.

Cohort Study (Prospective Observational Study)

A clinical research study in which people who presently have a certain condition or receive a particular treatment are followed over time and compared with another group of people who are not affected by the condition.

Case-control Study

Case-control studies begin with the outcomes and do not follow people over time. Investigator selects subjects with a particular result (the cases group) and interview the groups to ascertain what different experiences they had. They compare the odds ratio of having an experience with the outcome of interest to the odds of having an experience without the outcome of interest.

Cross-sectional study

The observation of a defined population at a single point in time or time interval. Exposure and outcome are determined / measured in a single occasion.

Recording data: For recording data, a standard Pro-forma, Schedule, format or Questionnaire has to prepared and Pretested in few cases

Recorders, Interviewers, interrogators and Investigators have to be trained in filling these schedules to reduce the personal bias and also prepare work Schedule for data collection by estimating work expected per hour, per day, per week or per month, per worker or per team.

PRESENTATION OF DATA

Research papers are depending on the amounts of data or information that can be summarized and easily read through tables and graphs. When we are **writing** a research paper, it is most important to remember that the data must be presented to the reader in a visually appealing way. Compile all data and verify accuracy and adequacy before processing further. Classify and tabulate as per the age, sex, class, profession and other desired characteristics. Prepare frequency table and Diagram table as per type of data

STATISTICAL ANALYSIS

Statistical methods involved in carrying out a study include planning, designing, collecting data, analyzing, drawing meaningful interpretation and reporting of the research findings. The statistical analysis gives meaning to the meaningless numbers, thereby breathing life into a lifeless data.

Put the results to unbiased statistical analysis by different methods like t-test, ANOVA, Man-Whiney, Kruskal Wallis test etc used to the level of significance, Null hypothesis, Interpretation of P-Value should be included (Parametric and Non-Parametric test), Degree of freedom at 5% and 1% level.

CONCLUSION

Draw Unbiased Conclusions based on the interpretations. The investigator conclusions summarize how your results support or contradict your original hypothesis. Summarize your research work results in a few sentences and that will be used to support your conclusion. Include key facts from your background research to help explain your results as needed.

State whether your results support or contradict your hypothesis. If appropriate, state the relationship between the independent and dependent variable. Summarize and evaluate your experimental procedure, making comments about its success and effectiveness. Suggest changes in the experimental procedure (or design) and/or possibilities for further study. Re-check the whole plan and its execution before making logical recommendations, preparation of thesis or Publication of scientific paper or reports

SUMMARY

An overview of content that provides a reader with the overarching theme, but does not expand on specific details. A summary describes a larger work (such as an entire book, speech, or research project), and should include noticeably less content then the original work. The purpose of a summary is to give a reader a condensed and objective account of the main ideas and features of a text. Usually, a summary has between one and three paragraphs or one hundred to three hundred words, depending on the length and complexity of the original essay and the intended audience and purpose.

Writing a summary is an important skill that students will use throughout their academic careers. In addition, summarizing improves reading skills and one can pick out the main ideas of a reading; it also helps to improve their vocabulary skills as investigator paraphrase a reading, alter the sentences wherever it required and also correct some grammatical errors.

PROTOCOL WRITING

The protocol is a document that describes how a **clinical trial** will be conducted (the objective(s), design, methodology, statistical considerations and organization of a **clinical trial**,) and ensures the safety of the **trial** subjects and integrity of the data collected.

Research is a document that describes the background, rationale, objectives, design, methodology, statistical considerations, and organization of a clinical research project. According to the ICH Good Clinical Practice guidelines, a protocol should include the following topics:

Protocol writing allows the researcher to review and critically evaluate the published literature on the interested topic, plan and review the project steps and serves as a guide throughout the investigation. The protocol is an inevitable document that enables the researcher to monitor the progress of the project.

Title of the Study: Title of proposal should be accurate, short, concise, and identify

What is the study about, **Who** are the targets, **Where** is the setting of the study and **When** it is launched, if applicable.

It should make the main objective clear, convey the main purpose of the research and mention the target population. To write a title maximum of 12-15 words should be used. It should give the complete idea about the area of research and what methods are going to be used in a compact, relevant, accurate, attractive, easy to understand, and informative way.

Administrative Details: The following administrative details and a protocol content summary should follow the title page:

Contents page list of relevant sections and sub-sections with corresponding page number.

Signature page is signed by senior members of the research team and dated to confirm that the version concerned has been approved by them.

Contact details for the research team members listing postal, e-mail addresses and telephone numbers.

Project Summary: The summary should be distinctive, concise and should sum up all the essentials of the protocol.

Introduction (Background): The background to the project should be concise and refer to the subject straight forwardly. In writing the review, attention should be drawn to the positives, negatives and limitations of the studies quoted.

Introduction is concluded by explaining how the present study will benefit the community. The literature review should logically lead to the statement of the aims of the proposed project and end with the aims and objectives of the study. The review should include the most recent publications in the field and the topic of the research is selected only after completing the literature review and finding some gaps in it.

The research question should be described precisely and concisely. It is going to be the basis of designing the project. The definition of the problem should be clear so that a reader can straight forwardly recognize the real meaning of it.

Study Objectives (Aims): The aims should be explicitly stated. These should be confined to the intention of the project and they should arise from the literature review. State the goal you need to achieve.

The study aims or objectives emerge from the study questions/ hypothesis. They are answers to what are the possible responses to the research question or hypothesis under analysis and measure. Aims should be logical and coherent, feasible, concise, realistic, considering local conditions, phrased to clearly meet the purpose of the study and related to what the specific research is intended to accomplish. For example, to evaluate knowledge level regarding dental caries in primary school children in KSA (this is not detailed). The following should be added: Causes, treatment, preventive measures, etc.

The objectives should be (SMART objective): Specific, Measurable, Achievable, Relevant and Time based.

Specific Aims: Details of each objective that will finally lead to the achievement of the goal should be stated. Specific aims one by one should be listed concisely. It is good practice not to include too many aims in the study (2-5 best); too many objectives often lead to inaccurate and poorly defined results. Furthermore, aims should be achievable, realistic and specific with no general and ambiguous statements. They should be stated in action verbs that illustrate their purpose: i.e., "to determine, to compare, to verify, to calculate, to reduce, to describe, etc."

Secondary Objectives (Optional): These are referred to as ancillary and minor objectives that could be studied during the course of the study.

The formulation of objectives helps to focus the study and to avoid the collection of any unnecessary data and hence organize the study in clear and distinct stages.

Hypothesis: It is a statement based on sound scientific theory that recognizes the predicted correlation between two or additional assessable variables [11]. It is always developed in response to the purpose statement or to answer the research questions posed. Furthermore, hypothesis transforms research questions into a format amendable to testing or into a statement that predicts an expected outcome.

Types of Hypothesis Statements

Null hypothesis: A null hypothesis is a statement that there is no actual relationship between variables (H0 or HN). It may be read as there is no difference between the groups to be compared and no relationship between the exposure and outcome under investigation. H0 states the contradictory of what the researchers expect. The final conclusion of the investigators will either keep a null hypothesis or reject it in support of an alternative hypothesis. It does not essentially mean that H0 is accurate when not rejecting it as there might not be an adequate proof against it.

Alternative hypothesis: An alternative hypothesis is a statement that suggests a potential outcome that the researcher may expect (H1 or HA). This hypothesis is derived from previous studies where an evident difference between the groups to be compared is present. It is recognized only when a null hypothesis is rejected. Practically, hypotheses are stated in the null form, because they have their inferential statistics. Such hypotheses of no difference will be challenged by researchers and the result of the statistical testing gives the probability that the hypothesis of no difference is true or false.

Aims should be logically linked and arranged according to the tested hypothesis statement.

Example:

Research question: Is there a difference in fluoride release between the **Compomer and Glass-ionomer cement?**

Null Hypothesis: There is no difference in fluoride release between the **Compomer and Glass-ionomer cement.**

Alternate Hypothesis: There is a difference in fluoride release between the Compomer and Glass-ionomer cement.

The statement of the problem should provide a summary of exactly what the project is trying to achieve.

What exactly do you want to study?

Why is it worth studying?

Does the proposed study have theoretical and/or practical significance?

Does it contribute to a new understanding of a phenomenon? (i.e., Does it address new or little known material or does it treat familiar material in a new way or does it challenge an existing understanding or extend existing knowledge?)

The justification of the research should be a convincing statement for the need to do it:

How does the research relate to the priorities of the region and the country?

What knowledge and information will be obtained?

What is the ultimate purpose that the knowledge obtained from the study will serve?

How will the results be disseminated?

How will the results be used, and who will be the beneficiaries?

Methods and Materials: It should be explained in detail about 'Where', 'Who', 'How' the research will be conducted. This will explains the study design and procedures and techniques used to achieve the proposed objectives. It explain in details about the proposed methodology for data gathering and processing.

Methodology composes an important part of the protocol. It assures that the hypothesis will be confirmed or rejected. It also refers to a thorough strategy to attain the objectives.

The methods and materials are divided into different subheadings:

a) **Study design (cross-sectional, case-control, intervention study, RCT, etc.):** Proper explanation should be given as to why a particular design was chosen (on the basis of proposed objectives and availability of resources).

A study design is the investigator plan to acquire the answer (s) to the hypothesis to be tested. Here, strategies will be applied to develop balanced, correct, objective and meaningful information. It also explains the methods that will be used to collect and analyze data. It is important to attain reliable and valid scientific results.

Ethics, logistic concerns, economic features and scientific thoroughness will determine the design of the study. Here, a chief concern is given to the legality of the results including potential bias mystifying issues.

Randomized controlled clinical trial is the best to document a causal relationship between an exposure and its outcome.

b) **Study population (Study subjects):** Study place where the investigator is going to conduct the research and who will be the study population (why doing research in this place and why selecting this population?) should be mentioned.

It gives the complete information about the study subjects, selection procedure and sample size calculation. Proper definition of eligibility, inclusion, exclusion and discontinuation criteria of the study subjects should be stated. Allocation of subjects to study arms should be explained and described in details keeping in mind about the concealment and randomization process.

c) **Sample size:** Sample size calculation is recommended for economical and ethical reasons. The calculation of the sample size must be explained including the power of the sample. The sampling technique should be mentioned in order to obtain a representative sample to reach your target population. The recruitment of the study subjects should be described according to the selection criteria (inclusion and exclusion criteria).

"Informed consent" should be mentioned (Permission granted in full knowledge of the possible consequences).

d) **Proposed intervention:** Full description of proposed intervention should be given. Here, all the activities and actions should be recorded and thoroughly explained in their order of occurrence.

When the investigator using drugs for clinical trials, both scientific and brand name should be mentioned followed by the name of the manufacturing company, city, and country. Drug route, dosage, frequency of administration, and total duration of treatment with the drug should be reported in detail.

When using apparatus its name should be given followed by the name of the manufacturer, city and country.

Involved personnel should precisely define: Who will be responsible for the interventions? What are the activities each person is going to perform and also with what frequency and intensity they are going to perform?

e) **Data collection methods, instruments used:**

Data collection tools are:

Retrospective data (medical records)

Questionnaires, interviews, Laboratory test (literature or personal knowledge should be referenced), Clinical examinations.

Description of instruments, tools used for data collection, as well as the methods used to test the validity and reliability of the instrument should be provided.

Data Management and Analysis Plan: This section should be written following statistical advice from a statistician. The analysis plan and which statistical tests will be used to verify the level of significance for the research question/hypothesis should be described. Names of variables that will be used in the analyses and the name of statistical analysis that will be performed to assess the outcome should be listed. The statistical software to be used for data analysis along with version should be mentioned.

Project Management: Work plan-A work plan is an outline of activities of all the phases of the research to be carried out according to an anticipated time schedule.

Proper time table for accomplishing each major step of the study should be defined. Assigning time frame to each step in the trial will be helpful in organizing the structure of the research trial. The personnel (investigators, assistants, laboratory technicians etc.) involved in the study or data collection should be properly trained.

Strengths and Limitations: It is important to mention the strengths or limitations of the study.

What study can achieve or cannot achieve is important, so as to prevent wasteful allocation of resources.

Ethical Considerations (Issues for Ethical Review and Approvals): It should indicate whether the procedures to be followed are in accord with the conditions of ethical committee requirement and procedure. In any case, study should not start unless approval from ethics committee is received

The following points should be explained:

The benefits and risks for the subjects involved. The physical, social and psychological implications of the research.

Details of the information to be given to the study patients including alternative treatments/approaches.

Information should be provided on the free informed consent of the participants. Information form should contain: Justification for research, outline of study, risks, confidentiality, and voluntary participation should be told patients about the freedom to withdraw from the study whenever they wish to. Confidentiality indicates how the personal information obtained from the patient will be kept secret (Data safety).

Operational Planning and Budgeting (Budget Summary): Outline the budget requirement showing head wise expenditure for the study-manpower, transportation, instruments, laboratory tests, and cost of the drug. Budget estimate is to be attached in the annexure. All costs including personnel, consumables, equipment, supplies, communication, and funds for patients and data processing are all included in the budget. Each item should be justified.

Reference System: Referencing is the regular method of recognizing information taken from other researchers' work. A proper citation will enable the readers to follow-up any reference of interest. Plagiarism refers to claiming and acquiring someone else's ideas, an action that is considered a criminal action.

Failure to reference an idea that you have found in your research, or to acknowledge the work of other team members in a team assignment falls under the category of plagiarism. The choice of referencing system is dependent upon the funding agencies where the research protocol is being submitted. These frequently identify their preferred system of referencing and this should be strictly adhered to.

Annexure

The following annexes are to be attached at the end of the protocol:

1. Informed consent form.
2. Letters from ethics committees.
3. Study questionnaire (copies of any questionnaires or draft questionnaires).
4. Case Record Forms (CRFs).
5. Budget details.
6. Curriculum Vitae (CV) of the chief investigator and co-investigator and their role in the study. It will ensure that the role of each investigator is well defined.

12 Non-Parametric Tests

PARAMETRIC TESTS

Most of the procedures / methods used or applied up to this point are classified as parametric statistics.

In case of parametric test investigator mainly focus on estimating or testing a hypothesis about one or more population parameter. In most of tests following features are common.

(i) The form of the frequency of parent population from which the samples have been drawn is assumed to be known and

(ii) Here the investigator concern is about testing statistical hypothesis about the parameters of this frequency function or estimating its parameters.

All the small samples tests of significance are based on the assumption that the parent population is normal and here the investigator mainly focus on the computation of mean, standard deviation/variance of the populations from which samples are drawn. Those tests which deal with the parameters of the population are called as parametric test.

NON – PARAMETRIC TEST

A parametric statistical test is a test whose model specifies certain conditions about the parameters of the population from which the samples are drawn. When the investigator need to perform a test, where the assumption about the form of the parent population is not taken into account. The statistical methods which are used to test about the experimental result without considering the mean standard deviation or variance is called as non-parametric test. A non-parametric (NP) test that does not depend on a particular form of the basic frequency function from the samples are drawn. Non-Parametric tests are most effectively used for data that consists of only classified variables or ranked variables that are considered to have an underlying continuous distribution.

Advantages and Disadvantages

Advantages

1. They allow the investigator for testing of hypothesis that are not stated about population parameter values.

2. Non-parametric tests may be used when the form of the sampled population is unknown.

3. Non-Parametric procedures tends to be computationally easier and more quicker than parametric procedure

4. Non-parametric tests are found to be more suitable for analyzing data when the observations are rated or ranked.

Disadvantages

1. Their primary drawback is that they tend to ignore much sample information that are gleaned by their parametric counterparts. This makes them generally less efficient.

2. The application of some of the non-parametric tests may be laborious for large samples.

WILCOXON SIGNED-RANK TEST

In case of Wilcoxon signed Rank test, here signs and amount variation of data values from the conjectured value and hence this test will be more powerful test..

In this test null hypothesis $\eta = \eta_0$, here one has to subtract η_0 form each of the experimental values or observed values.

If we find any difference as zero, there we omit that particular data or observation, then the investigator has to reduce the sample size n accordingly. The remaining differences which are retained, will be arranged in the increasing order of their absolute value. Then the ranks will be assigned according to position of each data value. After the assignment of ranks, with +ve or -ve signs, these ranks can be called as signed ranks.

The notation T^+ is called as sum of the positive ranks and T^- is called as sum absolute values of the negative ranks. Then T valued is obtained. This T – value is smaller value between T^+ and T^-.

Example: 7 6   4   1   2

Solution: For null hypothesis we can take $\eta = 4$ as median

X	Ascending order	X- η	Absolute difference	Arrangement of ranks in ascending
7	1	-3	3	0
6	2	-2	2	1
4	4	0	0	2
1	6	2	2	2
2	7	1	1	3

Median = η = 4

Sum of +ve rank = 3

Sum of -Ve ranks = 5

Smaller between these two values is 3

T = 3

WICOXON SIGNED – RANK TEST (FOR MATCHED PAIRS) n ≤ 30

To test the null hypothesis, that the population will have a specified value of median, call it as $\eta = \eta_0$. Here the investigator expects that the value of T+ and T- to be comparable size. If $T^+ < T^-$, then the observed values are farther below η_0 than above η_0 consequently, $\eta < \eta_0$. If T- < T+ , then the observed values are farther above η_0 than below η_0. Then $\eta > \eta_0$.

PROCEDURE FOR THE WICOXON SIGNED RANK TEST

Step 1. Set Hypothesis: The null hypothesis is set as

$H_0 : \eta = \eta_0$.; **H_1** : $\eta \neq \eta_0$. (Two Tailed)

$H_0 : \eta \geq \eta_0$.; **H_1** : $\eta < \eta_0$. (Left Tailed)

$H_0 : \eta \leq \eta_0$.; **H_1** : $\eta > \eta_0$. (Right Tailed)

H_0: Null hypothesis

H_1: Alternative Hypothesis

Step 2. Set the level of significance as $\alpha = 0.05$ or 0.01

Step 3: Subtract η_0 from each observed or experimental values, wherever the difference is zero, that will be discarded then ranks are assigned to each of the remaining differences.

$T^+ =$ The sum of the positive ranks

$T- = $ The absolute value of sum of $-ve$ ranks

Step 4: Test statistics : The test statistics is T. This is obtained by taking the smallest of them.

$$Z = \frac{R - N(N+1)/4}{\sqrt{\left[N\left(N+\frac{1}{2}\right)(N+1)\right]/12}}$$

Step 5: Critical value and Critical region:

Let n be the total number of observations after discarding the zeros or zero differences or difference.

For the small simple size ($n \leq 30$) the test value will be compared with the table for the corresponding level of significance.

Step 6: If test value T is less than critical value $T \leq T_c$, then H_0 will be rejected, otherwise H_0 may be regarded as true.

Step 7: Write the inference about the test result or draw the conclusion of test value T.

Example: The time to peak plasma concentration of paired which is obtained from Bioavailability experiment is as listed below. Verify the level of significance between these two paired data.

SLNO	Time to Peak (hr)	
	A	B
1	2.5	3.5
2	3	4
3	1.25	2.5
4	1.75	2
5	3.5	3.5
6	2.5	4
7	1.75	1.5
8	2.25	2.5
9	3.5	3
10	2.5	3
11	2	3.5
12	3.5	4

Solution:

SLNO	Time to Peak (hr)		Difference (B-A)	Absolute	Assigned ranks	Negative ranks	Positive ranks
	A	B					
1	2.5	3.5	1	1	7.5		7.5
2	3	4	1	1	7.5		7.5
3	1.25	2.5	1.25	1.25	9		9
4	1.75	2	0.25	0.25	2		2
5	3.5	3.5	0	0			
6	2.5	4	1.5	1.5	10.5		10.5
7	1.75	1.5	-0.25	0.25	2	2	
8	2.25	2.5	0.25	0.25	2		2
9	3.5	3	-0.5	0.5	5	5	
10	2.5	3	0.5	0.5	5		5
11	2	3.5	1.5	1.5	10.5		10.5
12	3.5	4	0.5	0.5	5		5
						Sum = 7	Sum = 59

Here N = 11 R = 59 = Sum of the ranks of large value

$$Z = \frac{R - N(N+1)/4}{\sqrt{\left[N\left(N+\frac{1}{2}\right)(N+1)\right]/12}} = \frac{59 - 11(11+1)/4}{\sqrt{\left[11\left(11+\frac{1}{2}\right)(11+1)\right]/12}} = 2.31 > 1.96,$$

Hence difference is significant

<table>
<tr><th colspan="6">Ranks</th></tr>
<tr><td colspan="2"></td><td>N</td><td>Mean Rank</td><td>Sum of Ranks</td></tr>
<tr><td rowspan="4">VAR00002 - VAR00001</td><td>Negative Ranks</td><td>2[a]</td><td>3.50</td><td>7.00</td></tr>
<tr><td>Positive Ranks</td><td>9[b]</td><td>6.56</td><td>59.00</td></tr>
<tr><td>Ties</td><td>1[c]</td><td></td><td></td></tr>
<tr><td>Total</td><td>12</td><td></td><td></td></tr>
</table>

a. VAR00002 < VAR00001

b. VAR00002 > VAR00001

c. VAR00002 = VAR00001

Test Statistics[a]	VAR00002 - VAR00001
Z	-2.323^{b}
Asymp. Sig. (2-tailed)	.020

a. Wilcoxon Signed Ranks Test

b. Based on negative ranks.

Problem: 1. A random sample of 6 ladies were selected to study the decrease in body after advising them to follow diet. Weight of of those subjects before and after diet are recorded and listed as below.

Weight Before: 170   180   175   173   176   185

  (lbs)

Weight After: 164   175   172   168   172   179

  (lbs)

Wilcoxon Signed – Rank test (Large Samples)

When the Size of the sample is large $(n > 30)$, then statistician will apply this test. Here we will compare the test values with the critical value Z at 5% (z = 1.96) and 1% level (Z= 2.58) of significance.

For large sample test, steps involved in computation test is similar to Wilcoxon-Signed Rank test and T^{+} and T^{-} are obtained.

Let n be the number of experimental data or observations left after discarding the zero(0) differences.

When sample is large $n > 30$, the statistics T will be approximately normal, Mean $(\mu_T) = \dfrac{n(n+1)}{4}$ and standard deviation $(\sigma_T) = \sqrt{\dfrac{n(n+1)(2n+1)}{24}}$

Test statistics Z is obtained by the equation $Z = \dfrac{T - \mu_T}{\sigma_T} \sim N(0\,,\,1)$

The computed value of Z is compared with the standard or critical value at 5% or 1% level of significance.

If $|Z|_{cal} > Z_{Table}$, H_0 is rejected, otherwise H_0 will be accepted. H_0 may be regarded as true value.

Example:

Ultrasounds were taken at the time of liver transplant and again after 5 to 10 year to determine the systolic pressure of the hepatic artery. Results of 21 transplants of 21 children are as shown in the table. Verify the level of significance between later and at transplant.

Child	Later	At Transplant
1	46	35
2	40	40
3	50	58
4	50	71
5	41	33
6	70	79
7	35	20
8	40	19
9	56	56
10	30	26
11	30	44
12	60	90
13	43	43
14	45	42
15	40	55
16	50	60
17	66	62
18	45	26
19	40	60
20	35	27
21	25	31

Solution:

Child	Later	At Transplant	Difference	Absolute Difference	Ranks	Signed Ranks	
1	46	35	11	11	13	13	0
2	40	40	0	0	2	0	0
3	50	58	-8	8	9		-9
4	50	71	-21	21	17.5	0	-17.5
5	41	33	8	8	9	9	0
6	70	79	-9	9	11	0	-11
7	35	20	15	15	15.5	15.5	0
8	40	19	21	21	20	20	0
9	56	56	0	0	2	0	0
10	30	26	4	4	5.5	5.5	0
11	30	44	-14	14	14	0	-14
12	60	90	-30	30	21	0	-21
13	43	43	0	0	2	0	0
14	45	42	3	3	4	4	0
15	40	55	-15	15	15.5	0	-15.5
16	50	60	-10	10	12	0	-12
17	66	62	4	4	5.5	5.5	0
18	45	26	19	19	17.5	17.5	0
19	40	60	-20	20	19	0	-19
20	35	27	8	8	9	0	-9
21	25	31	-6	6	7	0	-7
						90	-135

$$(\mu_T) = \frac{n(n+1)}{4} = \frac{(21)22}{4} = 115.5$$

And standard deviation $(\sigma_T) = \sqrt{\frac{n(n+1)(2n+1)}{24}} = \sqrt{\frac{21(21+1)(2*21+1)}{24}} = 28.77$

Test statistics Z is obtained by the equation $Z = \frac{T - \mu_T}{\sigma_T} = \frac{90 - 115.5}{28.77} = -0.89$

The absolute value of Z = 0.89 < 1.96 The difference is significant at 5%. Hence the null hypothesis is accepted.

1. Two instruments were used to measure the amount of dissolution in 30 minute. One is the original and another is new apparatus. Amount is dissolved in 30 minutes is as recorded below. Verify the level of significance difference between these two apparatus.

Amount dissolved (Original apparatus	53	61	57	50	63	62	54	52	59	57	64	
Amount dissolved (Modified apparatus	58	55	67	62	55	64	66	59	68	57	69	56

Ranks				
	VAR00002	N	Mean Rank	Sum of Ranks
VAR00001	1.00	12	10.17	122.00
	2.00	11	14.00	154.00
	Total	23		

MANN–WHITNEY TEST

The Wilcoxon Signed rank test can used to compare two populations, when two sets of sample data paired, then the investigator will introduce a test called Mann-Whitney. This test is useful to compare two independent samples by testing a hypothesis on the two population medians. This test was introduced by Wilcoxon and studied and used by Mann-Whitney. Some time Mann-Whitney test is called as Mann-Whitney-Wilcoxon test.

U-Statisitcs

Mann-Whitney –U- test. (Independent samples) for Small Samples

Consider two independent samples say $(x_1, x_2,-----x_{n1})$ and $(y_1, y_2,- - - -y_{n2})$ and these two random samples of sizes of n1 and n2 and randomly drawn from two populations respectively. Here the purpose of this test will be applied to test, whether these two samples are from the same population or different population.

The Mann-Whitney test, uses the Sum of the ranks (or rank sum) of each sample. To assign rank to each observation of the two samples are combined into a single sample and then the data's are arranged in the ascending order and the ranks, will be assigned to the combined sample data.

Let T_1 = Sum of the ranks of the observations of the first sample and T_2 = Sum of the ranks of the observations of the second sample (Y-values) in the combined samples..

Mann-Whitney U-Statistics are defined as

$$U_1 = T_1 - \frac{n1(n1+1)}{2} \qquad .....(1)$$

$$U_2 = T_2 - \frac{n2(n2+1)}{2} \qquad .....(2)$$

Then U = Smaller of (U_1, U_2)

OR

$$U_1 = n_1 n_2 + \frac{n2(n2+1)}{2} - T_2$$

$$U_2 = n_1 n_2 + \frac{n2(n2+1)}{2} - T_1$$

Note: $U_1 + U_2 = n_1 n_2$

$$T_1 + T_2 = \frac{(n2+n1)(n1+n2+1)}{2}$$

Example: A researcher designed an experiment to assess the effects of prolonged inhalation of cadmium oxide. Fifteen animals were selected as experimental subjects and another 10 similar animals are used as controls. The experiment was done to measure the variable hemoglobin level between experimental and control, to verify the effect of prolonged inhalation of cadmium oxide in reducing the hemoglobin level.

CLASSICAL METHOD

Step-1: Setup the hypothesis (Null)

Null Hypothesis: H0 : $\eta_x \geq \eta_y$ or $\eta_x \leq \eta_y$ or $\eta_x = \eta_y$

Step-2: Set Alternative Hypothesis:

H1 : $\eta_x < \eta_y$ (left Tailed) or H1 : $\eta_x > \eta_y$ (Right Tailed) or H1 : $n_x \neq n_y$ (Two-tailed) Respectively

Step-3: Level of Significance : Set up the level of significance α

Step-4: Combine the observations of both the samples to obtain a single sample and arrange the observations of the combined sample in ascending order of their magnitude. Assign ranks to the combined sample data so obtained and find the values of the of the statistical T1, T2 and U1 and U2 defined.

Step-5: Compute the test value U = Smaller of (U_1, U_2)

Step-6: The critical values of U for different values of (n1 and n2) and level of significance $\alpha = 0.05$ for single tailed and two tailed tests are compared with table.

Step-7: Reject H_0 if U lies in the critical region, otherwise, investigator fail to reject H_0

Step-8: Write the conclusion of the test in simple language.

Mann-Whitney-U-test. (Independent samples) for Large Samples: When the sample size is greater than 20 between two samples will be considered as large sample, then we may use the normal test for testing H0: $\eta1 = \eta2$. Here Mann-Whitney proves that under H_0 the sampling distribution of U is asymptotically normal with mean and Standard deviation, and those two equations are given by the equations

$$\text{Mean } (\mu_u) = \frac{n1\ n2}{2} \text{ and SD}(\sigma_u) = \sqrt{\frac{n1n2(n+n2+1)}{12}}$$

Then, for large samples, U~ $N(\mu_u, \sigma_u) \Longrightarrow$ $Z = \frac{U - \mu u}{\sigma u} \sim N(0, 1)$ for large samples and here we use normal test in the usual manner.

Assumptions for in case Mann-Whitney – U-test (Independent samples) for samples are

(i) We have to assume two samples are random.

(ii) Both the samples are independent

(iii) Sizes of both samples will be more 10 , that is $n_1 \geq 10$ and $n_2 \geq 10$

(iv) Investigator will not make any assumption about the form of the distributions from which the samples are drawn.

CLASSICAL METHOD

Step 1: Setup the hypothesis (Null)

Null Hypothesis: $H0 : \eta_x \geq \eta_y$ or $\eta_x \leq \eta_y$ or $\eta_x = \eta_y$

Step 2: Set Alternative Hypothesis:

H1 : $\eta_x < \eta_y$ (left Tailed) or H1 : $\eta_x > \eta_y$ (Right Tailed) or H1 : $n_x \neq n_y$ (Two-tailed) Respectively

Step 3: Level of Significance : $\alpha=0.01$

Step 4: Combine the observations of both the samples to obtain a single sample and arrange the observations of the combined sample in ascending order of their magnitude. Assign ranks to the combined sample data so obtained and find the values of the of the statistical T_1, T_2 and U_1 and U_2 defined.

Step 5: Compute the test value U = Smaller of (U_1, U_2)

Step 6: **Test Statistics:** Here we use normal approximation and normal test will be applied by considering H_0

Step 7: Z-Value is obtained and compared at $\alpha = 0.01$

Step 8: Write the conclusion of the test in simple language

The data below shows the salaries for the randomly selected advertisements in two different categories of drugs

X	Y	Rx	Ry
22	28	7	12
40	24	15	9
18	20	3	5
25	45	10	18
15	50	1	20
23	39	8	14
16	26	2	11
19	55	4	21
21	48	6	19
30	41	13	16
	42	69	17
			162

n1 = 10, n2 =11

UX = 14

Uy   96

U	Smaller of (Ux and Uy) = 14
μU	55
σu	14.20

Z = 2.89

KRUSKAL–WALLIS TEST OR H- TEST

Kruskal-Wallis test one of the non-parametric test which is alternative for ONE-Way ANOVA. This test is used to test the null hypothesis when more than two independent samples are drawn from the populations which have identical distributions and does not require the condition of normality of the populations.

The Kruskal-Wallis test is an extension of Mann-Whitney test to the situations where more than two populations are considered and is based on the ranks of sample observations.

Procedure:

1. In case Kruskal-Wallies test, k-samples of sizes n_1, n_2 - - - - - - n_k are drawn and these k-samples are combined to form a single of size n. . Then these n-items are assigned ranks from 1 to n from least value to highest. When two or more observations have the same value, each observation is given the mean of the ranks for which it is used.

2. Later the ranks assigned to observations in each of the k groups are added separately to give k rank sums.

3. Then the test statistic value is obtained using the equation

$$H = \frac{12}{N(n+1)} \sum_{j=1}^{k} \frac{R_j^2}{n_j} - 3(n+1) \qquad .....(12.1)$$

k = the number of samples

n_j = number of observations in the jth sample

n = the number of observations in all samples combined

R_j = the sum of the ranks in the jth sample

4. H value will be compared with the standard value of the degree of freedom (k − 1) of chi-squared value.

CLASSICAL METHOD

1. **Assumptions**: The samples drawn from different populations are independent. The distributions of the values in the sampled populations are identical except for the possibility that one or more of the populations are composed of values that tend to be larger than those of other populations.

2. **Hypothesis.:**

   H_0: Centres of the populations are equal
   H1 : Assume at least one of the population centre larger than at least one of the other Populations
   Let $\alpha = 0.01$

3 **Compute test statistics H**

4 Compare the test value H with the standard value of the table for $\alpha = 0.01$

5 **Drawing Conclusion**: The null hypothesis will be rejected if the computed value of H is so large that the probability of obtaining a value that large or larger when H_0 is true is equal to or less than the chosen significance level α.

Example: Three different types of drugs were experimented on three groups of subjects and concentration of drug after 4 hours in each subjects were measured and recorded as listed below. Do you find any significance difference between these three drugs.

Drug A Concentration (mg)	Drug B Concentration (mg)	Drug C Concentration (mg)
93	89	78
77	90	80
93	85	75
79	76	81
92	84	91
99	95	88
98	82	86
71	72	94
87	73	69
	68	100
Total		

Solution:

Drug A Concentration(mg)	Rank	Drug B Concentration(mg)	Rank	Drug C Concentration(mg)	Rank
93	23.5	89	19	78	9
77	8	90	20	80	11
93	23.5	85	15	75	6
79	10	76	7	81	12
92	22	84	14	91	21
99	28	95	26	88	18
98	27	82	13	86	16
71	3	72	4	94	25
87	17	73	5	69	2
		68	1	100	29
Total	R1 = 162		R2 = 124		R3 = 149

$$H = \frac{12}{n(n+1)} \sum_{j=1}^{k} \frac{R_j^2}{n_j} - 3(n+1)$$

$$H = \frac{12}{n(n+1)} \left(\frac{R_1^2}{n1} + \frac{R_2^2}{n2} + \frac{R_3^2}{n3} \right) - 3(n+1)$$

$$H = \frac{12}{29(29+1)} \left(\frac{162^2}{9} + \frac{124^2}{10} + \frac{149^2}{10} \right) - 3(29 + 1)$$

$$H = 2.05$$

The value of λ^2 for $k - 1 = 3 - 1 = 2$ degree of freedom at 5% level of significance is 5.99. $h = 2.05 < 5.99$, hence null-hypothesis cannot be rejected.

Example 2: Three types of weight reducing diets were advised to three homogeneous group of 22 patients and they were divided into three groups. The time period advised this diet plan was two months. The reduce in weight in kilograms during these two months were as recorded below.

Diet 1	Diet 2	Diet 3
4.2	5.3	1.4
3.3	7.4	2.0
2.8	8.3	2.8
6.1	5.6	3.0
5.0	6.5	1.5
3.9	7.3	0.8
	8.5	4.2
		3.5
		0.4

Apply the Kruskal-Wallis test to test the null-hypothesis, that the effectiveness of the three weight reducing diet plans are the same at 5% level of significance.

Solution: The result is analyzed using SPSS statistical software

Ranks			
	GROUPS	N	Mean Rank
DIETS	1.00	6	11.67
	2.00	7	18.71
	3.00	9	5.78
	Total	22	

Test Statistics[a,b]	
	Diets
Chi-Square test value = λ^2	15.650
Degree of freedom = DOF	2
P-Value	.000
a. Kruskal Wallis Test	
b. Grouping Variable: Groups	

The value of λ^2 for $k - 1 = 3 - 1 = 2$ degree of freedom at 5% level of significance IS 5.99. $h = 15.650 > 5.99$, hence null-hypothesis is rejected. The diet plans are not same

FRIEDMAN's TEST FOR K RELATED SAMPLES:

The **Friedman test** is a non-parametric test, alternative to the one-way ANOVA with repeated measures. It is used to **test** for differences between groups when the dependent variable being measured is ordinal.

If we extended the idea of the Wilcoxon test for paired data to the case where each related set has n observations, then we can test the hypothesis that k samples came from identical populations by means of Friedman test

When you choose to analyze your data using a Friedman test, part of the process involves checking to make sure that the data you want to analyze can actually be analyzed using a Friedman test. You need to do this because it is only appropriate to use a Friedman test if your data "passes" the following four assumptions:

1: One group that is measured on three or more different occasions.

2: Group is a random sample from the population.

3: Your dependent variable should be measured at the ordinal or continuous level.

4: Samples do NOT need to be normally distributed.

Here data may be arranged into a two-way table with N rows and k columns. Each row ranked from 1 for the smallest to the largest, its rank being the number of samples. If the populations from which samples have been drawn were identical then the ranks could be expected to occur in about equal numbers in each columns. The null-hypothesis of equality of population is rejected if the calculated is greater than critical value of chi-square (λ^2) at $(k - 1)$ degree of freedom at the level of significance. The test value is calculated using the equation

$$S = \frac{12}{NK(k+1)} [R_1^2 + R_2^2 + R_3^2 + - - - - - -] - 3N(k + 1)$$

Example: The quality control departments were asked to analyze five chemical substances in order to see level of significant, if all laboratories are performing the analysis in the same manner. Apply Friedman's test and verify the level of significance for the data analyzed and ranked are assigned as follow.

Laboratories

	1	2	3	4	5	6
Chemical A	1	5	3	2	4	6
B	3	2	1	4	6	5
C	3	4	2	5	1	6
D	4	4	6	3	2	5
E	1	5	1	2	3	6
Total of Ranks	R1=12	R2=20	R3=13	R4=16	R5=16	R6=28

$$S = \frac{12}{NK(k+1)}[R_1^2 + R_2^2 + R_3^2 + ------] - 3N(k+1)$$

$$S = \frac{12}{5*6(6+1)}[12^2 + 20^2 + 13^2 + 16^2 + 16^2) - 3*5(6+1)$$

$$S = \frac{12}{210}[144 + 400 + 169 + 256 + 256) - 105$$

$$S\ 114.8 - 105 = 9.8$$

The Chi-squared value for degree of freedom (k − 1) = 6 − 1 = 5 at 5% level of significance is 11.07.

9.8 < 11.07.

Hence null-hypothesis cannot be rejected, Laboratories are different.

13 Epidemiology

Epidemiology is the method used to find the causes of health outcomes and diseases in populations. The first known epidemiologist, also known as father of medicine. He taught about causal factors, how disease affect people, and how disease spread. In epidemiology, the patient is the community and individuals are viewed collectively. By definition, epidemiology is the study (scientific, systematic, and data-driven) of the distribution (frequency, pattern) and determinants (causes, risk factors) of health-related states and events (not just diseases) in specified populations (neighbourhood, school, city, state, country, global). It is also the application of this study to the control of health problems. The word epidemiology is based on three Greek word: epi, the prefix, meaning "on, upon, or befall"; demo, the root, meaning "the people"; and logos, the suffix, meaning, "the study of".

PROPORTION

In an experiment, the outcomes may be classified as one of the two possible categories. For example the presence or absence of disease. One of these categories is taken as outcome of primary interest.

Example: When patient is diagnosed the possible outcome may be presence or absence of disease.

In general one can relay on the two categories as positive(+) and negative(-ve). The preferable outcome is positive, when the primary category is taken into consideration.

It is always necessary to summarize the characteristics of observations made on a group or subjects or patients. To summarize the data the number of positive outcomes x is not sufficient, but also the size of sample or total number of subjects or observation n chosen for study should also be considered for further statistical calculation/analysis. The number x which we consider gives or tells us very little information and becomes very meaningful only after adjusting for the size n of the group.

In general the figure x and n are often combined to get a value or compute a value; is called as Proportion.

That is written as $P = \dfrac{x}{n}$

The value P always lies between 0 and 1($0 \leq P \leq 1$). The proportion P can also be expressed as percentage and it can be obtained by the equation $P = \left(\dfrac{x}{n}\right)*100$

Definition: In general the proportion can be defined as a number used to describe a group of people or subjects accordingly to dichotomous or binary characteristics under investigation.

It has been told , that characteristics with multiple categories can be dichotomized by pooling some categories to form a new one, and the concept of proportion can be applied.

CASE

Cases are the subjects who have a particular characteristic of interest. They may be the subjects or patients who have developed or have a particular disease of interest or those who are coming under a particular treatment or subjects who have received a particular treatment.

A case definition in epidemiology is a set of standard criteria for diagnosing a particular disease or health related condition, by specifying clinical criteria and limitations on person, place and time factors.

CONTROL

Control are the corresponding subjects who don't have or don't possess a particular characteristic of our interest. The control group, receiving no intervention, is used as a baseline to compare groups and assess the effect of that intervention.

Cases and controls are compared to find, if one or more factors are commonly present in one group than other and one can draw the conclusion accordingly.

SELECTION OF CASES

1. Cases are generally selected from the group who are seeking medical treatment for the disease under study.
2. It is preferable to include those who have been diagnosed recently , which will be more helpful for the investigator to avoid difficulty in distinguishing the exposures that precedes the disease, from those very often the disease occurred or the disease developed.
3. Use established criteria for diagnoses
4. It is desirable to include all consecutive incident cases occurring in a defined population over a specified period of time.

SELECTION OF CONTROLS

1. Controls are selected from a random sample, those subjects without any diseases and from the same population, where cases have been selected.
2. Control group subjects in generally are matched for essentially confounding factors such as socio-economic status and the environmental condition they live.
3. Matched for too many factors, which can lead to overmatching, that should be avoided.

4. Control can be randomly selected from a larger population when the entire population of eligible control is known. Selection of controls can also be made systematically (i.e., every nth person listed), assuming that the order of potential controls is not related to factors such as age, gender and education.

RATE

As the name implies, rate signifies speed or the frequency of occurrence. The term rate usually is reserved to refer to those calculations that involve the frequency of occurrence of some events. The rate can be expressed in the form of $\left(\frac{a}{a+b}\right)$*k, where a = the frequency with which an event has occurred during some specified period of time , (a + b) is the number of subjects or persons exposed to the of the event during the same period of time and k is some number like 10, 100, 1000 etc.

As indicated in the expression $\left(\frac{a}{a+b}\right)$*k, the numerator of a rate is a component part of the denominator. The purpose of the multiplier, k called the base, is to avoid results involving the very small numbers that may arise in the calculation of rates and to facilitate comprehension of the rate. The value chosen for k will depend on the magnitude of the numerator and denominator.

Example:

Urinary creatinine excretion in males is nearly 200 mg/24 hrs. The duration such as per minute, per week or per year could be an ingredient of the rate.

As mentioned the rate has three important values, they are

1. Numerator
2. Denominator
3. Standard multiplier

Most mortality and fertility indicators are rates.

INCIDENCE RATE

The incidence is rate, that can be defined as

$$\text{Incidence} = \frac{Number\ of\ persons\ who\ developed\ the\ diseae\ over\ a\ defined\ period\ of\ time}{Number\ of\ persons\ itially\ without\ the\ disease\ ,who\ are\ followed\ for\ the\ defined\ period\ of\ time}$$

In general the incidence is aimed to investigate possible time trends. Generally the incidence is the number of new-cases of a particular disease arising in a specified period.

If 80 new cases of coronary artery disease (CAD) occurred in a city, in a period of one year, this is the incidence of CAD during that year in that particular city. It can become rate, when incidence is calculates per unit of population and time.

The denominator is the number of persons at risk for developing that outcome. Thus those who are not at risk, such that, they are already suffering due to that disease, they are excluded from the denominator.

Incidence can be calculated or obtained only, when the exact time onset is known. The period should be long enough to allow representative number of new cases to occur.

Example: 1: The incidence of rheumatic heart disease (RHS) is 5 per 1000 per year in children of age 6 – 16 years.

$$\text{Incidence} = \left(\frac{5}{1000}\right)$$

$$\text{Incidence rate} = \left(\frac{5}{1000}\right)*100$$

Example 2: Compute the incidence rate of oral cancer per 100 persons/year among regular tobacco chewers for the data given below

SLNO	1	2	3	4	5	6	7	8
Duration of follow-up	3.0	2.8	4.4	1.7	0.5	2.5	3.5	4.0
Oral cancer development	No	Yes	Yes	No	No	Yes	No	No

Solution:

Total = 23.3

Number who develop the oral cancer disease = 3

Then the incidence rate of oral cancer per 100 persons / year among regular tobacco chewers is

$$\text{Incidence rate} = \left(\frac{3}{22.3}\right)*100 = 13.5\%$$

PREVALENCE:

In general people may develop a particular disease, may remain sick for some time and bigger is the pool of diseased persons. Then the prevalence can be defined as

$$\text{Prevalence} = \left(\frac{\text{Number of diseased persons at the time of investivation}}{\text{Total number of persons examined}}\right)$$

When we conclude per 100 or per 1000 or per million persons at risk, then it is called as prevalence rate.

Example: If the prevalence rate of cataract blindness is nearly 1.8 percent in people of age 50 years or more in the year 2012. It means that on the average 18 blinds existed in every 1000 persons in that year.

DURATION OF SICKNESS

People with acute diseases like diarrhoea and cold may last in few days, where as some chronic diseases such as cancer and blindness can go on for the life time after onset.

The duration of sickness, may be lifetime or one year or two year etc, can be considered as another indicator of the magnitude of morbidity.

This is very important for calculating incidence and prevalence also. To calculate these two, the duration of sickness is most important.

The duration of sickness for any disease, will vary from person to person. To obtain the summary about the disease, the mean duration of the disease will be obtained.

When the condition is stable, then the incidence, duration of disease and recovery/mortality remain constant for a substantial period, then the relationship between incidence, prevalence and duration can be written as

Prevalence = Incidence × Average duration of disease

The incidence and average duration should be taken in same unit. If incidence computed in year, then the duration also should be taken in the year only.

Example: If the incidence of diarrhoea among children's of age between 1 yr and 3 yrs is 4 episodes per child per year. The average duration in days is 0.0137 in year, then

the Prevalence = 4 × 0.0137 = 0.055.

At any point of time, nearly 5.5% of children may suffer diarrhoea in that particular population.

CHANGE RATE

The change rate can be defined as $\text{Change rate} = \left(\dfrac{New\ value\ -old\ value}{Old\ value}\right)*100$

The change rate may exceed 1000 also. The change rate is not a proportion (Proportion lies between 0 1nd 1) . In general change rates are used primarily for description and are not involved in common statistical analysis.

Example: The total number of patients who were suffering from cancer were 2000 in the year 2010 in a particular city. The total number has been increased to 3000 in the year 2011. Compute the change in rate of getting cancer disease in one year duration.

Solution:

Given that in the year 2010, total number of patients suffering due to cancer is 2000, then the old value = 2000

In the year 2011 the number 3000. The new value = 3000

$$\text{Change rate} = \left(\frac{New\ value\ -old\ value}{old\ value}\right) * 100$$

$$\text{Change rate} = \left(\frac{3000\ -2000}{2000}\right) * 100 = 0.5 * 100 = 50\%$$

The change rate of patients suffering due to cancer is increased by 50% in one year duration.

MEASURES OF MORBIDITY and MORTALITY

In general morbidity is any condition that restricts the daily life in any manner. The term generally restricted to physical conditions although those mental conditions that affect physical activity are also included.

Measures of **morbidity** frequency characterize the number of persons in a population who become ill (incidence) or are ill at a given time (prevalence).

At an individual levels the extent of morbidity can be measured in terms of illness or disability and duration of illness

MORTALITY RATE

A mortality rate is a measure of the frequency of occurrence of death in a defined population during a specified interval. Mortality measures are often the same mathematically; it's just a matter of what you choose to measure, illness or death.

The formula for calculating the mortality rate is as follows:

$$\text{Mortality Rate} = \left(\frac{\text{The number of deaths in a given period of time}}{\text{Population from which the deaths occurred in the given period of time}}\right)*10^n$$

$10^n = ?$

Morbidity refers to the unhealthy state of an individual, while **mortality** refers to the state of being mortal.

For example, a **morbidity** rate looks at the incidence of a disease across a population and/or geographic location during a single year. **Mortality** rate is the rate of death **in a** population.

SCREENING TEST

The proportion has been used in the evaluation of screening test or diagnostic procedures. The screening test will be done for the people who come to clinics, they will be classified as healthy or as falling into one of a number of disease categories. These types of tests more important in medicine and in epidemiologic studies and may become a basis of early interventions. In some cases screening tests may be imperfect, that the healthy persons will occasionally may be wrongly diagnosed as being not healthy or ill; while some people who are really ill may fail to be detected. Suppose that each person in large population can be classified as truly positive or negative for a particular disease, this diagnosis may be based on more refined methods that are used in the test.

There are two fundamental proportions for evaluating diagnostic procedure are Sensitivity and Specificity.

SENSITIVITY

Sensitivity is defined as the proportion of diseased people detected as positive by the diagnostic test .

$$\text{Sensitivity} = \frac{\text{Number of diseased persons who screen +ve}}{\text{Total number of diseased personf who have been choosen for diagnosis}}$$

The corresponding errors are called as false negative.

SPECIFICITY:

Specificity is the proportion of healthy people detected as negative by diagnostic test.

$$\text{Specificity} = \frac{\text{Number of healthy persons who screen } -ve}{\text{Total number of healt hy person who have been choosen for diagnosis}}$$

And the corresponding errors are false positive.

In most of studies, the desirable test or screening procedure be highly sensitive and highly specific.

Sometimes, these two types of errors may go in opposite directions, that is an effort to increase sensitivity may lead to more false positives, and vice versa.

True	TEST	
	+	−
+	True Positive	False Positive
-	False Negative	True Negative
Total	True Positive + False Negative	False Positive + True Negative

Example: X-ray result in 83 cases with lesion and 277 similar subjects subjects without that Lesions as listed in the table.

X-ray (Critenon) result	Lesion (Actual)	
	Present +	Absent −
+	66(True Positive)	72(False Positive)
-	17(False Negative)	205(True Negative)
Total	83 True Positive + False Negative	277 False Positive + True Negative

$$\text{Sensitivity} = \frac{TP}{TP+FN} = \frac{66}{83} = 0.80 = 80\%, \quad \text{Specificity} = \frac{TN}{TN+FP} = \frac{205}{277} = 0.74 = 74\%,$$

This measure the degree of uncertainty (or rather the degree of certainty) inherent in this criterion.

Equivalently, in medical tests sensitivity is the extent to which actual positives are not overlooked (so false negatives are few), and specificity is the extent to which actual negatives are classified as such (so false positives are few). Thus a highly sensitive test rarely overlooks an actual positive (for example, showing "nothing bad" despite something bad existing); a highly specific test rarely registers a positive classification for anything that is not the target of testing (for example, finding one bacterial species and mistaking it for another closely related one that is the true target); and a test that is highly sensitive *and* highly specific does both, so it "rarely overlooks a thing that it is looking for" *and* it "rarely mistakes anything else for that thing." Because most medical tests do not have sensitivity and specificity values above 99%, "rarely" does *not* equate to certainty. But for practical reasons, tests with sensitivity and specificity values above 90% have high credibility, albeit usually no certainty, in differential diagnosis.

Sensitivity therefore quantifies the avoiding of false negatives, and specificity does the same for false positives. For any test, there is usually a trade-off between the measures – for instance, in airport security since testing of passengers is for potential threats to safety, scanners may be set to trigger alarms on low-risk items like belt buckles and keys (low specificity), in order to increase the probability of identifying dangerous objects and minimize the risk of missing objects that do pose a threat (high sensitivity). This trade-off can be represented graphically using a receiver operating characteristic curve. A perfect predictor would be described as 100% sensitive, meaning all sick individuals are correctly identified as sick, and 100% specific, meaning no healthy individuals are incorrectly identified as sick. In reality, however, any non-deterministic predictor will possess a minimum error bound known as

Application to Screening Study

Imagine a study evaluating a new test that screens people for a disease. Each person taking the test either has or does not have the disease. The test outcome can be positive (classifying the person as having the disease) or negative (classifying the person as not having the disease). The test results for each subject may or may not match the subject's actual status. In that setting:

True positive: Sick people correctly identified as sick

False positive: Healthy people incorrectly identified as sick

True negative: Healthy people correctly identified as healthy

False negative: Sick people incorrectly identified as healthy

In general, Positive = identified and negative = rejected. Therefore:

True positive = correctly identified, False positive = incorrectly identified

True negative = correctly rejected, False negative = incorrectly rejected

RELATIVE RISK

In general medicine can be considered as a qualitative science. As per medical science the blood pressure is quantitative. Some time it is more convenient to talk the presence or absence hypertension or the degree of hypertension. Here quantities are converted into qualities. In epidemiological study, the events such as disease, recovery and death are considered as qualities. The degree or magnitude of association between two qualitative characteristics is measured in terms of relative risk or odd ratio. These ratio helps to make decision in the face of uncertainties.

The relative risk, is also called as risk ratio, and it is an important index in epidemiological studies, because in such studies, it is also more useful to measure the increased risk (if any) of incurring a particular disease, if certain factor is present.

This is most useful to compare two groups or population with respect to a certain unwanted event (ex: disease or death). the traditional method of expressing it in prospective studies is simply the ratio of incidence rates.

This is a statistical term used to describe the chances of a certain event occurring among one group versus another. It is commonly used in epidemiology and evidence based medicine, where relative risk helps to identify the probability of developing a disease after an exposure (e.g, a drug treatment or an environmental event) versus the chance of developing the disease in the absence of that particular exposure. The relative risk is computed using the formula.

$$\text{The Relative risk} = \frac{\text{Incidence rate among the exposed}}{\text{Incidence rate among the non exposed}}$$

A **relative risk** [RR] is 1.0, **means** you are average – there is no difference in **risk** between the control and experimental groups. A **relative risk** of 0.5 **means** that your **risk** is 1/2 that of average or a 50% lower **risk**. A **relative risk** of 1.5 **means** you have a 50% higher **risk** than average.

ODD RATIO

The odds ratio is the ratio in one group (Disease group) to another group (Control group). The odd ratio is approximately the same as relative risk, when disease is rare, but not otherwise.

In cohort studies such an index is obtained readily by observing the experience of groups of subjects with and without the factor. In a case-control study the data don't present an immediate answer to this type of questions.

In a large study, at a particular time, data will be classified as positive or negative according to some risk factor and as having or not having a certain disease under investigation.

For this type study, we prepare a 2×2 contingency table. The data will be presented as listed below.

	Disease		Total
Factor	+	–	
-	A	B	A+B
+	C	D	C+D
Total	A+C	B+D	N= A+B+ C+D

The relative risk (RR) is calculated using the equation

$$RR = \frac{\frac{A}{A+B}}{\frac{C}{C+D}} = \frac{Incidence \ in \ exposed}{Incidence \ in \ Nonexposed}$$

$$= \frac{A(C+D)}{C(A+B)}$$

In many situations, the number of subjects classified as disease positive is small compared to the number classified as –ve, i.e., $C+D \sim D$, $A+B \sim B$

$$\therefore \quad R.R = OR = \frac{\frac{A}{B}}{\frac{C}{D}} = \frac{AD}{BC}$$

$$OR \qquad = \frac{AD}{BC}$$

This odd ratio (OR) helps to measure the strength of association between the outcome and antecedent. If OR = 1, then there is no association between outcome and antecedent. If OR > 1, indicates that the antecedent is more in cases than in controls and indicating a positive association. It also explains that the exposed group have more risk than unexposed group. Similarly OR < 1 indicates a negative association in the sense that the presence of antecedent is less in the control groups. Higher the OR, stronger the association.

$$OR = \frac{\frac{n(Exposed \ cases)}{n(unexpos \ ed \ cases)}}{\frac{n(exposed \ non \ cases)}{n(Unexposed \ non -cases)}}$$

Example : Compute the Odd ratio for the data listed given in the 2x2 – contingency table

Smoking	Lung Cancer		Total
	Present(Yes)	Absent(NO)	
Smoking (Yes)	30	70	100
Smoking (No)	10	90	100
Total	40	160	N= 200

Solution:

$$OR = \frac{AD}{BC} = \frac{30*90}{10*70} = = \frac{270}{700} = 0.3$$

CONDITIONING ON AN EVENT

Kolmogorov definition

Given two events A and B, from the sigma-field of a probability space, with the unconditional probability of B (that is, of the event B occurring) being greater than zero – $P(B) > 0$ – the conditional probability of A given B is defined as the quotient of the probability of the joint of events A and B, and the probability of B

$$P(A \mid B) = \frac{P(A \cap B)}{P(B)},$$

where P(A∩B) is the probability that both events A and B occur. This may be visualized as restricting the sample space to situations in which B occurs. The logic behind this equation is that if the possible outcomes for A and B are restricted to those in which B occurs, this set serves as the new sample space.

Note that this is a definition but not a theoretical result. We just denote the quantity $\frac{P(A \cap B)}{P(B)}$ as P(|B) and call it the conditional probability of A given B.

Example:

		Diabetes	Refractive Error	Total
Cholecystitis	C	3000	29700	327000
	Not C	97000	960300	1057300
	Total	100000	990000	1090000

Here in the we written three conditions, cholecystitis, diabetes and refreactive error as C,D and D

P(C|RE) =3000/100000 = 0.0300

P(C|CR)= 29700/990000= 0.0300

P(NotC|RE) =97000/100000 = 0.97

P(Not C|CR)= 960300/990000= 0.97

Relative Risk

The relative Risk for an outcome D associated with binary risk factor E, denoted by RR it is defined as

$$RR = \frac{P(D|E)}{P(D|\bar{E})} = \frac{P(D|E)}{P(D|Not\ E)}$$

Here the relative risk must be positive number, if the value of RR=1 , this is a null value and indicates that P(D|E) = P(D|$\bar{E}$). That is both D and E are independent. If RR>1 then this indicates that there is greater risk or probability of D when exposed (E) than when unexposed ($\bar{E}$) and the vice versa is also possible.

The relative is one of the useful data and is a basis of a multiplicative model for, that is to obtain the risk of disease for an exposed individual, we can use baseline – unexposed risk and multiply it with RR.

	Unmarried	Married	Total
Death	300	500	800
Live at 1 Year	1000	2000	3000
Total	1300	2500	3800

$$RR = \frac{P(D|E)}{P(D|\bar{E})} = \frac{\left[\frac{300}{1300}\right]}{\left[\frac{500}{2500}\right]} = \frac{0.23}{0.20} = 1.15$$

ODD RATIO: We the investigator **have** been measuring the risk of the outcome D through the risk or probability P(D); an alternative quantity is the odds of D and it can be obtained by $\frac{P(D)}{P(Not\ D)}$. Just like Relative risk Odds Ratio measures the association by comparing odds of D in exposed and unexposed subgroups. The odds Ratio for D associated E is defined as

$$OR = \frac{P(D|E)}{P(Not\ D|E)} = \frac{\frac{P(D|E)}{P(Not\ D|E)}}{\frac{P(D|NotE)}{P(Not\ D|Not\ E)}}$$

In the same as relative risk, the null value of the Odd Ratio is OR = 1, this indicates D and E are independent. If OR>1, this indicates that the risk D is more with the exposure E and if OR< 1 when there is a lower risk of D if E is present.

Infant Mortality		Mother's marital Status		
		Unmarried(D)	Married(NotD)	Total
	Death (E)	300	500	800
	Live at 1 year(Not E)	1000	2000	3000
	Total	1300	2500	3800

$$OR = \frac{P(D|E)}{P(Not\ D|E)} = \frac{\frac{P(D|E)}{P(Not\ D|E)}}{\frac{P(D|NotE)}{P(Not\ D|Not\ E)}} = \begin{bmatrix} \frac{\frac{300}{1300}}{\frac{1000}{1300}} \\ \frac{\frac{500}{2500}}{\frac{2000}{2500}} \end{bmatrix} = \frac{0.30}{0.25} = 1.20$$

ATTRIBUTABLE RISK

In order explain disease D in the population, can be explained due the presence of the risk factor E. This can answered by Attributable risk. The attributable Risk is a measure of association designed to provide an answer to the question and defined as the fraction of all cases of D in the population that can be attributed to E. In general the attributable risk can be defined as

$$AR = \frac{P(D) - P(D|\bar{E})}{P(D)}$$

But $P(D) = P(D|E)P(E) + P(D|\bar{E})P(\bar{E})$

$$AR = \frac{P(D|E)P(E) + P(D|\bar{E})P(\bar{E}) - P(D|\bar{E})}{P(D)}$$

$$AR = \frac{P(D|E)P(E) + P(D|\bar{E})(P(\bar{E})-1)}{P(D)}$$

$$AR = \frac{P(D|E)P(E) - P(D|\bar{E})P(E)}{P(D)}$$

$$AR = \frac{P(E)(P(D|E) - P(D|\bar{E}))}{P(D|E)P(E) + P(D|\bar{E})P(\bar{E})}$$

$$AR = \frac{P(E)[RR-1]}{P(E)RR + P(\bar{E})}$$

$$AR = \frac{P(E)[RR-1]}{1 + P(E)(RR-1)}$$

The above expression clears that the attributable Risk depends on both the strength of association between D and E and the prevalence of the risk factor E.

		Mother's marital Status		
		Unmarried(D)	Married(NotD)	Total
	Death (E)	300	500	800
Infant Mortality	Live at 1 year(Not E)	1000	2000	3000
	Total	1300	2500	3800

$$AR = \frac{P(E)[RR-1]}{1 + P(E)(RR-1)}$$

$$RR = \frac{P(D|E)}{P(D|\bar{E})} = \begin{bmatrix} \frac{300}{1300} \\ \frac{500}{2500} \end{bmatrix} = \frac{0.23}{0.20} = 1.15$$

$$P(E) = \frac{300}{3800} = 0.34$$

$$AR = \frac{P(E)[RR-1]}{1 + P(E)(RR-1)} = \frac{0.34[1.15-1]}{1 + 0.34[1.15-1]} = \frac{0.34*0.15}{1 + 0.34*0.15} = \frac{0.05}{1.05} = 0.05$$

COHORT STUDY

A cohort study is a particular form of longitudinal study that sample a cohort (a group of people who share a defining characteristic, typically those who experienced a common event in a selected period, such as birth or graduation), performing a cross-section at intervals through time. While a cohort study is a panel study, a panel study is not always a cohort study as individuals in a panel study do not always share a common characteristic.

Cohort studies represent one of the fundamental designs of epidemiology which are used in research in the fields of medicine, nursing, psychology, Pharmaceutical science, and in any field reliant on 'difficult to reach' answers that are based on evidence (statistics). In medicine for instance, while clinical trials are used primarily for assessing the safety of newly developed pharmaceuticals before they are approved for sale, epidemiological analysis on how risk factors affect the incidence of diseases is often used to identify the causes of diseases in the first place, and to help provide pre-clinical justification for the plausibility of protective factors (treatments). Cohort studies differ from clinical trials in that no intervention, treatment, or exposure is administered to participants in a cohort design; and no control group is defined. Rather, cohort studies are largely about the life histories of segments of populations, and the individual people who constitute these segments. Exposures or protective factors are identified as pre-existing characteristics of participants. The study is controlled by including other common characteristics of the cohort in the statistical analysis. Both exposure/treatment and control variables are measured at baseline. Participants are then followed over time to observe the incidence rate of the disease or outcome in question. Regression analysis can then be used to evaluate the extent to which the exposure or treatment variable contributes to the incidence of the disease, while accounting for other variables that may be at play.

In medicine, a cohort study is often undertaken to obtain evidence to prove the existence of a association between cause and effect that is associated; failure to prove the hypothesis often strengthens confidence in it. Generally the cohort is identified before the subjects under investigation get the disease. The study groups follow a group of subjects those who do not have the disease for a period of time and later record the number subjects who develops the disease (new incidence). The cohort cannot therefore be defined as a group of subjects who already have the disease. Prospective (longitudinal) cohort studies between exposure and disease strongly aid in studying causal associations, though distinguishing true causality usually requires further corroboration from further experimental trials.

PROSPECTIVE COHORT STUDY

A prospective cohort study is a longitudinal cohort study that follows over time a group of similar individuals (cohorts) who differ with respect to certain factors under study, to determine how these factors affect rates of a certain outcome. For example, one might follow a cohort of middle-aged truck drivers who vary in terms of smoking habits, to test the hypothesis that the 20-year incidence rate of lung cancer will be highest among heavy smokers, followed by moderate smokers, and then non-smokers.

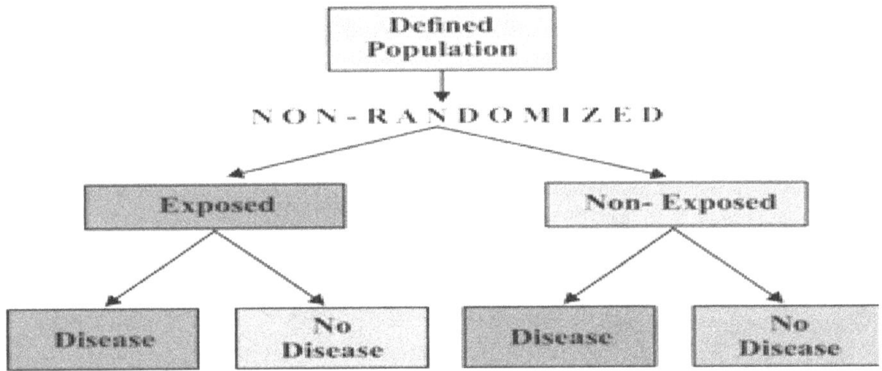

The prospective study is important for research on the etiology of diseases and disorders. The distinguishing feature of a prospective cohort study is that at the time that the investigators begin enrolling subjects and collecting baseline exposure information, none of the subjects have developed any of the outcomes of interest. After baseline information is collected, subjects in a prospective cohort study are then followed "longitudinally," i.e. over a period of time, usually for years, to determine if and when they become diseased and whether their exposure status changes outcomes. In this way, investigators can eventually use the data to answer many questions about the associations between "risk factors" and disease outcomes. For example, when we identify smokers and non-smokers at baseline and between those groups measure rate of incidence in developing the heart problem or heart disease. Prospective cohort studies are typically ranked higher in the hierarchy of evidence than retrospective cohort studies.

One of the advantages of prospective cohort studies is they can help determine risk factors for being infected with a new disease because they are a longitudinal observation over time, and the collection of results is at regular time intervals, errors will be minimized to the maximum extent.

RETROSPECTIVE COHORT STUDY

A **retrospective cohort study**, also called a **historic cohort study**, is a longitudinal cohort study used in medical and psychological research. A cohort of individuals that share a common exposure factor is compared with another group of equivalent individuals not exposed to that factor, to determine the factor's influence on the incidence of a condition such as disease or death. Retrospective cohort studies have existed for approximately as long as prospective cohort studies.

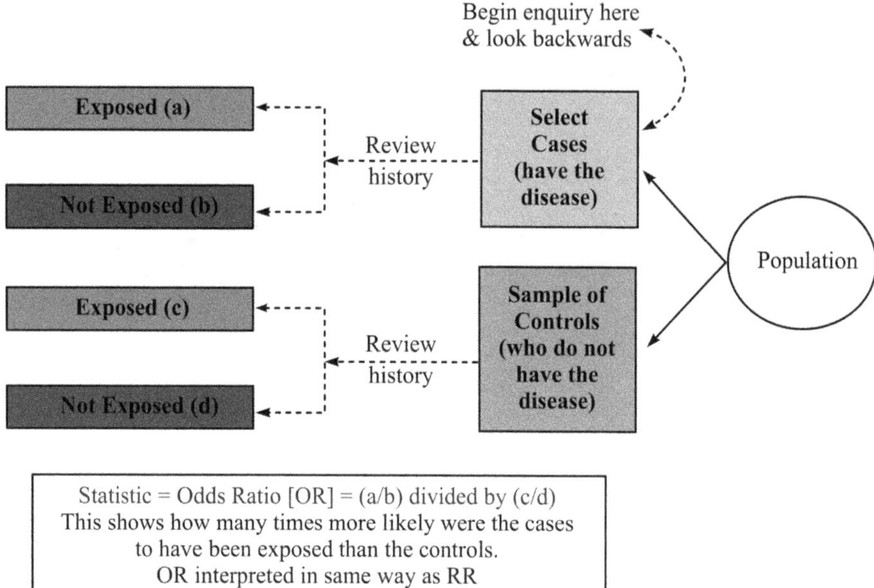

The retrospective cohort study compares groups of individuals who are alike in many ways but differ by a certain characteristic (for example, female nurses who smoke and ones who do not smoke) in terms of a particular outcome (such as lung cancer). Data on the relevant events for each individual (the form and time of exposure to a factor, the latent period, and the time of any subsequent occurrence of the outcome) are collected from existing records and can immediately be analyzed to determine the relative risk of the cohort compared to the control group.

This is fundamentally the same methodology as for a prospective cohort study, except that the retrospective study is performed post-hoc, looking back. The prospective study looks forward, enrolling patients unaffected by the outcome and observing them to see whether the outcome has occurred. However, both kinds of cohort studies share the same starting point (considering data from before the occurrence of the outcome). The first objective is still to establish two groups - exposed versus non-exposed - which are then assessed retrospectively to establish the most likely temporal sequence of events leading to the current disease state in both the exposed and unexposed groups.

Retrospective cohort studies require particular caution because errors due to confounding and bias are more common than in prospective studies.

Advantages

Retrospective cohort studies exhibit the benefits of cohort studies and have distinct advantages relative to prospective ones:

1. They are conducted on a smaller scale.

2. They typically require less time to complete.

3. They are generally less expensive, because resources are mainly devoted to collecting data.
4. They are better for analyzing multiple outcomes.

In a medical context, they can potentially address rare diseases, which would necessitate extremely large cohorts in prospective studies.[5]

Retrospective studies are especially helpful in addressing diseases of low incidence, since affected people have already been identified. The fact that retrospective studies are generally less expensive than prospective studies may be another key benefit. Additionally, it has essentially all the benefits of a cohort study.

Disadvantages

1. Retrospective studies have disadvantages vis-a-vis prospective studies:
2. Some key statistics cannot be measured, and significant biases may affect the selection of controls.
3. Researchers cannot control exposure or outcome assessment, and instead must rely on others for accurate recordkeeping. When relying on individual recall of former exposure to risk variables, recall may be inaccurate and subject to biases. It can be very difficult to make accurate comparisons between the exposed and the non-exposed.
4. The retrospective aspect may introduce selection bias and mis-classification or information bias. With retrospective studies, the temporal relationship is frequently difficult to assess.
5. Retrospective studies may need very large sample sizes for rare diseases like cancer, heart diseases, AIDs etc.

OBSERVATIONAL STUDY – CROSSS SECTIONAL

Cross-sectional study design is a type of observational study design. In a cross-sectional study, the investigator measures the outcome and the exposures in the study participants at the same time. Unlike in case–control studies (participants selected based on the outcome status) or cohort studies (participants selected based on the exposure status), the participants in a cross-sectional study are just selected based on the inclusion and exclusion criteria set for the study. Once the participants have been selected for the study, the investigator follows the study to assess the exposure and the outcomes. Cross-sectional designs are used for population-based surveys and to assess the prevalence of diseases in clinic-based samples. These studies can usually be conducted relatively faster and are inexpensive. They may be conducted either before planning a cohort study or a baseline in a cohort study. These types of designs will give us information about the prevalence of outcomes or exposures; this information will be useful for designing the cohort study. However, since this is a onetime measurement of exposure and outcome, it is difficult to derive causal relationships from cross-sectional analysis. We can estimate the prevalence of disease in cross-sectional studies. Furthermore, we will also be able to estimate the odds ratios to study the association between exposure and the outcomes in this design.

In a cross-sectional study, the investigator measures the outcome and the exposures in the study participants at the same time. Unlike in case–control studies (participants selected based on the outcome status) or cohort studies (participants selected based on the exposure status), the participants in a cross-sectional study are just selected based on the inclusion and exclusion criteria set for the study. Once the participants have been selected for the study, the investigator follows the study to assess the exposure and the outcomes.

After the entry into the study, the participants are measured for outcome and exposure at the same time. The investigator can study the association between these variables. It is also possible that the investigator will recruit the study participants and examine the outcomes in this population. The investigator may also estimate the prevalence of the outcome in those surveyed.

Cross-sectional studies involve data collected at a defined time. They are often used to assess the prevalence of acute or chronic conditions, but cannot be used to answer questions about the causes of disease or the results of intervention. Cross-sectional data cannot be used to infer causality because temporality is not known. They may also be described as censuses. Cross-sectional studies may involve special data collection, including questions about the past, but they often rely on data originally collected for other purposes. They are moderately expensive, and are not suitable for the study of rare diseases. Difficulty in recalling past events may also contribute bias.

How and When Cross-Sectional Studies Are Used

This type of study uses different groups of people who differ in the variable of interest but who share other characteristics such as socioeconomic status, educational background, and ethnicity. Cross-sectional studies are often used in developmental psychology, but this method is also utilized in many other areas including social science and education.

For example, researchers studying developmental psychology might select groups of people who are remarkably similar in most areas but differ only in age. By doing this, any differences between groups can presumably be attributed to age differences rather than to other variables.

Advantages

1. Cross-sectional studies can usually be conducted relatively faster and are inexpensive – particularly when compared with cohort studies (prospective)

2. The study takes place at a single point in time

3. It does not involve manipulating variables

4. It allows researchers to look at numerous characteristics at once (age, income, gender, etc.)

5. It's often used to look at the prevailing characteristics in a given population

6. It can provide information about what is happening in a current population

7. These studies are conducted either before planning a cohort study or a baseline in a cohort study. These types of designs will give us information about the prevalence of outcomes or exposures; this information will be useful for designing the cohort study

8. These study designs may be useful for public health planning, monitoring, and evaluation. For example, sometimes the National AIDS Programme conducted cross-sectional sentinel surveys among high-risk groups and ante-natal mothers every year to monitor the prevalence of HIV in these groups.

9. While cross-sectional studies cannot be used to determine causal relationships, they can provide a useful springboard to further research. When looking at a public health issue, such as whether a particular behaviour might be linked to a particular illness, researchers might

utilize a cross-sectional study to look for clues that will serve as a useful tool to guide further experimental studies.

Disadvantages

1. Since this is a onetime measurement of exposure and outcome, it is difficult to derive causal relationships from cross-sectional analysis

2. These studies are also prone to certain biases. For example, we wish to study the relation between diet and exercise and being overweight/obese. We conduct a cross-sectional study and recruit 250 individuals. We assess their dietary habits, exercise habits, and body mass index at one point of time in a cross-sectional survey. However, individuals who are overweight/obese have started to exercise more or altered their feeding habits (eat more salads). Hence, in a cross-sectional survey, we may find that overweight/obese individuals are also more likely to eat salads and exercise more. Thus, we have to be careful about interpreting the associations and direction of associations from a cross-sectional survey

3. The prevalence of an outcome depends on the incidence of the disease as well as the length of survival following the outcome. For example, even if the incidence of HIV (number of new cases) goes down in one particular community, the prevalence (total number of cases – old as well as new) may increase. This may be due to cumulative HIV positive cases over a period. Thus, just performing cross-sectional surveys may not be sufficient to understand disease trends in this situation.

4. However, in modern epidemiology it may be impossible to survey the entire population of interest, so cross-sectional studies often involve secondary analysis of data collected for another purpose.

Case Control Study

Definition

A study that compares subjects who have a disease or outcome of interest (cases) with subjects who do not have the disease or outcome (controls), and looks back retrospectively to compare how frequently the exposure to a risk factor is present in each group to determine the relationship between the risk factor and the disease.

Case control studies are observational because no intervention is attempted and no attempt is made to alter the course of the disease. The goal is to retrospectively determine the exposure to the risk factor of interest from each of the two groups of individuals: cases and controls. These studies are designed to estimate odds.

Case control studies are also known as "retrospective studies" and "case-referent studies."

The case–control is a type of epidemiological observational study. An observational study is a study in which subjects are not randomized to the exposed or unexposed groups, rather the subjects are *observed* in order to determine both their exposure and their outcome status and the exposure status is thus not determined by the researcher.

Porta's **Dictionary of Epidemiology** defines the case–control study as an observational epidemiological study of persons with the disease (or another outcome variable) of interest and a suitable control group of persons without the disease (comparison group, reference group). The potential relationship of a suspected risk factor or an attribute to the disease is examined by comparing the diseased and non diseased subjects with regard to how frequently the factor or attribute is present (or, if quantitative, the levels of the attribute) in each of the groups (diseased and non diseased).

For example, in a study trying to show that people who smoke (the *attribute*) are more likely to be diagnosed with lung cancer (the *outcome*), the *cases* would be persons with lung cancer, the *controls* would be persons without lung cancer (not necessarily healthy), and some of each group would be smokers. If a larger proportion of the cases smoke than the controls, that suggests, but does not conclusively show, that the hypothesis is valid.

The case–control study is frequently contrasted with cohort studies, wherein exposed and unexposed subjects are observed until they develop an outcome of interest

Control Group Selection

Controls need not be in good health; inclusion of sick people is sometimes appropriate, as the control group should represent those at risk of becoming a case.[1] Controls should come from the same population as the cases, and their selection should be independent of the exposures of interest.

Controls can carry the same disease as the experimental group, but of another grade/severity, therefore being different from the outcome of interest. However, because the difference between the cases and the controls will be smaller, this results in a lower power to detect an exposure effect.

As with any epidemiological study, greater numbers in the study will increase the power of the study. Numbers of cases and controls do not have to be equal. In many situations, it is much easier to recruit controls than to find cases. Increasing the number of controls above the number of cases, up to a ratio of about 4 to 1, may be a cost-effective way to improve the study.

Case–control studies are a relatively inexpensive and frequently used type of epidemiological study that can be carried out by small teams or individual researchers in single facilities in a way that more structured experimental studies often cannot be. They have pointed the way to a number of important discoveries and advances. The case–control study design is often used in the study of rare diseases or as a preliminary study where little is known about the association between the risk factor and disease of interest.

Compared to prospective cohort studies they tend to be less costly and shorter in duration. In several situations, they have greater statistical power than cohort studies, which must often wait for a 'sufficient' number of disease events to accrue.

Advantages and Disadvantages

When conditions are uncommon, case-control studies generate a lot of information from relatively few subjects. When there is a long latent period between an exposure and the disease, case-control studies are the only feasible option. Consider the practicalities of a cohort study or cross sectional study in the assessment of new variant CJD and possible etiologies. With less than 300 confirmed cases a cross sectional study would need about 200 000 subjects to include one symptomatic patient. Given a postulated latency of 10 to 30 years a cohort study would require both a vast sample size and take a generation to complete.

In case-control studies comparatively few subjects are required so more resources are available for studying each. In consequence a huge number of variables can be considered. This type of study is therefore useful for generating hypotheses that can then be tested using other types of study.

This flexibility of the variables studied comes at the expense of the restricted outcomes studied. The only outcome is the presence or absence of the disease or whatever criteria was chosen to select the cases.

The major problems with case-control studies are the familiar ones of confounding variables and bias. Bias may take two major forms.

Sampling Bias

The patients with the disease may be a biased sample (for example, patients referred to a teaching hospital) or the controls may be biased (for example, volunteers, different ages, sex or socioeconomic group).

Observation and Recall Bias

As the study assesses predictor variables retrospectively there is great potential for a biased assessment of their presence and significance by the patient or the investigator, or both.

Overcoming Sampling Bias

Ideally the cases studied should be a random sample of all the patients with the disease. This is not only very difficult but in many instances is impossible because many cases may not have been diagnosed or have been misdiagnosed. For example, many cases of non-insulin dependent diabetes will not have sought medical attention and therefore be undiagnosed. Conversely many psychiatric diseases may be differently labeled in different countries and even by different doctors in the same country. As a result they will be misdiagnosed for the purposes of the study. However, in reality you are often left studying a sample of those patients who it is possible to recruit. Selecting the controls is often a more difficult problem.

To enable the controls to represent the same population as the cases, one of four techniques may be used.

1. A convenience sample sampled in the same way as the cases, for example, attending the same outpatient department. While this is certainly convenient it may reduce the external validity of the study.

2. Matching the controls may be a matched or unmatched random sample from the unaffected population. Again the problems of controlling for unknown influences is present but if the controls are too closely matched they may not be representative of the general population. "Over matching" may cause the true difference to be underestimated.

    The advantage of matching is that it allows a smaller sample size for any given effect to be statistically significant.

3. Using two or more control groups. If the study demonstrates a significant difference between the patients with the outcome of interest and those without, even when the latter have been sampled in a number of different ways (for example, outpatients, in patients, GP patients) then the conclusion is more robust.

4. Using a population based sample for both cases and controls. It is possible to take a random sample of all the patients with a particular disease from specific registers. The control group can then be constructed by selecting age and sex matched people randomly selected from the same population as the area covered by the disease register.

Overcoming Observation and Recall Bias

Overcoming retrospective recall bias can be achieved by using data recorded, for other purposes, before the outcome had occurred and therefore before the study had started. The success of this strategy is limited by the availability and reliability of the data collected. Another technique is blinding where neither the subject nor the observer know if they are a case or control subject. Nor are they aware of the study hypothesis. In practice this is often difficult or impossible and only partial blinding is practicable. It is usually possible to blind the subjects and observers to the study hypothesis by asking spurious questions. Observers can also be easily blinded to the case or control status of the patient where the relevant observation is not of the patient themselves but a laboratory test or radiograph.

INTERVENTIONAL STUDY

Interventional study (clinical trial) a type of clinical study in which participants are assigned to groups that receive one or more intervention/treatment (or no intervention) so that researchers can measure the effects of the interventions on biomedical or health-related outcomes.

An interventional study is one in which the participants receive some kind of intervention, such as a new medicine, in order to evaluate it. In the medicines development process, medicines are evaluated through interventional studies known as clinical trials.

There are many variations in how clinical trials are designed, but they are commonly randomized (participants are allocated to different arms in the study randomly) and controlled (the study medicine is given to one arm, and the outcomes are compared with an alternative treatment or placebo given to another arm). These are called randomized controlled trials, or RCTs.

Resource text

Intervention studies are considered to provide the most reliable evidence in epidemiological research. Intervention studies can generally be considered as either preventative or therapeutic .

Therapeutic trials are conducted among individuals with a particular disease to assess the effectiveness of an agent or procedure to diminish symptoms, prevent recurrence, or reduce mortality from the disease.

Preventative trials are conducted to evaluate whether an agent or procedure reduces the risk of developing a particular disease among individuals free from that disease at the beginning of the trial, for example, vaccine trials. Preventative trials may be conducted among individuals or among entire communities.

Types of experimental interventions may include:

- Therapeutic agents
- Prophylactic agents
- Diagnostic agents

- Surgical procedures
- Health service strategies

Characteristics of an intervention study

A distinguishing characteristic of an intervention study is that the intervention (the preventative or therapeutic measure) being tested is allocated by the investigator to a group of two or more study subjects like individuals, households, communities. Subjects are followed prospectively to compare the intervention with control (standard treatment, no treatment or placebo).

The main intervention study design is the randomized controlled trial (RCT).

Cross-over Trials

A pre-post clinical trial/cross-over trial is one in which the subjects are first assigned to the treatment group and, after a brief interval for cessation of residual effect of the drug, are shifted into the placebo /alternative group. Thus, the subjects act as their own control at the end of the study. However, such studies are not feasible if there is mortality, or if the disease is easily cured by one of the interventions.

Randomized Controlled Trials

The randomized controlled trial is considered as the most rigorous method of determining whether a cause-effect relationship exists between an intervention and outcome. The strength of the RCT lies in the process of randomization that is unique to this type of epidemiological study design.

Generally, in a randomized controlled trial, study participants are randomly assigned to one of two groups: the experimental group receiving the intervention that is being tested and a comparison group (controls) which receives a conventional treatment or placebo. These groups are then followed prospectively to assess the effectiveness of the intervention compared with the standard or placebo treatment.

The random allocation of subjects is used to ensure that the intervention and control groups are similar in all respects (distribution of potential confounding factors) with the exception of the therapeutic or preventative measure being tested. The choice of comparison treatments may include an existing standard treatment or a placebo (a treatment which resembles the intervention treatment in all respects except that it contains no active ingredients).

General outline of a two armed randomized controlled trial.

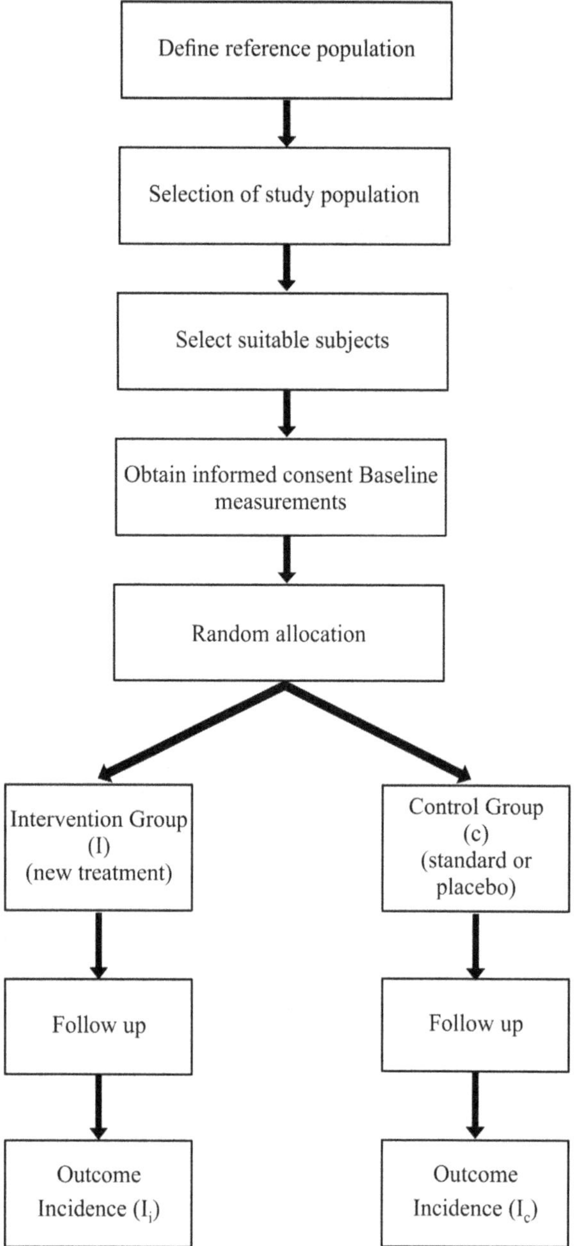

Basic outline of the design of a randomized controlled trial

1. Development of a comprehensive study protocol. The study protocol will include:

    - Aim and rationale of the trial
    - Proposed methodology/data collection
    - Definition of the hypothesis
    - Ethical considerations

- Background/review of published literature
- Quality assurance and safety
- Treatment schedules, dosage, toxicity data etc.

2. Formulation of hypothesis.

3. Objectives of the trial.

4. Sample size calculations.

5. Define reference population.

6. Choice of a comparison treatment - placebo or current available best treatment.

7. Selection of intervention and control groups, including source, inclusion and exclusion criteria, and methods of recruitment.

8. Informed consent procedures.

9. Collection of baseline measurements, including all variables considered or known to affect the outcome(s) of interest.

10. Random allocation of study participants to treatment groups (standard or placebo vs. new).

11. Follow-up of all treatment groups, with assessment of outcomes continuously or intermittently.

12. Monitor compliance and losses to follow-up.

13. Interim analysis.

14. Analysis - comparison of treatment groups.

15. Interpretation (assess the strength of effect, alternative explanations such as sampling variation, bias).

16. Publication.

RANDOMIZATION

The aim of randomization is to ensure that any observed differences between the treatment groups are due to differences in the treatment alone and not due to the effects of confounding (known or unknown) or bias. That is, that the groups are similar in all respects with the exception of the intervention under investigation.

Methods of random allocation are used to ensure that all study participants have the same chance of allocation to the treatment or control group, and that the likelihood of receiving an intervention is equal regardless of when the participant entered the study. Therefore, the probability of any participant receiving the intervention or the standard treatment/placebo is independent of any other participant being assigned that treatment.

The assignment of study subjects to each intervention is determined by formal chance process and cannot be predicted or influenced by the investigator or participant. In a well designed RCT, random allocation is determined in advance.

Methods of randomization - allocation of subjects to intervention and control groups

1. Simple randomization

For example, computer generated random number tables. Simple randomization is rarely used.

2. Block randomization

Block randomization is a method used to ensure that the numbers of participants assigned to each group is equally distributed and is commonly used in smaller trials.

3. Stratified randomization

Stratified randomization is used to ensure that important baseline variables (potential confounding factors) are more evenly distributed between groups than chance alone may assure. However, there are a limited number of baseline variables that can be balanced by stratification because of the potential for small numbers of subjects within each stratum.

4. Minimized randomization

This method may be used when the study is sufficiently small and simple randomization will not result in balanced groups. Note that deterministic methods of allocation such as by date of birth or alternate assignment to each group are not considered as random.

Advantages of Randomization

Eliminates confounding - tends to create groups that are comparable for all factors that influence outcome, known, unknown or difficult to measure. Therefore, the only difference between the groups should be the intervention.

Eliminates selection bias.

Gives validity in statistical tests based on probability theory.

Any baseline differences that exist between study groups are attributable to chance rather than bias. Though this should still be considered as a potential concern.

Disadvantages of Randomization

Does not guarantee comparable groups as differences in confounding variables may arise by chance.

Blinding in Randomized Controlled Trials

Blinding is a process where the critical information on allocation of treatment is hidden either from the patients, or from observer or the evaluator in the study. The method of blinding in RCT is used to ensure that there are no differences in the way in which each group is assessed or managed, and therefore minimize bias. Bias may be introduced, for example, if the investigator is aware of which treatment a subject is receiving, as this may influence (intentionally or unintentionally) the way in which outcome data is measured or interpreted. Similarly, a subject's knowledge of treatment assignment may influence their response to a specific treatment.

Blinding also involves ensuring that the intervention and standard or placebo treatment appears the same.

Double blinding is when neither the investigator nor the study participant is aware of treatment assignments. However, this design is not always possible.

A single blind RCT is when the investigator but not the study participants know which treatment has been allocated.

Strengths of a Randomized Controlled Trial

A well designed randomized control trial provides the strongest evidence of any epidemiological study design that a given intervention has a postulated effectiveness and is safe.

A RCT provides the best type of epidemiological study from which to draw conclusions on causality.

Randomization provides a powerful tool for controlling for confounding, even by factors that may be unknown or difficult to measure. Therefore, if well designed and conducted, a RCT minimizes the possibility that any observed association is due to confounding.

Clear temporal sequence - exposure clearly precedes outcome.

Provides a strong basis for statistical inference.

Enables blinding and therefore minimizes bias.

Can measure disease incidence and multiple outcomes.

Weaknesses of a Randomized Controlled Trial

Ethical constraints - for example, it is not always possible or ethical to manipulate exposure at random.

It is more Expensive and time consuming.

Requires complex design and analysis if unit of allocation is not the individual.

Inefficient for rare diseases or diseases with a delayed outcome.

Generalisability - subjects in a RCT may be more willing to comply with the treatment regimen and therefore may not be representative of all individuals who might be given the treatment.

Classification of Clinical Trials

Clinical studies form a class of all scientific approaches to evaluating medical disease prevention, diagnostic techniques, and treatments. Among this class, trials, often called clinical trials, form a subset of those clinical studies that evaluate investigational drugs.

PHASE 0

What happens in phase 0?

Phase 0 of a clinical trial is done with a very small number of subjects, usually in this phase less than 15 subjects will be selected. Investigators use a very small dose of medication to make sure it is not harmful to humans before they start using it in higher doses for later phases.

If the medication acts differently than expected, the investigators will likely to do some additional preclinical research before deciding whether to continue the trial.

PHASE I

What happens in phase I?

The Phase 1 trials focus on safety of new investigational medicine. These are the first human trials after the successful trials on animals. During phase I of a clinical trial, investigators spend several months looking at the effects of the medication on about 20 to 80 people who have no underlying health conditions.

This phase aims to figure out the highest dose humans can take without serious side effects. Investigators monitor participants very closely to see how their bodies react to the medication during this phase. Phase I trials to patients from standard treatment failure who are at high risk of death in the short term.

While preclinical research usually provides some general information about dosing, the effects of a medication on the human body can be unpredictable.

In addition to evaluating safety and ideal dosage, investigators also look at the best way to administer the drug, such as orally, intravenously, or topically. The goal in the Phase I trial is to identify a maximum tolerance dose, a dose that has reasonable efficacy.

According to the FDA, approximately 70 percent of medications move on to phase II.

PHASE II

What happens in phase II?

Phase II of a clinical trial involves several hundred participants who are living with the condition that the new medication is meant to treat. They're usually given the same dose that was found to be safe in the previous phase.

Investigators monitor participants for several months or years to see how effective the medication is and to gather more information on about any side effects it might cause.

The drug, at the optimal dos (MTD) found in a Phase I trial is given to a small group of patients who meet predetermined inclusion criteria.

While phase II involves more participants than earlier phases, it's still not large enough to demonstrate the overall safety of a medication. However, the data collected during this phase helps investigators come up with methods for conducting phase III.

The FDA estimates that about 33 percent of medications move on to phase III.

What happens in phase III?

Phase III trials are conducted before regulatory approval. Phase III of a clinical trial usually involves up to 3,000 participants who have the condition that the new medication is meant to treat. Trials in this phase can last for several years.

The purpose of phase III is to evaluate how the new medication works in comparison to existing medications for the same condition. To move forward with the trial, investigators need to demonstrate that the medication is at least as safe and effective as existing treatment options.

To do this, investigators use a process called randomization, which is most suitable for clinical trials. In this investigators randomly choosing some participants to receive the new medication and others to receive an existing medication.

Phase III trials are usually double-blind, which means that neither the participant nor the investigator knows which medication will administered to the participants. This helps to eliminate bias while drawing interpreting results.

The FDA usually requires a phase III clinical trial before approving a new medication. Due to the larger number of participants and longer duration of phase III, rare and long-term side effects are more likely to show up during this phase.

If investigators demonstrate that the medication is at least as safe and effective as others already on the market, the FDA will usually approve the medication.

Roughly 25 to 30 percent of medications move on to phase IV.

PHASE IV

What happens in phase IV?

Phase IV clinical trials happen after the FDA has approved medication. This phase involves thousands of participants and may take many years or longer periods to draw inference.

Investigators use this phase to get more information about the medication's long-term safety, effectiveness, and any other benefits.

The bottom line

Clinical trials and their individual phases are a very important part of clinical research. They allow the safety and effectiveness of new drugs or treatments to be properly assessed before being approved for use in the general public.

Experimental Design

Experimental design refers to how participants are allocated to the different conditions (or IV levels) in an experiment.

Probably the commonest way to design an experiment in psychology is to divide the participants into two groups, the experimental group, and the control group, and then introduce a change to the experimental group and not the control group.

The researcher must decide how he/she will allocate their sample to these IV level. For example, if there are 10 participants, will all 10 participants take part in both conditions (e.g., repeated measures) or will the participants be split in half and take part in only one condition each?

14 Sample Size Calculation

Quality of clinical trials has improved steadily over last two decades, but certain areas in trial methodology still require special attention like in sample size calculation. The sample size is one of the basic steps in planning any clinical trial and any negligence in its calculation may lead to rejection of true findings and false results may get approval.

The determination of sample size is critical planning clinical research, because sample size is usually the most important factor determining the time and funding necessary to perform the research. The sample has a profound impact on the likelihood of finding statistical significance.

Although statisticians play a major role in sample size estimation basic knowledge regarding sample size calculation is very sparse among most of the anesthesiologists related to research including under trainee doctors. Members of committees are responsible for evaluating and funding clinical studies look closely at assumptions used to estimate the numbers of study subjects needed and at the way in which calculations of sample size is to determine whether the proposed research is realistic (e.g., whether there are adequate subjects included in the intervention and control groups in a randomized clinical trial, or in the groups of cases and controls in a case-control Study). In Clinical research sample explains sometimes apparently useful clinical results are not statistically significant.

Researchers are often surprised to find out that the answer depends on a number of factors, and they have to give the statistician some information before they can get an answer. Thus calculating the sample size for a trial requires four basic components that are following.

P VALUE OR (OR ALPHA)

Everybody is familiar with the term of P value. This is also known as level of significance and in a clinical trial investigator set an acceptable limit for P value. It may be the $P < 0.05$ is significant, it means that we are accepting that probability of difference in studying target due to chance is 5% or there are 5% chances of detection in difference when actually there was no difference exist (false positive results). This is also known as Type I error or alpha. This Type-I is inversely proportional to the sample size chosen for study.

POWER

Sometimes we may commit another type of error, that when we may fail to detect the difference when actually there is the difference. This is type of error is Type-II error that detects false negative results, exactly opposite to mentioned above where we find false positive results when actually there was no difference. To accept or reject null hypothesis by adequate power, acceptable limit for the false negative rate must be decided before conducting the study. In another term, Type II error is the probability of failing to find the difference between two study groups when actually a difference exist and it is termed as beta (β). The statistically the maximum acceptable value for β in bio-statistics is 0.20 or a 20% chance that null hypothesis is falsely accepted. The "power" of the study then is equal to ($1-\beta$) and for a β of 0.2, the power is 0.8, which is the minimum power required to accept the null hypothesis. Usually, most of clinical trial uses the power of 80% which means that we are accepting that one in five times (i.e., 20%) we will miss a real difference. The power of a study increases as the chances of committing a Type-II decreases.

THE EFFECT SIZE

Effect size (ES) is the minimal difference that investigator wants to detect between study groups and is also termed as the minimal clinical relevant difference. We can estimate the ES by three techniques that is, pilot studies, previously reported data or educated guess based on clinical experiences.

To understand the concept of ES, here we take one example. Suppose that treatment with Drug A results in a reduction of mean blood pressure (MBP) by 10 mm of Hg and with Drug B results in a reduction of MBP by 20 mm of Hg. Then, absolute ES will be 10 mm of Hg in this case. ES can be expressed as the absolute or relative difference.

As in above example, relative difference/reduction with drug intervention is 10/20 or 50%. In other word, for continuous outcome variables the ES will be numerical difference and for binary outcome e.g., effect of drug on development of stress response (yes/no), researcher should estimate a relevant difference between the event rates in both treatment groups and could choose, for instance, a difference of 10% between both the groups as ES. In statistics, the difference between the value of the variable in the control group and that in the test drug group is known as ES. Even a small change in the expected difference with treatment has a major effect on the estimated sample size, as the sample size is inversely proportional to the square of the difference. For larger ES, smaller sample size would be needed to prove the effect but for smaller ES, sample size should be large.

THE VARIABILITY

Finally for the sample size calculation, investigator need to know the population variance of a given outcome variable which is estimated using standard deviation (SD). Investigators often use an estimate obtained from information in previous studies because the variance is usually an unknown quantity. For a homogenous population, we need smaller sample size as variance or

SD will be less in this population. Suppose for studying the effect of diet program A on the weight, we include a population with weights ranging from 35 to 100 kg. Now, it is easy to understand that the SD in this group will be more and we would need a larger sample size to detect a difference between interventions, else the difference between the study groups would be concealed by the inherent difference between them because of the SD. If, on the other hand, we take a sample from a population with weights between 55 and 75 kg we would naturally get a more homogenous group, thus reducing the SD and, therefore, the sample size required will reduced. Other factors affecting the sample size calculation are dropout rate and underlying event rate in the population

DROPOUT RATE

Dropout rate means that estimate of a number of subjects those can leave out the study/clinical trial due to some personal reason or nor meeting the inclusive criteria. Normally the sample size calculation will give a number of study subjects required for achieving target statistical significance for a given hypothesis. However in clinical practice, we may need to enroll more subjects to compensate the potential dropout.

If n is the sample size required as per formula and if d is the dropout rate then adjusted sample size N1 is obtained as $N1 = n/(1\text{-}d)$.

Event Rate in Population

Prevalence rate or underlying event rate of the condition under study in population is very important while calculating sample size. It is usually estimated from previous literature. For example studying the association of smoking and brain tumour, the prevalence rate for a brain tumour in studying population should be known prior to the study. Sometimes, we have to readjust the sample size after starting the trial because of unexpectedly low event rate in the population.

Statisticians are probably consulted very frequently by investigator, because they wants know the sample size needed for a study than for a for any other reason. Before going to start any clinical trial study investigator will try to answer the main questions, they are

1. What size sample – large or small – would be needed if there was a very large variance in the outcome variable?

2. What sample would be needed if the investigator wanted the answer to be very close to the true value (i,e., have very narrow confidence limits or very small p-value)?

3. What size sample would be needed if the difference that the investigator wanteded to be able to detect was extremely small?

The factors which are affecting the sample size or subjects required for clinical trials are 1. Whether the research design involves paired data (e.g ., each subjects has a pair of observations from two points two points in time – before and after treatment) or unpaired data (e.g., observations are compared between an experimental groups and control group); 2. Whether the investigator anticipates a large or small variance in the variable of interest; 3. Whether investigator considers Type-II error or Type-I error. 5. The alpha chosen is one-sided or two-sided and 6. Whether the investigator wants to be able to detect a fairly small or extremely small difference between the means or proportions of the outcome variable.

SIZE OF THE RANDOM SAMPLE FOR SPECIFIED PRECISION

Chose a large sample from infinite large population.

Let $\bar{x}$ be the mean of large sample, and the mean of large population is $= \mu$. The $\bar{x}$ is an unbiased estimate of the population.

Let E be the permissible error in estimation of population mean μ and confidence coefficient is $(1 - \alpha)$, then we the investigator have to determine the size of sample which is written as n, such that

$$P[|\bar{x} - \mu| \leq E] = 1 - \alpha \qquad .....(1)$$

But for normal population or for large sample of any population, $\bar{x} \sim N(\mu, \sigma^2/n)$

When we chose 95% confidence coefficient, then

$$P\left[\left|\frac{\bar{x}-\mu}{\frac{\sigma}{\sqrt{n}}}\right| \leq 1.96\right] = 0.95$$

$$P\left[|\bar{x} - \mu| \leq 1.96 \frac{\sigma}{\sqrt{n}}\right] = 0.95 \qquad .....(14.1)$$

Equate 1 and 2, then

$$E = 1.96 \frac{\sigma}{\sqrt{n}}$$

$$\sqrt{n} = 1.96 \frac{\sigma}{E}$$

Squaring both side

$$n = \frac{(1.96)^2 \sigma^2}{E^2} = \frac{(Z\alpha/2)^2 \sigma^2}{E^2}$$

Similarly we can obtain the sample size, when proportional values of sample and population are known is $n = \frac{PQ(Z\alpha/2)^2}{E^2}$

When P is not known, then $n = \frac{pq(Z\alpha/2)^2}{E^2}$, where p and q proportions of success and failure of sample.

Example: In a clinical trial studies a random sample of 64 subjects are selected for study, the mean of B.P. was found to be 160 and variance is 100.

(i) Compute the 95% confidence limits for population mean

(ii) If the investigator wants in the 95% confidence, that the error in estimate of population mean should not exceed ± 1.4, how many additional number of patients are required?

Solutio: a) Given that n = 64 , $\bar{x}$(Mean) = 160 and $s^2 = 100$

$$\therefore S = \sqrt{S^2} = \sqrt{100} = 10$$

Then the confidence limits are

$$\bar{x} \pm (1.96)\frac{S}{\sqrt{n}} = 160 \pm (1.96)\frac{10}{\sqrt{64}}$$

$$= 157.55 \quad 162.45$$

(b) To find n, given that E = ±1.4

$$\therefore \quad E^2 = (1.4)^2 = 1.96$$

$$n = \frac{(Z\alpha/2)^2 s^2}{E^2}$$

$$n = \frac{(1.96)^2 10^2}{1.4^2} = 196$$

Hence the additional number of patients required = 196 – 64 = 132.

Steps in the Calculation of Sample Size:

The first step in calculating sample size to choose the appropriate formula to use , based on the type of study and the type of error to be considered. Four common formulas for calculating sample size are as listed below

1. Whenever paired t-test is applied to know the level of significance difference between and after treatment of subjects using a particular drug in clinical trials.

$$n = \frac{(Z\alpha)^2 s^2}{d^2}$$

   $Z\alpha$=Gaussian Value, s= Standard deviation of the before – after difference and n is the sample size.

   If the level of significance is %5 and Type-I error is considered, then $Z\alpha$ is taken as 1.96 and for 1% level of significance $Z\alpha$ is considered as 2.58.

2. If we are applying randomized controlled trials with one experimental group and one control group and type-I error is considered , then n = $\frac{(Z\alpha)^2 2 s^2}{d^2}$, since the investigator selects two groups of subjects (Experimental and Controlled) for the clinical trial studies, then the numerator value should be multiplied by 2.

3. If we are applying randomized controlled trials with one experimental group and one control group and type-I error(α) and Type-II(β) are considered , then n = $\frac{(Z\alpha+Z\beta)^2 2 s^2}{d^2}$, since the investigator selects two groups of subjects (Experimental and Controlled) for the clinical trial studies, then the numerator value should be multiplied by 2.

4. If we are applying randomized controlled trials for proportional values with one experimental group and one control group and type-I error(α) and Type-II error (β) are considered, then n = $\frac{(Z\alpha+Z\beta)^2 2 (\bar{p})(1-\bar{p})}{d^2}$, since the investigator selects two groups of subjects (Experimental and Controlled) for the clinical trial studies, then the numerator value should be multiplied by 2. In case proportional the proportion of patient who survive for 6 years, the variance is easier to calculate. The investigator need to estimate only the proportion that would survive 6 years with the new treatment (which is p1 and that is taken as 60%) and proportion expected to survive with control group's treatment (which is p2 and that is taken

as 40%). If we consider two study groups are of approximately same size, then the investigator must obtain the average (mean) survival in the combined group that will written as $\bar{p}$ *that will* = 50% if both the study groups are equal in size.

Example 1: Clinical trial study was using an antihypertensive drug to see the effect that drug in reducing systolic blood pressure and standard deviation s = 15mm Hg. The 5% (type-I Error-α) level of significance, with two tail has been considered and average of the difference between before and after treatment is 10 mm HG. Calculate the sample size needed for this clinical trial study.

Solution: Equation is n = $\dfrac{(Z\alpha)^2 s^2}{d^2}$ = $\dfrac{(1.96)^2\, 15^2}{10^2}$ = 8.64 = 9

Only nine subjects are needed for this study, because each paired subject serves as his or her own control in a before and after study. When the estimated value of n is a fraction, then n should be rounded up to the safe.

Example 2:

Clinical trial study was using an antihypertensive drug to see the effect that drug in reducing systolic blood pressure between treatment group and control group, the combined standard deviation between these two groups is 15mm Hg. The 5% (type-I Error-α) level of significance, with two tail has been considered and average of the difference between treatment and control is 10 mm HG. Calculate the sample size needed for this clinical trial study.

Solution: Equation is n = $\dfrac{(Z\alpha)^2 2*s^2}{d^2}$ = $\dfrac{(1.96)^2 *2*15^2\, 15}{10^2}$ = 17.28 = 18

$$= 18 \text{ subjects per group x } 2 = 36 \text{ subjects}$$

Example 3:

Clinical trial study was using an antihypertensive drug to see the effect that drug in reducing systolic blood pressure between treatment group and control group, the combined standard deviation between these two groups is 15mm Hg. The 5% (type-I Error-α and Type-II Error – β) level of significance, with two tail has been considered and average of the difference between treatment and control is 10 mm HG. Calculate the sample size needed for this clinical trial study.

Solution: Equation is n = $\dfrac{(Z\alpha+z\beta)^2 2*s^2}{d^2}$ = $\dfrac{(1.96+0.84)^2\, 2*15^2}{10^2}$ = 35.28 = 36

$$= 36 \text{ subjects per group x } 2 = 72 \text{ subjects}$$

Example 4: In measuring reaction time, a psychologist estimates that the standard deviation is of 0.95 sec. How large a sample of measurements must be taken in order to be 95% that the error of his estimate of mean will not exceed 0.01 sec?

Solution: The equation is n = $\dfrac{(Z\alpha)^2 s^2}{d^2}$ = $\dfrac{(1.96)^2\, 0.95^2}{0.01^2}$ = 96

Effect size is a standard measure that can be calculated from any number of statistical outputs. *Recall from the Correlation review r can be interpreted as an effect size using the same guidelines. If you are comparing groups, you don't need to calculate Cohen's d. If you are asked for effect size, it is r.

Sample Size required per Group When using t-test to compare Means of Continuous Variables

Effect size equations. To calculate the standardized mean difference between two groups, subtract the mean of one group from the other (M1 – M2) and divide the result by the standard deviation (SD) of the population from which the groups were sampled.

EFFECT SIZE EQUATIONS

The standardized mean difference (*d*)

To calculate the standardized mean difference between two groups, subtract the mean of one group from the other (M1 – M2) and divide the result by the standard deviation (SD) of the population from which the groups were sampled. If the population standard deviation is unknown, we can estimate it in different ways. Three different methods for estimating the population standard deviation give rise to three of the better-known effect size indexes, as follows:

$$\text{Cohen's } d = \frac{M_1 - M_2}{SD_{Pooled}}$$

$$\text{Glass's } \Delta = \frac{M_1 - M_2}{SD_{Control}}$$

$$\text{Hedges' } g = \frac{M_1 - M_2}{SD \times Pooled}$$

Sample size required per group when using t-test to compare means of continuous variables

Sample Size per group for Comparing two means

| One-Sided α = | 0.005 | | | 0.025 | | | 0.05 | | |
| Two-Sided α = | 0.01 | | | 0.05 | | | 0.10 | | |
E/S* β =	0.05	0.10	0.20	0.05	0.10	0.20	0.05	0.10	0.20
0.10	3565	2978	2338	2600	2103	1571	2166	1714	1238
0.15	1586	1325	1040	1157	935	699	963	762	551
0.20	893	746	586	651	527	394	542	429	310
0.25	572	474	376	417	338	253	347	275	199
0.30	398	33	262	290	235	176	242	191	139
0.40	225	188	148	164	133	100	136	108	78
0.50	145	121	96	105	86	64	88	70	51
0.60	101	85	67	74	60	45	61	49	36
0.70	75	63	50	55	44	34	45	36	26
0.80	58	49	39	42	34	25	35	28	21
0.90	46	39	21	34	27	21	28	22	14
1.0	38	32	26	27	23	17	23	18	14

Sample Size Required per Group when Using the Chi-Squared Statistic or Z test to Compare Proportions of Dichotomous Variables

Sample Size per Group for Comparing Two Proportions

Upper number: α=0.05(One-sided) or α = 0.10 (Two-sided); β=0.20

Middle number: α=0.025(One-sided) or α = 0.05 (Two-sided); β=0.20

Lower number: α=0.025(One-sided) or α = 0.05 (Two-sided); β=0.10

Difference Between P1 and P2

Smaller of P1 and P2	0.05	0.10	0.15	0.20	0.25	0.30	0.35	0.40	0.45	0.50
0.05	381	129	72	47	35	27	22	18	15	13
	473	159	88	59	43	33	26	22	18	16
	620	267	113	75	54	41	33	27	23	19
0.10	578	175	91	58	41	31	24	20	16	14
	724	219	112	72	51	37	29	24	20	17
	958	296	146	92	65	48	37	30	25	21
0.15	751	217	108	67	46	34	26	21	17	15
	944	270	139	82	57	41	32	26	21	18
	1252	354	174	106	73	53	42	33	26	22

Table *contd...*

Smaller of P1 and P2	0.05	0.10	0.15	0.20	0.25	0.30	0.35	0.40	0.45	0.50
0.20	900	251	121	74	50	36	28	22	18	15
	1133	313	151	91	62	44	34	27	22	18
	1540	412	197	118	80	57	44	34	27	23
0.25	1024	278	132	79	53	38	29	23	18	15
	1289	348	165	98	66	47	35	28	22	18
	1714	459	216	127	85	60	46	35	28	23
0.30	1123	300	141	83	55	39	29	23	18	15
	1415	376	175	103	68	48	36	28	22	18
	1893	496	230	134	88	62	47	36	28	23
0.35	1197	315	146	85	56	39	29	23	18	15
	1509	395	182	106	69	48	36	28	22	18
	2009	522	239	138	90	62	47	35	27	23
0.40	1246	325	149	86	56	39	29	22	17	14
	1572	407	186	107	69	48	35	27	21	17
	2093	538	244	139	90	62	46	34	26	21
0.45	1271	328	149	85	55	38	28	21	16	13
	1603	411	186	106	68	47	34	26	20	16
	2135	543	244	138	88	60	44	33	25	19
0.50	1271	325	146	83	53	36	26	20	15	--
	1603	407	182	103	66	44	32	24	18	--
	2135	538	239	134	85	57	42	30	23	--
0.55	1246	315	141	79	50	34	24	18	--	--
	1572	395	175	98	62	41	29	22	--	--
	2093	522	230	127	80	53	37	27	--	--
0.60	1197	300	132	74	46	31	22	--	--	--
	1509	376	165	91	57	37	26	--	--	--
	2009	496	216	118	73	48	33	--	--	--
0.65	1123	278	121	67	41	27	--	--	--	--
	1415	438	151	82	51	33	--	--	--	--
	1883	459	197	106	65	41	--	--	--	--

Table *contd...*

Smaller of P1 and P2	0.05	0.10	0.15	0.20	0.25	0.30	0.35	0.40	0.45	0.50
0.70	1024	251	108	58	35	--	--	--	--	--
	1289	313	133	72	43	--	--	--	--	--
	1714	412	174	92	54	--	--	--	--	--
0.75	900	217	91	47	--	--	--	--	--	--
	1133	270	112	59	--	--	--	--	--	--
	1504	354	146	75	--	--	--	--	--	--
0.80	751	175	72	--	--	--	--	--	--	--
	944	219	88	--	--	--	--	--	--	--
	1252	286	113	--	--	--	--	--	--	--
0.85	578	129	--	--	--	--	--	--	--	--
	724	159	--	--	--	--	--	--	--	--
	958	207	--	--	--	--	--	--	--	--
0.90	381	--	--	--	--	--	--	--	--	--
	473	--	--	--	--	--	--	--	--	--
	620	--	--	--	--	--	--	--	--	--

Sample Size for determining whether a correlation coefficient differs from zero

One Sided α=	0.005			0.025			0.05		
Two-Sided α=	0.01			0.05			0.0101		
β=	0.05	0.10	0.20	0.05	0.10	0.20	0.05	0.10	0.20
r									
0.05	7118	5947	4663	5193	4200	3134	4325	3424	2469
0.10	1773	1481	1162	1294	1047	782	1078	854	616
0.15	783	655	514	572	463	346	477	378	273
0.20	436	365	287	319	259	194	266	211	153
0.25	276	231	182	202	164	123	169	134	98
0.30	189	158	125	139	113	85	116	92	67
0.35	136	114	90	100	82	62	84	67	49
0.40	102	86	68	75	62	47	63	51	37
0.45	79	66	53	58	48	36	49	39	29
0.50	62	52	42	46	38	29	39	31	23
0.60	40	34	27	30	25	19	26	21	16
0.70	27	23	19	20	17	13	17	14	11
0.80	18	15	13	14	12	9	12	10	8

The general equation that can be used to obtain sample size when coefficient of correlation r is known is $N = \left(\frac{z\alpha + Z\beta}{C}\right)^2 + 3$

N = Total number of subjects required and C = 0.5*ln[(1 + r)/(1 − r)]

For estimating the sample size when we are going verify the level of difference between two correlation coefficients r1 and r2, then the sample size can be obtained by using the equation

$$N = \left(\frac{z\alpha + Z\beta}{C1 - C2}\right)^2 + 3$$

$C_1 = 0.5\text{*ln}[(1 + r_1)/(1 − r_1)]$

$C_2 = 0.5\text{*ln}[(1 + r_2)/(1 − r_2)]$

Sample Size for a descriptive study of a continuous variable

Sample Size form for common values of W/S

W/S	90%	95%	99%
0.10	1083	1537	2665
0.15	482	683	1180
0.20	271	385	664
0.25	174	246	425
0.30	121	171	295
0.35	89	126	217
0.40	66	97	166
0.50	44	62	107
0.60	31	43	74
0.70	23	32	55
0.80	17	25	42
0.90	14	19	33
1.0	11	16	27

The Value of W/S is taken as standardized width of the confidence interval, where W is difference of the means and S is standard deviation of the sample, then the sample size can be obtained by using the equation $N = \frac{(Z\alpha)^2 s^2}{W^2}$.

Sample Size for a Descriptive study of a Dichotomous Variable

Upper Number: 90% Confidence level

Middle Number: 95% confidence level

Lower number: 99% confidence level

Total Width of Confidence interval (W)

Expected Proportion(P)	0.10	0.15	0.20	0.25	0.30	0.35	0.40
0.10	98	44					
	138	61					
	239	106					
0.15	139	62	35	22			
	196	87	49	31			
	339	151	85	54			
0.20	174	77	44	28	19	14	
	246	109	61	39	27	20	
	426	189	107	68	47	35	
0.25	204	91	51	33	23	17	13
	288	128	72	46	32	24	18
	499	222	125	80	55	41	31
0.30	229	102	57	37	25	19	14
	323	143	81	52	36	26	20
	559	249	140	89	62	46	35
0.40	261	116	65	42	29	21	16
	369	164	92	59	41	30	23
	639	284	160	102	71	52	40
0.50	272	121	68	44	30	22	17
	384	171	96	61	43	31	24
	666	296	166	107	74	54	42

To estimate the sample size, one has to read the expected proportion (P) of the interested variables and the desired confidence interval width. The sample size can be considered for 90%, 95% and 99% confidence levels.

The general that can be used to calculate sample size for the values P, W and confidence level $(1 - \alpha)$ is

$$N = \frac{4z_{\alpha}^{2}P(1-P)}{W^2}$$

Where P – Proportional Value and W – width of the confidence interval

Zα Gaussian Value for two sided test α, $(1-\alpha)$ is the confidence level. Here Zα is I, 96 for 95% confidence level and 2.58 for 99% confidence level.

15 Graphs

GRAPHS OF FREQUENCY DISTRIBUTION

The theoretical meaning of graph is the pictorial representation of data which has been collected and tabulated in table. The frequency distribution graphs are designed to reveal more effectively the characteristic features of a frequency data. Such types of graphs are more appealing to the eye and are more perceptible to the mind than the data which are written in table. The most commonly used graphs in clinical studies and Pharmaceutical industries are

a. Histogram b. Frequency Polygon c. Frequency curve d, Ogive e. E. Semilog graph, f. Pie chart, g. Stem and leaf graph etc.

HISTOGRAM

It is one of the most popular and commonly used device for constructing graph of continuous frequency distribution. The can be considered as a useful presentation of a frequency table.

The frequency or proportion of observations in each class-interval is plotted as a rectangle. For the construction of Histogram, class-interval should be of equal width. Each class-interval drawn on X-axis and by a section (base of the rectangle) which is equal to the magnitude of the clas-interval. On each class-interval (as base) series of rectangles are erected with corresponding frequency of each interval as height of rectangles. The series of adjacent rectangles (one for each class) so formed gives the histogram of the frequency distribution and its area represents the total frequency of the distribution as distributed throughout the different classes.

The choice of interval for histogram depends on the nature of data, the distribution of data and what purpose we are presenting the data in the form of graph.

Example: The frequency distribution of heights of 30 patients in centimetre is as listed below. Construct histogram for the given data.

Height in cms Class – Interval		Number of Patients f
139	149	6
149	159	9
159	169	7
169	179	5
179	189	2
189	199	1
		30

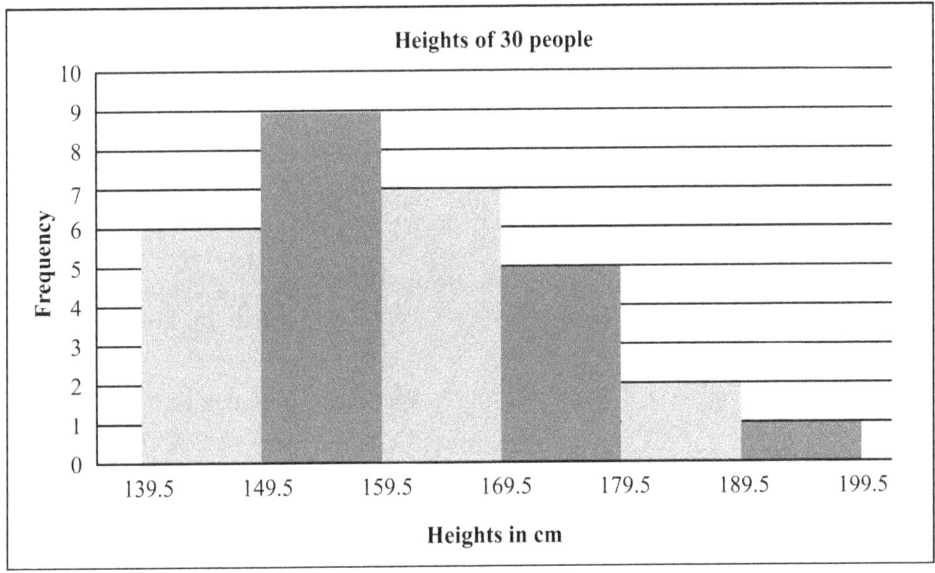

2. Frequency Polygon

The frequency polygon is another method for presentation of data of the frequency distribution like continuous and discrete series. For grouped or continuous frequency distribution, may be drawn in two methods.

Method 1: After the construction of histogram for the given continuous frequency distribution, the mid-points of the tops (Upper horizontal sides) of the adjacent rectangles of the histogram by straight line graph. Then the graph obtained by joining those mid-points is called as a frequency polygon. After the construction of the frequency polygon some portion of a triangular strip lies outside the frequency polygon of some rectangles, but at the same time, another triangular strip of the same area which outside the histogram will be included under the polygon. The area of the frequency polygon is equal to the area of the frequency distribution.

Method 2: The frequency polygon of a continuous frequency distribution can also be constructed by joining the frequencies of different classes (along Y-axis) against the mid-values of the corresponding classes (along x-axis) by series of straight lines between each intervals.

Class - Interval		Mid values	F Frequency
0	20	10	1
20	40	30	6
40	60	50	16
60	80	70	30
80	100	90	40
100	120	110	40
120	140	130	15
140	160	150	2

OGIVE

(Cumulative Frequency Plot or Graph)

Ogive is a graphical presentation of cumulative frequency distribution of continuous series. In this method the cumulative frequency values will be plotted on Y-axis and the class boundaries along X-axis.

The ogive can be classified as 1. Less than ogive and 2. More than ogive

LESS THAN OGIVE

This method consists of plotting downward or less than cumulative frequency against the upper or more than values of each class-interval. The points so obtained are joined by a smooth curve. The less than is an increasing curve, sloping upwards from left to right and the shape that will be elongated S – Shape.

Cholesterol Level(mg/100 ml)		Number of men
80	120	13
120	160	20
160	200	50
200	240	100
240	280	37
280	320	20
320	360	10

More Than Values	Downward cf
80	13
120	33
160	83
200	183
240	220
280	240
320	250

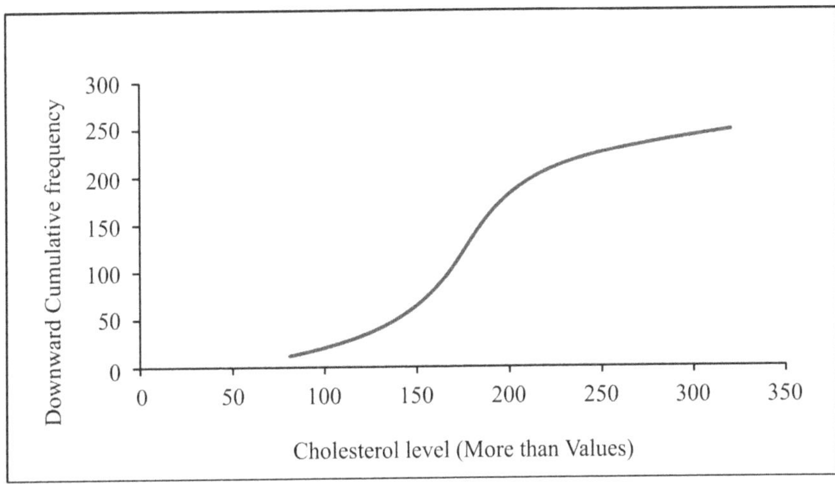

Less than Ogive Curve

More than Ogive: The more than ogive graph constructed by plotting more than cumulative or upward cumulative frequency on Y-axis against lower limit or boundary of respective class interval.

The more than ogive is a decreasing curve and slopes downwards from left to right and has the shape of elongated S upside down.

Less than Values	Upward cf
120	250
160	237
200	217
240	167
280	67
320	30
360	10

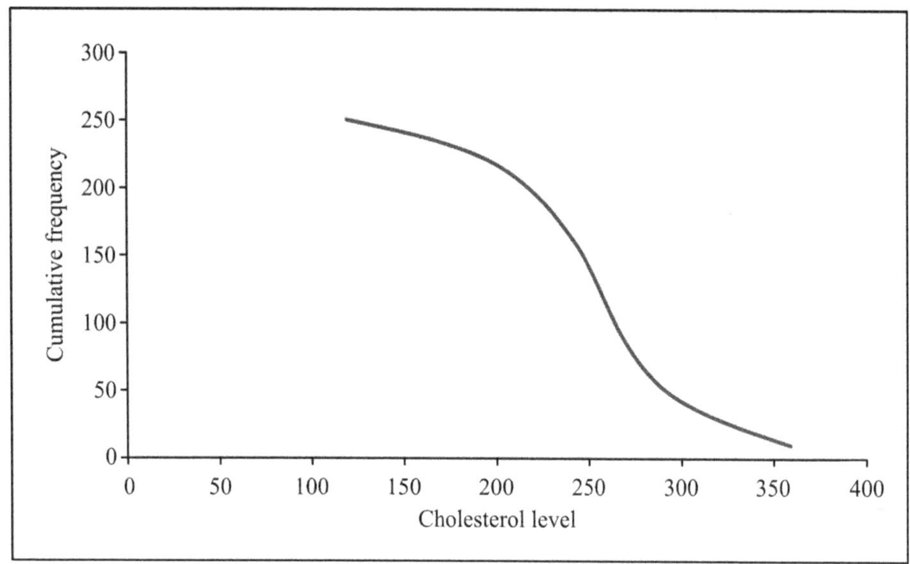

More than Ogive Curve

PIE CHART

Pie Charts are popular ways of presenting categorical data. The pie or circle represents 100% or all of the results. Here circle will be divided into different sections or segments, they are also called as sectors representing certain proportions or percentage of various component parts to the total. Such a sub-divided circle diagram is known as Pie-chart or Pie – diagram.

These charts are frequently used in pharmaceutical industry to present the scientific data in appropriate circumstances.

Example: A batch of tablets were shown to have 70% with no defects, 15% slightly chipped, 10% are discoloured and 5% are dirty. Construct the Pie chart

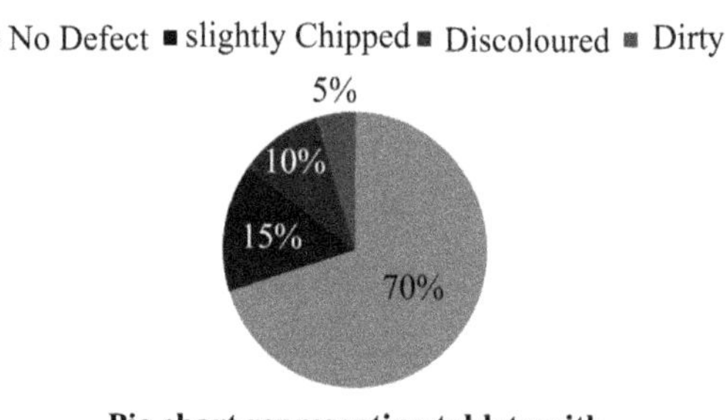

**Pie chart representing tablets with
different conditions**

SEMI-LOG GRAPH

In general to construct graph we use natural scale in which equal distances represent equal absolute magnitude on both of the axes. But in case of phenomena under study increase or decrease in the value of the variable is very rapid. In such a situation we are primarily we focus on the study of relative changes rather than the absolute changes. When we encounter these type of problems, semi-logarithmic or logarithmic or ratio scale graph used to highlight or emphasize relative changes. In Pharmaceutical and medical science, a **semi-log graph** or **semi-log plot** is a way of visualizing data that are related according to an exponential relationship. One **axis** is plotted on a **logarithmic** scale. The type of curve which obtained by plotting absolute scale on X-axis and logarithmic values on Y-axis is called as Semi-logarithmic graph. Many experiments in the pharmaceutical studies, the results of the data when is taken in logarithm, that will relate to the independent variable X. Semi-logarithmic graph paper has the usual absolute or natural scale on X-axis and logarithmic scale on Y-axis. In this graph the equal interval represent ratio. This graph is most useful in the first-order kinetic process, often apparent in drug degradation and pharmacokinetic systems, there exist a linear relationship when the investigator plots log(C) on Y-axis and time on X-axis (Absolute scale or arithmetic scale).

The first order kinetic equation can be written as $\log(C) = \log(C_0) - \dfrac{kt}{2.303}$ where C is concentration of drug at time t-hour and Co is concentration of drug when time is zero hour

Shape of the curve on semi-logarithmic scale and natural Scale:

1. The values of data under study is increasing by a constant amount (difference between different interval of time is constant) will give a straight line rising upward when the data is plotted on natural scale, but when same data plotted on semi-logarithmic scale graph, we will get an upward rising curve. The slope of the curve will be steadily decreasing. That indicates that the decreasing rate is very steady. The curve is concave to the base.

Example: 1 The concentration of drug in solution, which is measured as a function of time is as listed below. Construct the graph on natural scale and also semi-logarithmic scale graph

Time(Weeks)	Concentration	Log(Concentration)
0	0	0
2	10	1
4	20	1.30
6	30	1.48
8	40	1.60
10	50	1.70

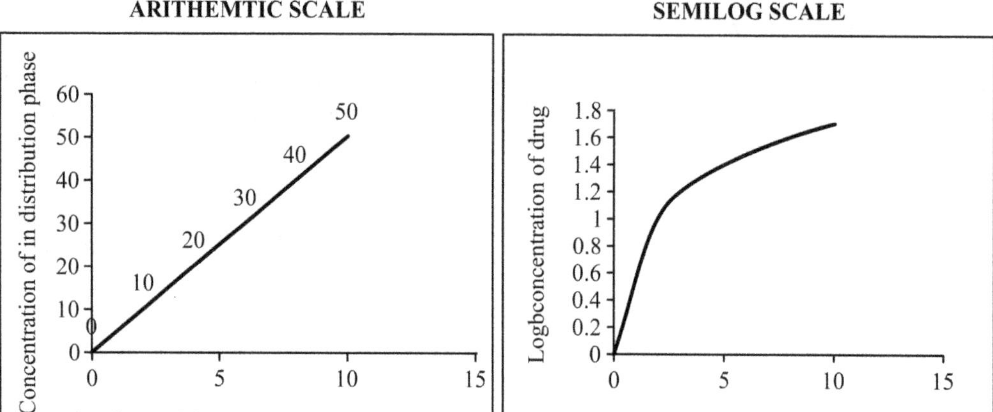

2. The values of data under study is increasing by a constant rate (the ratio between the phenomenon under study at different interval of time is constant) will give a curve convex to the base when data plotted on natural scale and the slope of the curve will be steadily increasing. The same data when they are plotted on semi-logarithmic scale graph, we will get an upward rising straight line.

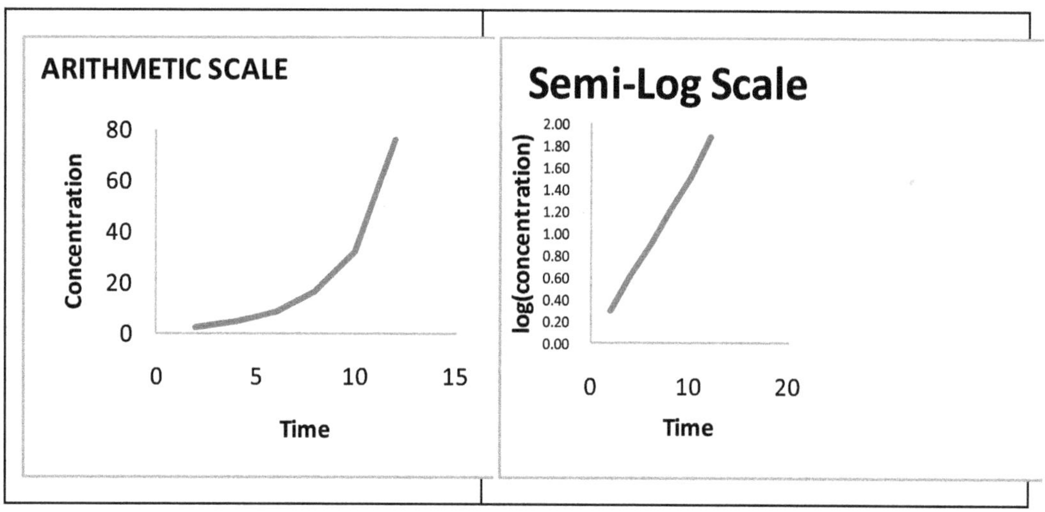

3. The values of data under study is decreasing by a constant amount (difference between different interval of time is constant) will give a straight line falling downward when the data is plotted on natural scale, but when same data are plotted on semi-logarithmic scale graph, we will get an downward falling curve to the right. The slope of the curve will be steadily increasing.

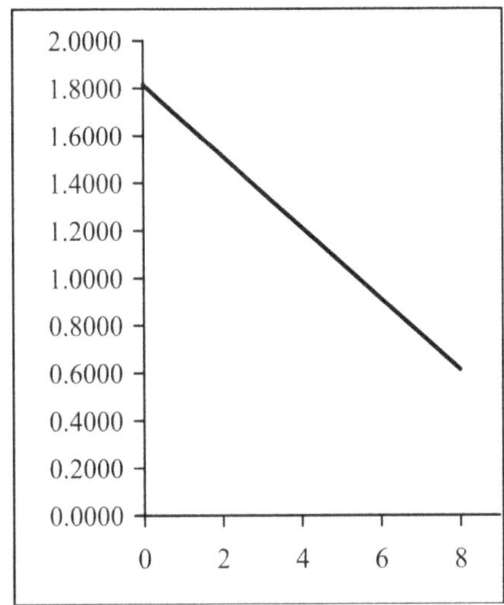

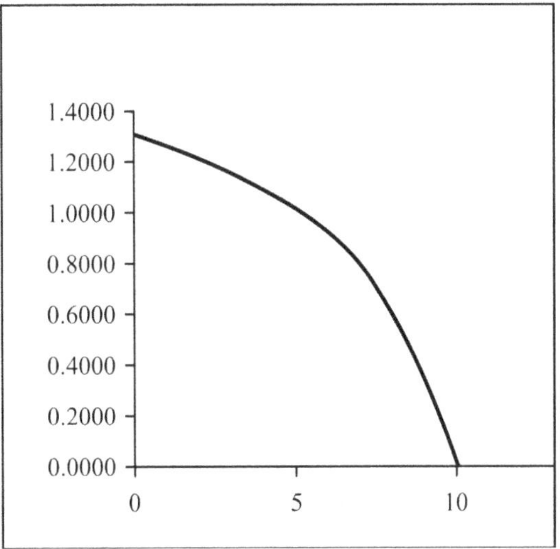

4. The values of data under study is decreasing by a constant rate (the ratio between the phenomenon under study at different interval of time is constant) will give a curve moving downwards with a declining slope when data are plotted on natural scale, but when same data are plotted on semi-logarithmic scale graph, we will get a straight line moving downward.

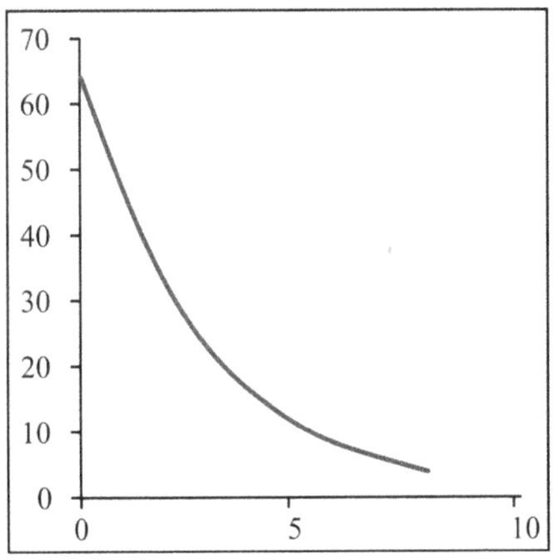

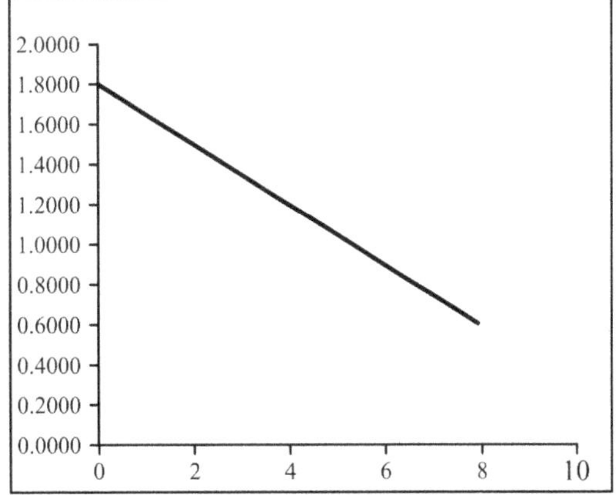

The general format of semi-log graph sheet

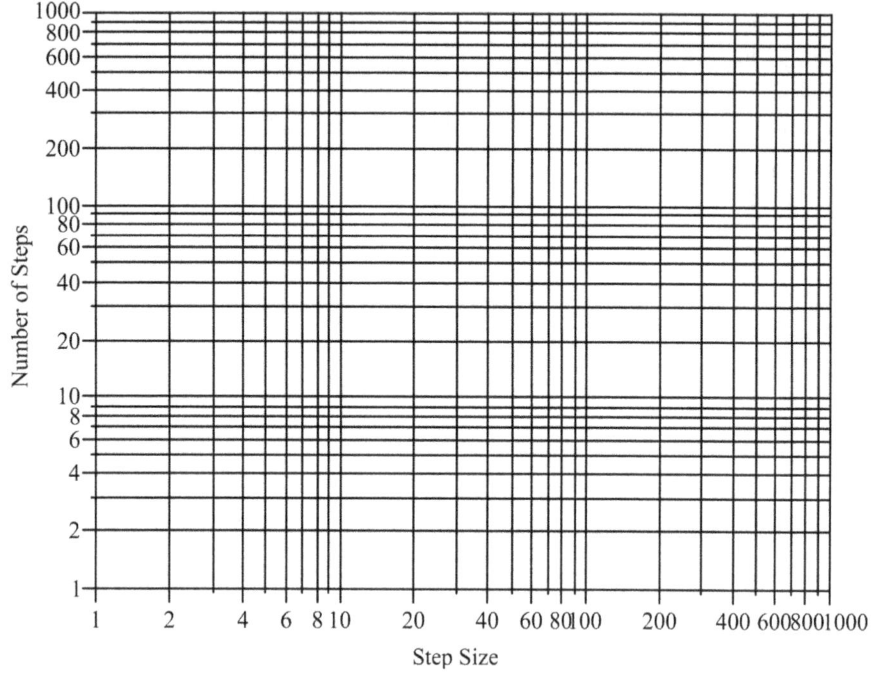

Interpretation of Semi-logarithmic or Ratio Curves

1. If the curve is rising upwards, the rate of growth of phenomenon under study is increasing positively and if curve falls downward that indicates rate of growth phenomenon is decreasing

2. If the curve is nearly a straight line which is moving upward, indicates the rate of change of phenomenon under study is more or less constant. Similarly , if the curve is nearly a straight line and moving downward indicates that the rate of change of phenomenon is decreasing at a uniform rate.

3. If the curve rises (falls) steeply at one point of time, than any another point of time, indicates that there is a rapid rate of increase or decrease at that point of time than any other point of time

4. If two curves of different data on the same semi-logarithmic graph are parallel to each other, then they represent equal percentage of change between both the phenomenon under study.

5. If the first is steeper than the second curve on the same ratio chart, that indicates, the changing rate first is faster than the second

Example:

A 3 year old, 15 kg patient was brought in for surgery and was given a 100 mcg/kg iv bolus injection of a muscle relaxant. The plasma concentrations were measured post injection and noted in the table below. Construct a semi-log graph

Time (h)	Plasma Conc. (mcg/L)
0.5	100
1	85
3	57
5	37
7	22

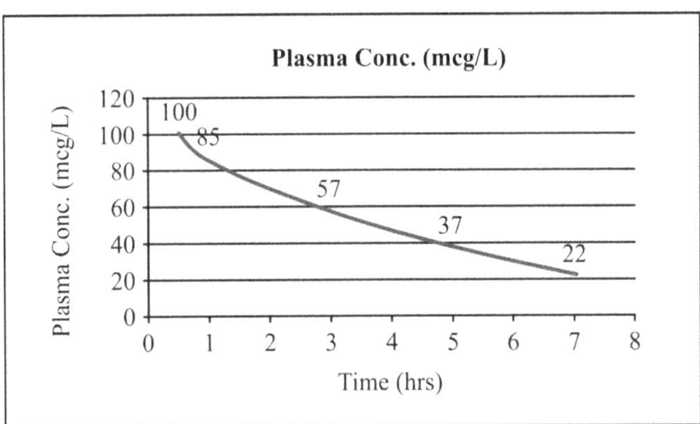

Stem-and – Leaf Diagrams

A stem-and-leaf diagram is a graphical representation in which the data points are grouped in such a way that we can see the shape of the distribution while retaining the individual values of the data points. It is more useful for small data.

A stem-and-leaf diagram consists of a series of rows of numbers. The number used to label a row is called as a stem and other numbers in the row are called as leaves.

Example: The age of 27 patients who have chosen for a pilot study is as listed below. Construct stem-and-leaf diagram for the same data.

SLNO	1	2	3	4	5	6	7	8	9	10	11	12	13	14	15	16	17	18
AGE	20	23	18	29	35	37	29	41	45	50	53	55	60	48	39	47	58	60

1	1	8
2	2	0 3 9 9
3	3	5 7 9
4	4	1 5 7 8
5	5	0 3 5 8
6	6	0 0
	Stems	Leafs

This device is not practicable for use with larger data sets, because stems are too longs

Exercise 1: The area under the curve $(AUC_{0\to\infty})$ First start by getting the concentration at constant time intervals say 0, 4, 8, 12, 16, and 20 hrs. Construct semi-log graph.

Time (hrs)	Concentration (mcg/L)
0	110
4	50
8	22
12	10
16	5
20	2

CUBIC GRAPH

In the mathematical field of graph theory, a cubic graph is a graph in which all vertices have degree three. In other words, a cubic graph is a 3-regular graph. Cubic graphs are also called trivalent graphs.

Cube plots can be used to show the relationship between factors and a response. Each cube can show three factors. If there are only two factors, Minitab displays a square plot. Minitab draws as many cubes as necessary to show up to eight factors. You can draw a cube plot for two types of means:

Data means - the means of the response variable for the combinations of factor levels that are in the design.

Fitted means - after you analyze the design for a response, you can plot the fitted means for all combinations of factor levels.

Data Means versus Fitted Means

Data means are the average of the raw data.

Fitted means are the means for each factor level or combination of factor levels that you would expect to get if your design were balanced.

To calculate the fitted means:

1 Find the fitted value for every possible combination of factor levels (or cell) when all covariates are set at their overall mean.

2 Using only one fitted value per cell, find the average of the fitted values from step 1 for each factor level or combination of factor levels. These averages are the least squares means.

For a balanced design with no covariates, the fitted mean for each factor level or combination of factor levels is the same as the average of the response values for that level or combination.

Note: You can create a cube plot with or without a response measure. Viewing the factors without the response allows you to see what a design looks like.

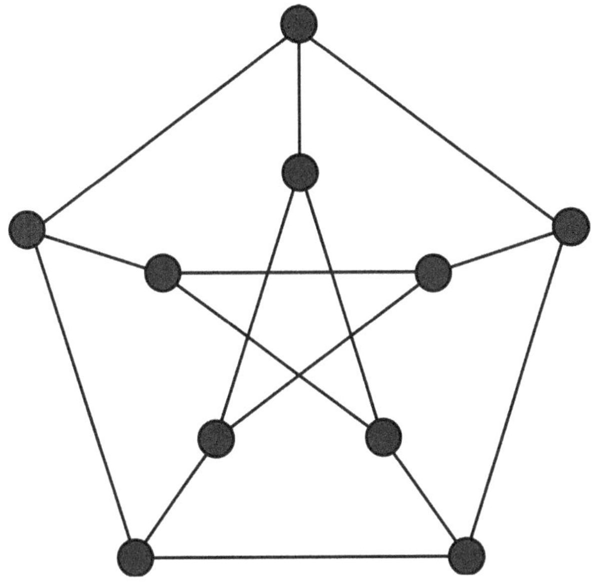

CONTOUR PLOT / GRAPH:

The contour plot is a two-dimensional (2D) representation of the response plotted against combinations of numeric factors and/or mixture components. It can show the relationship between the responses, mixture components and/or numeric factors.

A contour plot is a graphical technique for representing a 3-dimensional surface by plotting constant z slices, called contours, on a 2-dimensional format. That is, given a value for z, lines are drawn for connecting the (x, y) coordinates where that z value occurs.

A contour line (also isoline, isopleth, or isarithm) of a function of two variables is a curve along which the function has a constant value, so that the curve joins points of equal value. The contour interval of a contour map is the difference in elevation between successive contour lines.

Calculating Contour Intervals

A map's legend usually identifies the contour interval on the map, but sometimes only part of a map is available. Knowing how to calculate the contour interval becomes a useful skill.

On most maps, every fifth contour line, shown as a heavier or darker line, is an index line or index contour. These index lines will be marked with their elevation. Find the elevations of two adjacent index lines. The higher number shows the uphill elevation. Find the difference between the two elevations. For example, if the uphill elevation equals 1,000 feet above mean sea level and the lower elevation equals 800 feet above mean sea level, the difference in elevation equals 200 feet.

To calculate the contour interval, start by counting the contour lines from one index line to the next index line. Maps usually count five contour lines from one index line to the next, including that next index line. As when counting from one number to the next, like from five to 10, start with the next line up from the index line, counting each contour line up to and including the next index line.

To find the elevation interval between contour lines, divide the elevation difference between index lines by the number of contour lines from one index line to the next. In the example above, the distance, 200, is divided by the number of lines, 5. The contour interval equals $200 \div 5 = 40$, or 40-foot contour intervals. If, on the other hand, the elevation difference between index lines had been 100 feet, the contour interval would be $100 \div 5 = 20$, or a 20-foot contour interval.

Example 1: Construct a Contour and Cubic Graph graphs for the input and response data which are listed in the table

TRAIL	LIPID	SURFACTENT	TIME	RESPONSE (Y)
1	1	0.5	5	123
2	2.5	1.5	5	176
3	1	0.5	10	131.8
4	2.5	1.5	10	133
5	1	1.5	5	170
6	2.5	0.5	5	497
7	2.5	0.5	10	388.8
8	1	1.5	10	219

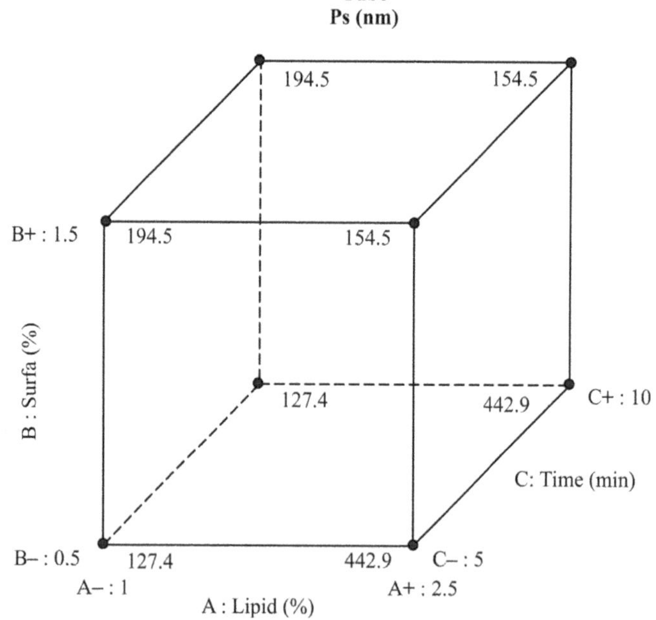

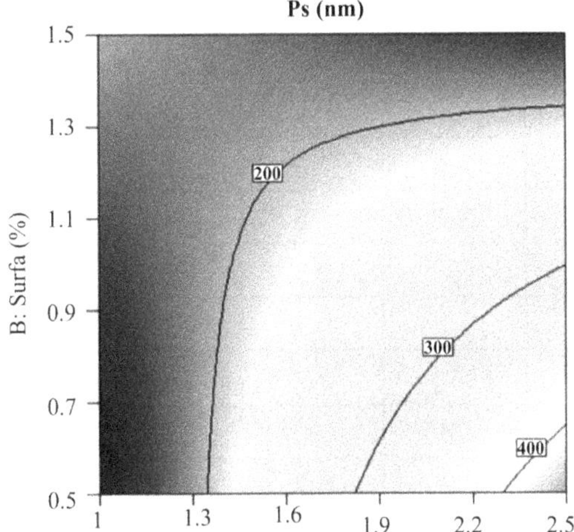

Example 2: Composition of mixture of ethanol, propylone glycol and water and solubility of compound in these mixture at 20^0C is as listed below. Construct Contour Graph

Mixture	Ethanol	Propylene Glycol	Water	Solubility
1	0	0	0	6.1
2	0	1	0	3.3
3	0	0	1	1.1
4	0.5	0	0.5	2.6
5	0.5	0.5	0	4.6
6	0	0.5	0.5	2.3
7	0.33	0.33	0.33	1.7
8	0.67	0.17	0.17	3.6
9	0.17	0.67	0.17	3.3
10	0.17	0.17	0.67	1.3

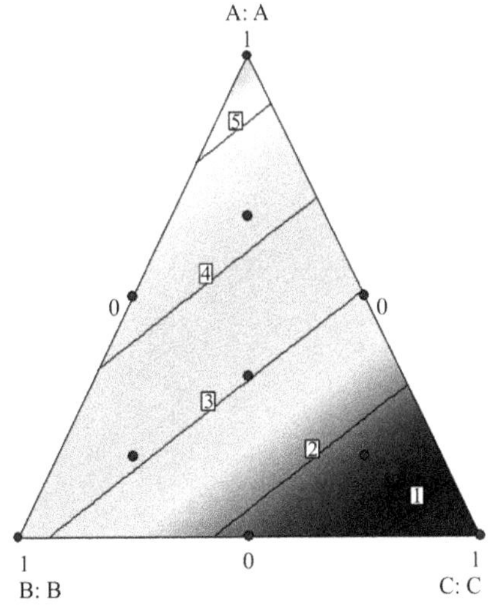

Example 3: Construct a Cubic Graph for the data which is tabulated as follows

Trials	Factor A	Factor B	Factor C	Factor D	Factor E	Response
1	6	2.4	7.3	27.8	0.01	40
2	6	3.2	8.8	29.4	0.01	40
3	6	5	9.5	28.4	0.01	50
4	6	6.2	9.1	28.7	0.01	50
5	6	16.6	9.7	28.2	0.01	70
6	6	48	9	28.8	0.01	30
7	6	4927	8.2	23.3	0.01	40
8	6	7382	8.6	23.1	0.01	60
9	6	113.384	10.5	22.8	0.01	80
10	9	136	8.1	24.4	0.01	30

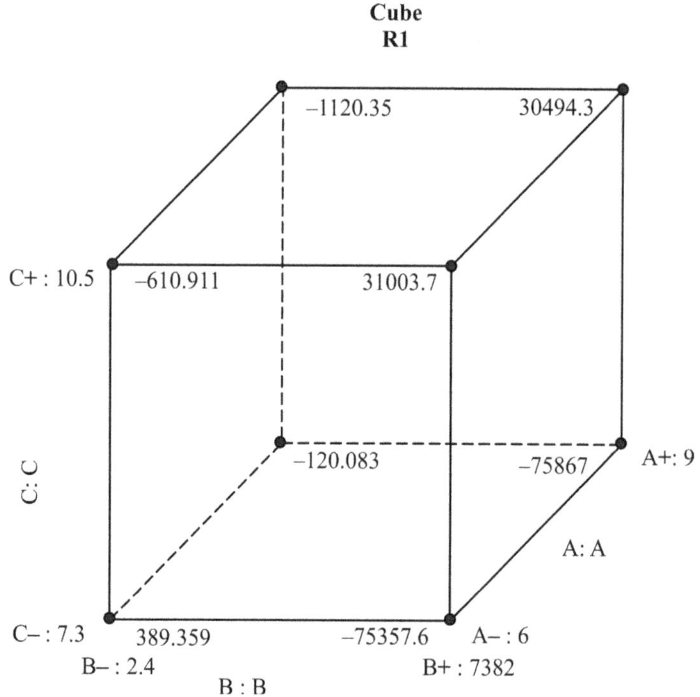

Statistical Package for the Social Sciences

It is a comprehensive and flexible statistical analysis and data management tool. It is one of the most popular statistical package which can perform highly complex data manipulation and analysis with ease. It is designed for both interactive and non interactive users.

Features of SPSS

1. It is easy for you to learn and use
2. SPSS includes a lot of data management system and editing tools
3. It offers you in-depth statistical capabilities
4. It offers an excellent plotting, reporting and presentation features
5. Here are few key points why SPSS is considered the best tool to use
6. Effective data management
7. SPSS in data analysis easier and quicker for you as the program knows the location of the cases and the variables. It reduces the manual work of the user to a great extent
8. Wide range of options
9. SPSS offers a wide range of methods, graphs and charts to you. It also comes with better screening and cleaning option of the information as a preparation for further analysis.
10. Wide range of options
11. In SPSS the output is kept separate from the data itself. It stores the data in a separate file.

Variable View

It is the sheet where you define the Variable of the Data that you have, The Variable View Consists of the Following Column heading,

Name : Enter the Unique Identifiable and Sorting Variable Name, Eg: In the Data of Students, The Variables can be ID, Sex, Age, Class, Etc, Note : This will not allow any special character or Space while describing the variables of the Data, and Once you enter the First Variable, Immediately you can see SPSS generating all the other information regarding how you want to set that Variable that you have entered to be,

Type : You can change the Type of Variable, Whether Numeric, Alphabets or Alpha Numeric by selecting the respective Type in this column, this will restrict the use of any other type being used under this variable column

Width: Defines the Character Width this Variable Should allow, Especially helpful while entering Mobile number which allow only 10 character

Decimal: Defines the Decimal point the you required to display, Eg: Used in case of percentages

Label: Since the Name Column Doesn't allow you to use any Special Character or Space, here you can give any name as an Label for that Variable you wanted to assign

Value: This is to define/ Label a Value Wherever you see in the Data, Eg: You can Label "0" in the data as ABSENT for Exam, So when you find 0 in the data, it will be labelled as ABSENT for Exam, You Can also Label the Employee ID Number with their Name, So that Using the value Label Switch Button you can view the Name of the employee, but in report the Name will not appear, only the EMP ID number will appear, This helps in reading the data better in data view

Missing: You can mention the Data which you don't want the SPSS to consider while analyzing, Like "0" Value is considered as Absent, so for analysis it will neglect "0" if its mentioned in Missing, which will be helpful in Mean, Mode Etc,

- **Align:** You can mention the alignment of the data in the data sheet, Left, Right of Middle,

- **Measure:** This is where you will define the measure of the Variable that you have entered, Whether Scale, Ordinal or Nominal type of Variable

DATA VIEW

The Data View is a Spreadsheet which contains rows and columns, The Data Can be entered in the Data View Sheet Either Manually or the data can be imported from the data file, SPSS can read the data file in any of the one format, which can be Excel, Plain text files or relational (SQL) Databases, Before importing the excel sheet change the excel file format to (.xls)

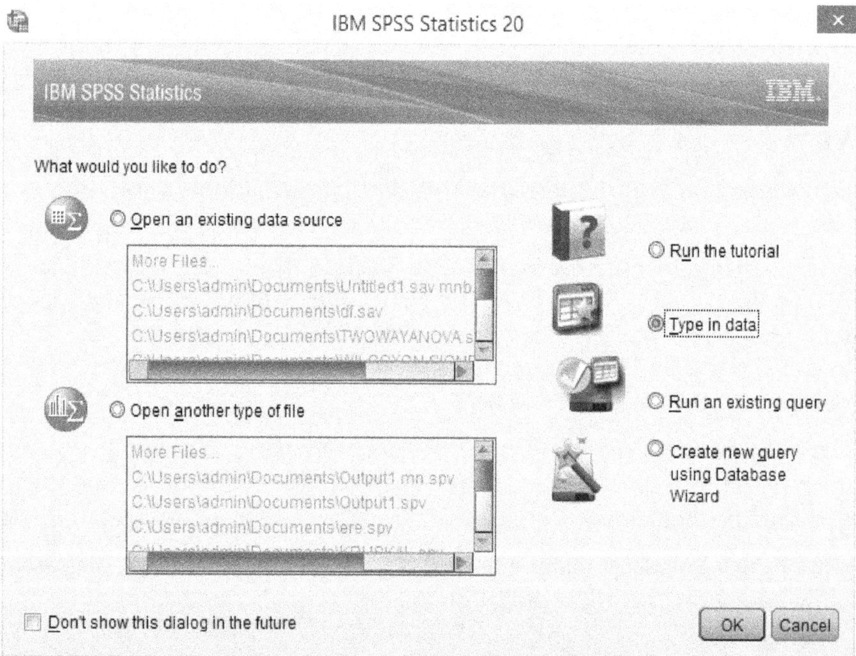

SPSS for Windows Dialogue Box

When SPSS is opened, by default dialogue box appears and that gives or display the different options for users. This dialogue box can be prevented from opening in the future by clicking the option Don't show this dialogue in the future. The other way is if we click Cancel option then the SPSS data editor appears as an empty spreadsheet. At the top of the screen the menu bar and at the bottom a status bar appears.

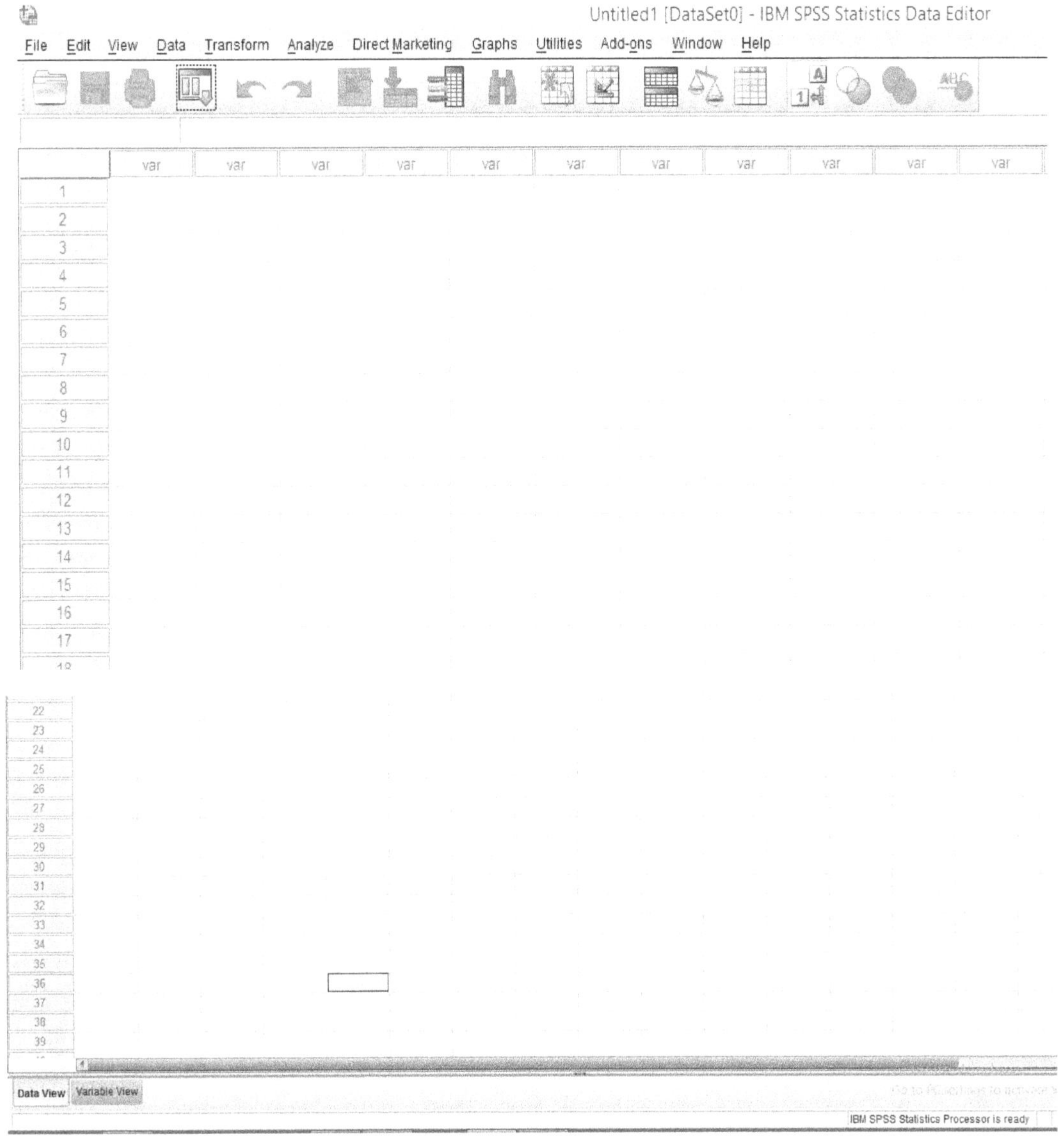

The status bar explains about the facilities currently available or which is active and also display that SPSS Processor is ready.

DATA VIEW SPREADSHEET

The data View sheet, which allows the user to enter and view. The other window is variable as shown in variable view spreadsheet. Here the user can toggle between the windows by clicking on the appropriate tabs on the bottom left of the screen. User can enter the data in the Data View spreadsheet. For the analysis of data SPSS represents or assumes that row as cases and columns variables. By default SPSS uses a period/full stop to indicate missing numerical values. String variable cells are simply left empty

VARIABLE VIEW SPREADSHEET

The variable view spreadsheet helps to define the variable as shown in the variable view display.

As soon as data is entered under a column in data view sheet, then by default name of the column appears in a row at the top of each column in the variable view.

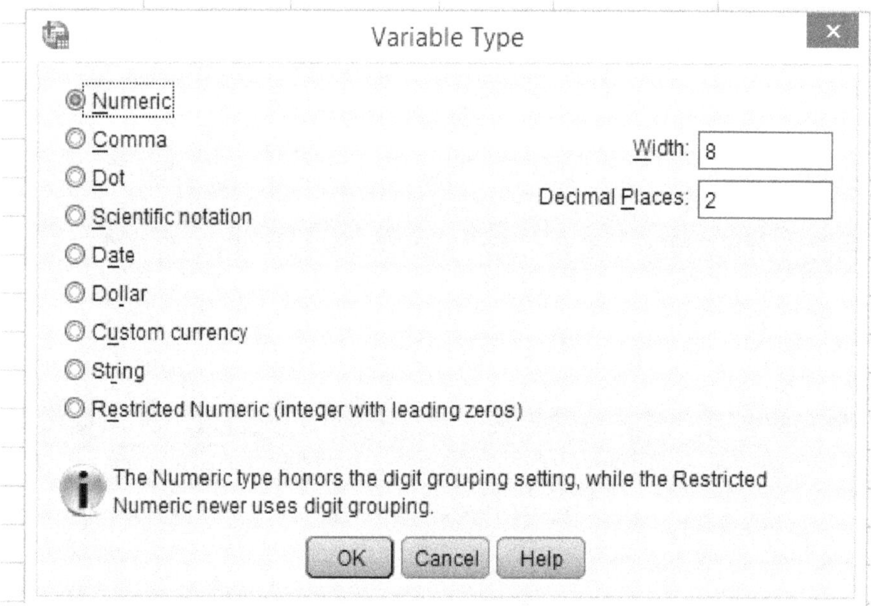

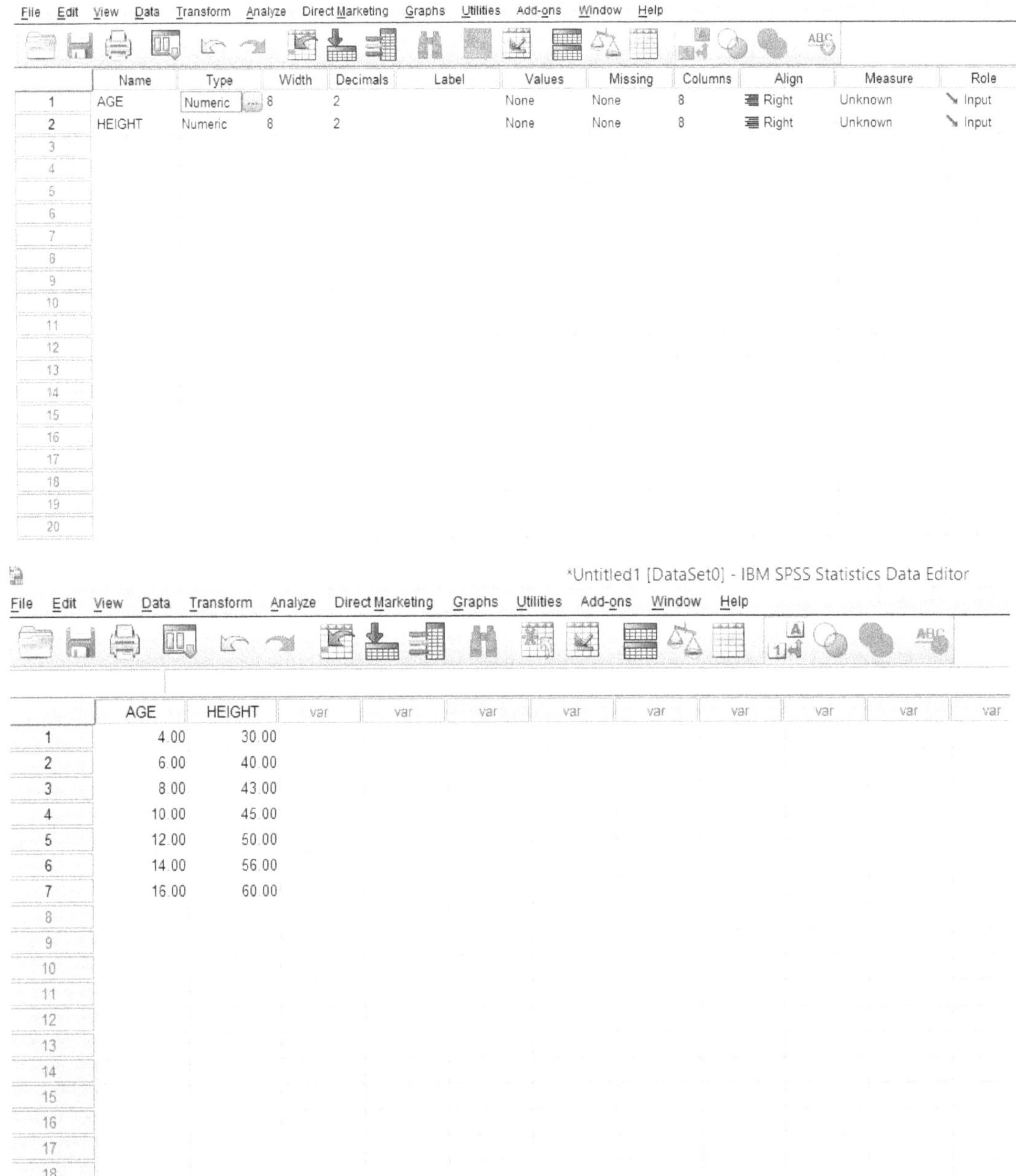

Methods of Analysis

As the name suggests SPSS is statistics software is used to perform only statistical operations. To improve your data analysis skills and simplify your decisions, one has to execute these five steps in your data analysis process:

1. Define Your Questions. 2. Set Clear Measurement to be made. 3. Collect Data. 4. Analyze Data. 5. Interpret Results.

In Pharmaceutical calculation to analyze the data, depending on the type experimental (clinical trial or Pharmaceutical problems) different statistical tools will be used to analyze the data.

Computation of Average (Arithmetic Mean) and Standard deviation:

To compute the mean and standard deviation data should be entered in the data view sheet Click "Analyze" on the toolbar and then move mouse over "Descriptive Statistics." Click "Descriptive" to open the variables dialog box. Then select the variables you want to find descriptive statistics. The detail of the calculation procedure is explained below.

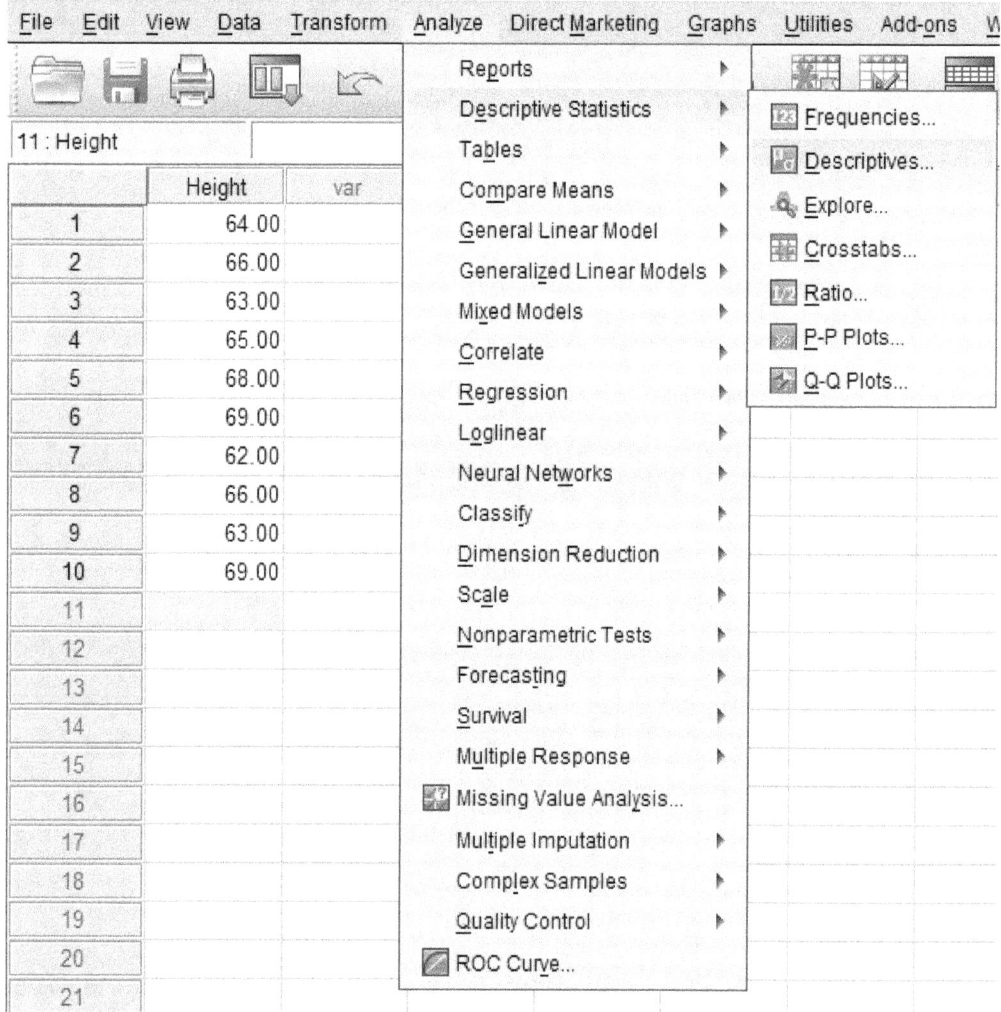

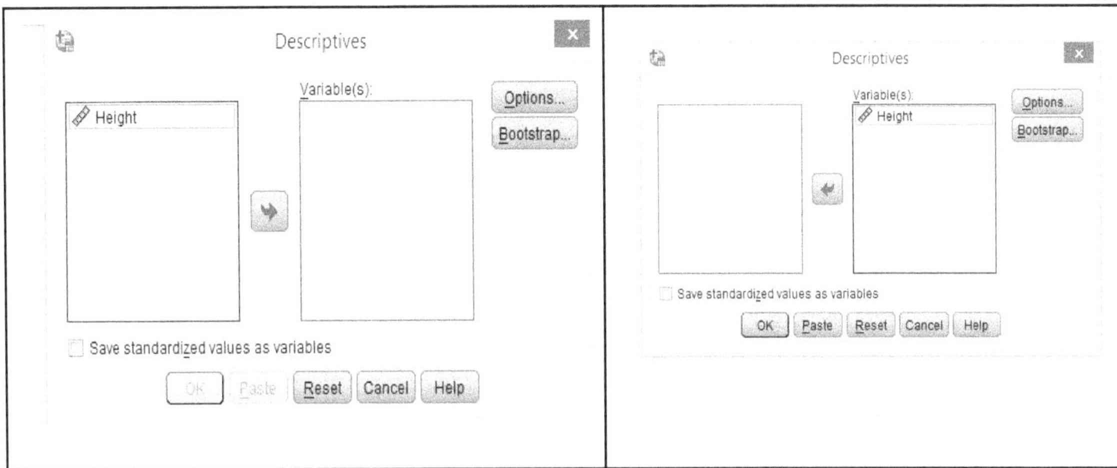

At the end user has to select and click ok option to compute the value of mean and standard deviation of the selected data in a tabular form.

Descriptive Statistics					
	N	Minimum	Maximum	Mean	Std. Deviation
Height	10	62.00	69.00	65.5000	2.54951
Valid N (listwise)	10				

Computation of Coefficient of Correlation between Two Variables

To compute Pearson coefficient of Correlation, in the tool bar select Analyze > Correlate > Bivariate. Select the variables X and Y and move them to the Variables box. In the Correlation Coefficients area, then select Pearson. Then to verify the level of Significance, select your desired significance test, i.e., two-tailed or one-tailed and click OK to perform calculation and to present the output in a desired format.

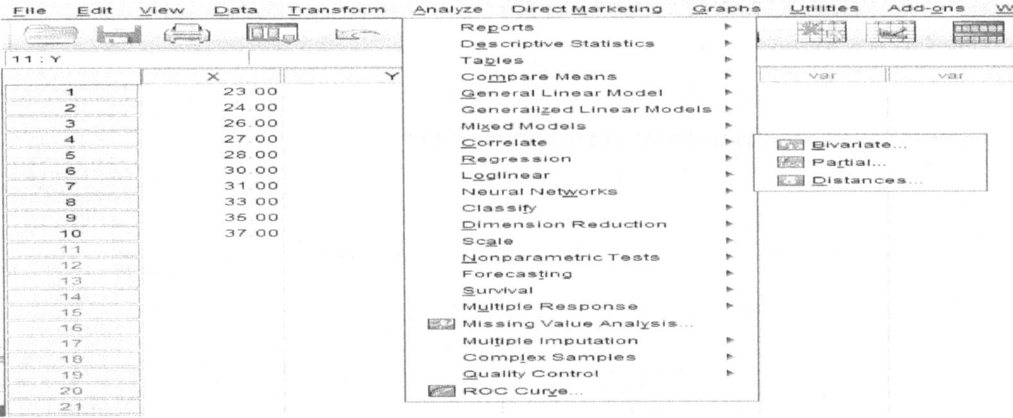

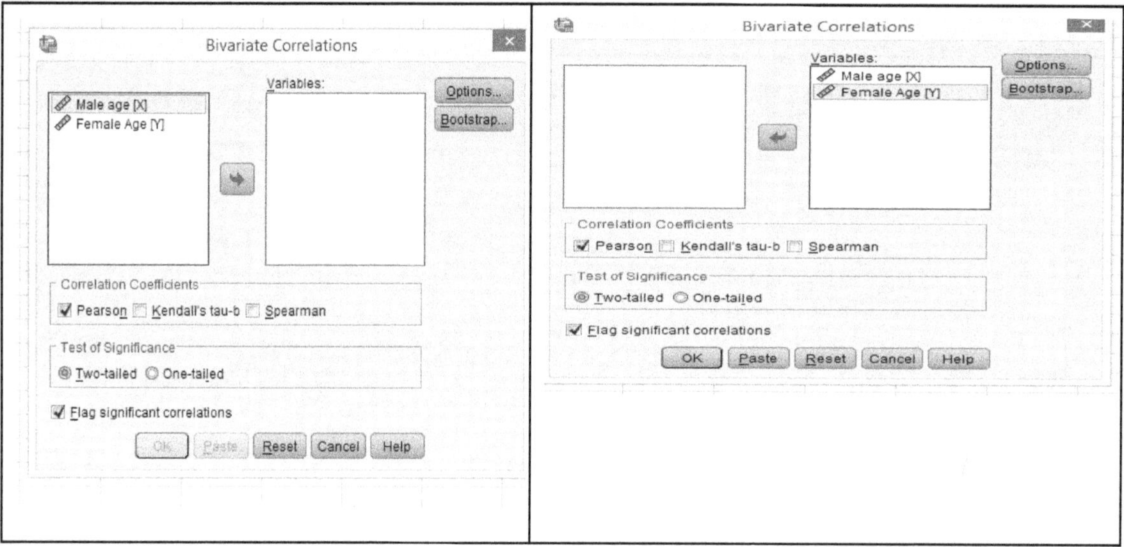

CORRELATIONS

		Male age	Female Age
Male age	Pearson Correlation	1	.980**
	Sig. (2-tailed)		.000
	N	10	10
Female Age	Pearson Correlation	.980**	1
	Sig. (2-tailed)	.000	
	N	10	10
**. Correlation is significant at the 0.01 level (2-tailed).			

Formation of Regression Equation Y on X:

SPSS will be used for Linear Regression Analysis not only to just fitting a **linear** line through a cloud of data points. It also consists of 3 **steps, they are**

(1) analyzing the correlation and directionality of the data,

(2) Estimating the regression model, i.e., fitting the line, and

(3) Finally evaluation will be done to verify the validity and to know the importance of model

The analysis of data will be done in different steps, as explained below.

Enter the data in the data view spread sheet

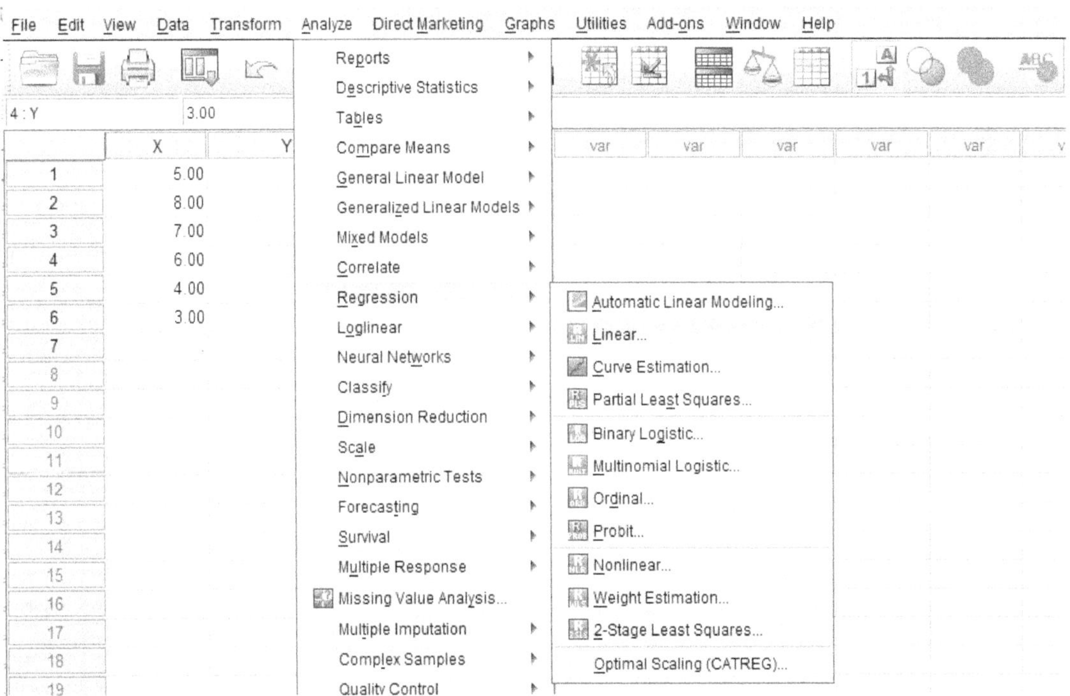

In the tool bar select Analyze > Regression > Linear > Transfer data to respective place >Click OK and the result will be displayed in a table

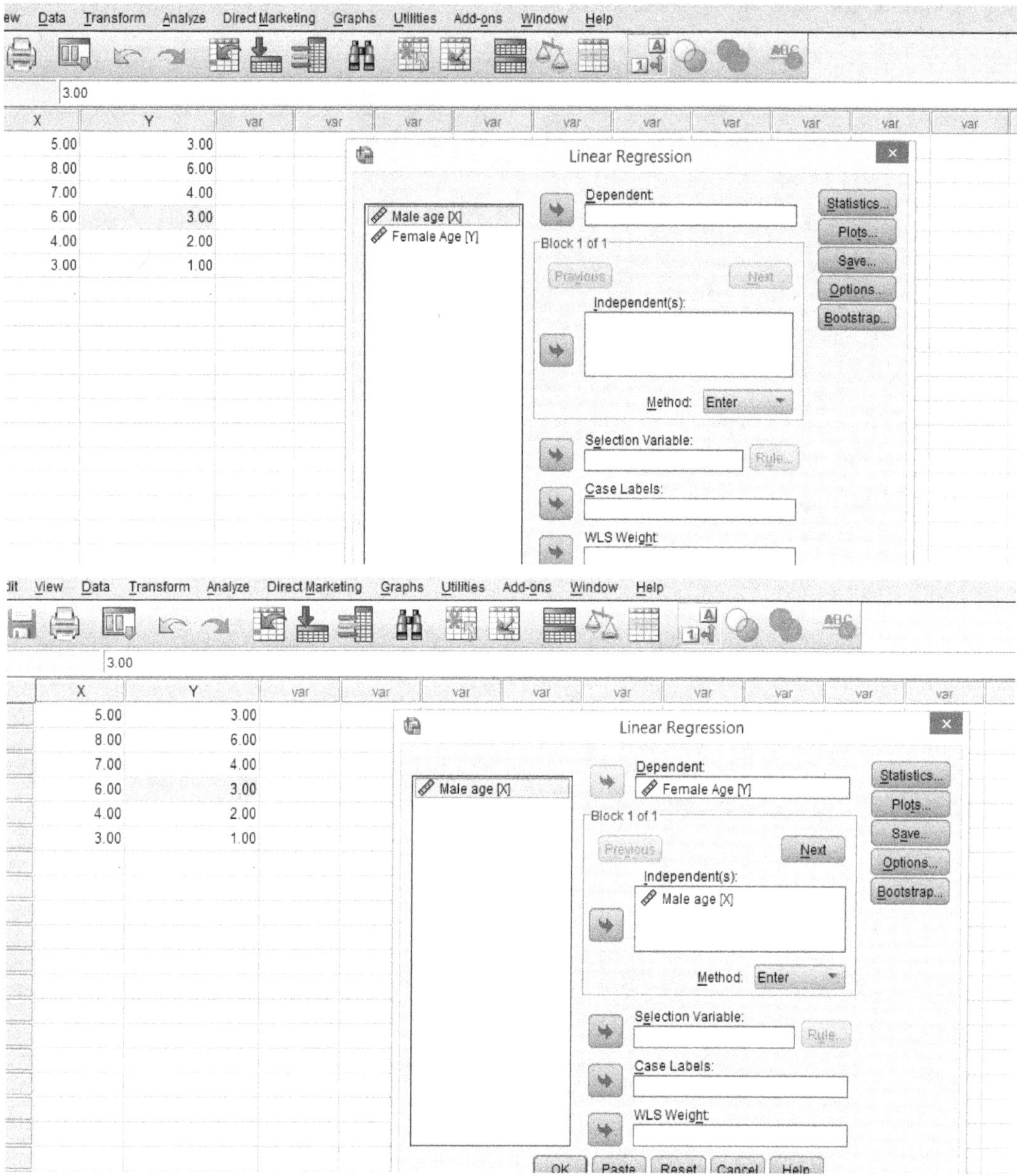

Variables Entered/Removed

Mode 1	Variables Entered	Variables Removed	Method
1	Male age[b]	.	Enter

a. Dependent Variable: Female Age

b. All requested variables entered.

Model Summary				
Model	R	R Square	Adjusted R Square	Std. Error of the Estimate
1	.962[a]	.926	.907	.52554

a. Predictors: (Constant), Male age

ANOVA

	Model	Sum of Squares	df	Mean Square	F	Sig.
1	Regression	13.729	1	13.729	49.707	.002[b]
	Residual	1.105	4	.276		
	Total	14.833	5			

a. Dependent Variable: Female Age

b. Predictors: (Constant), Male age

Coefficients

	Model	Unstandardized Coefficients		Standardized Coefficients	t	Sig.
		B	Std. Error	Beta		
1	(Constant)	-1.705	.723		-2.356	.078
	Male age	.886	.126	.962	7.050	.002

a. Dependent Variable: Female Age

Computation of t-value using One–Sample t-test using SPSS

The one-sample t-test is used to determine whether a sample comes from a population with a specific mean. This population mean is not always known, but sometimes that is hypothesized. For a one-sample t-test, there will be only one variable's data to be entered into SPSS Statistics and entered data will be displayed in the data sheet as shown below.

	SAMPLE	var	var	var	var	var	var	var	var	var	var
1	50.00										
2	49.00										
3	52.00										
4	44.00										
5	45.00										
6	48.00										
7	46.00										
8	45.00										
9	49.00										
10	45.00										
11											
12											

To compute the value of t-value using **One Sample t Test in SPSS**, user has to click Analyze > Compare Means > **One-Sample T Test**. The **One-Sample T Test** window opens, there the user will specify the variables to be used in the analysis.

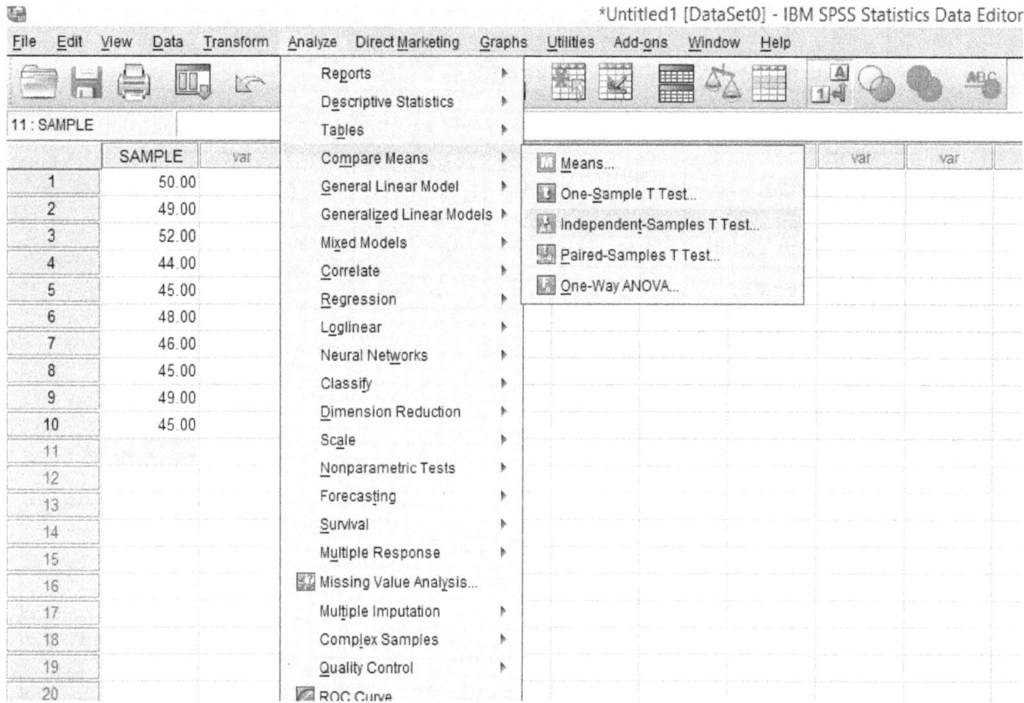

You will be presented with the **One-Sample T Test** dialogue box, as shown below:

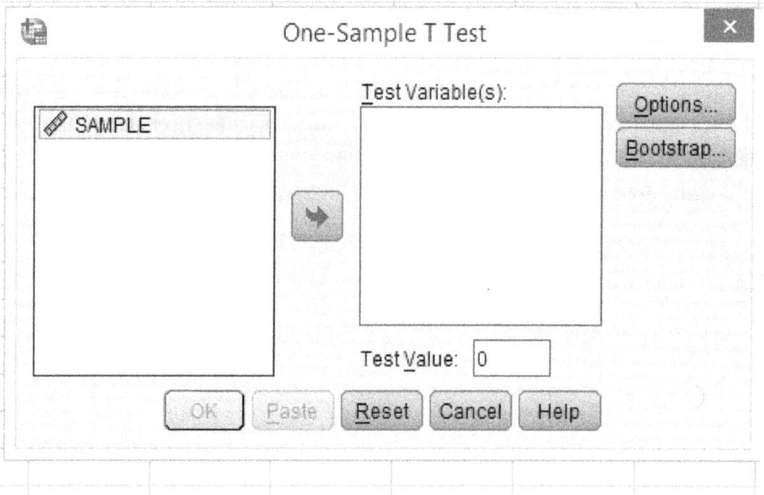

Transfer the dependent variable, into the test variable(s) box by selecting it (by clicking on it) and then clicking on the button. Enter the population mean that we are comparing the sample mean against in the test value box, by changing the current value of "0" to "50". Here 50 will be the population mean from which the sample has been taken. You will end up with the following screen:

Click on the option button, then the One-Sample T Test dialogue will appear on the screen as shown below

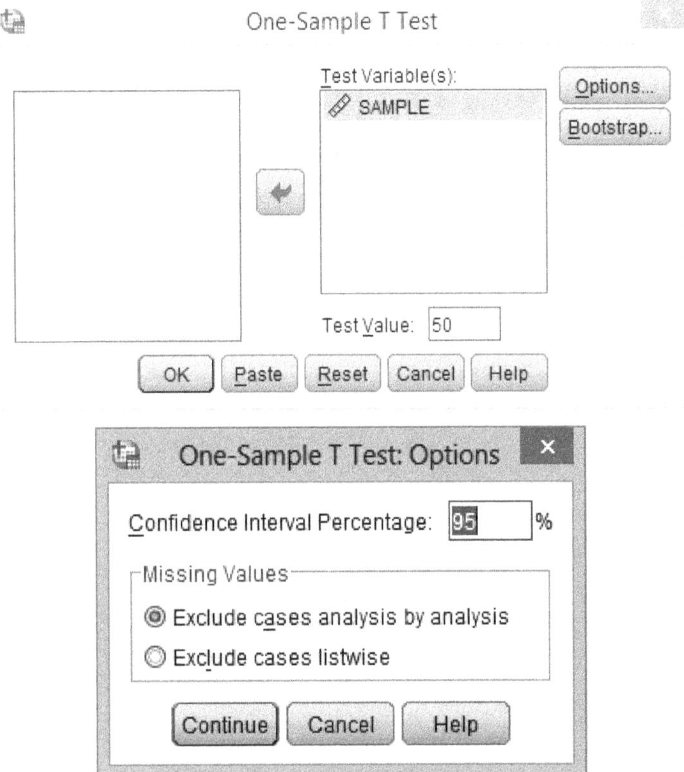

Click the continue button again user will come back to **One-Sample T Test** dialogue box.

Click the ok button to generate the result. The generated result will be displayed in different tables as shown below.

One-Sample Statistics

	N	Mean	Std. Deviation	Std. Error Mean
SAMPLE	10	47.3000	2.66875	.84393

One-Sample Test

	Test Value = 50					
	t	df	Sig. (2-tailed)	Mean Difference	95% Confidence Interval of the Difference	
					Lower	Upper
SAMPLE	-3.199	9	.011	-2.70000	-4.6091	-.7909

Computation of t-Value using Independent Samples t Test. Using SPSS

To compute t-value using Independent Samples t Test in SPSS,

click Analyze > Compare Means > Independent-Samples T Test. The Independent-Samples T Test window opens where you will specify the variables to be used in the analysis

Click **Analyze > Compare Means > Independent-Samples T Test...** on the top menu, as shown below:

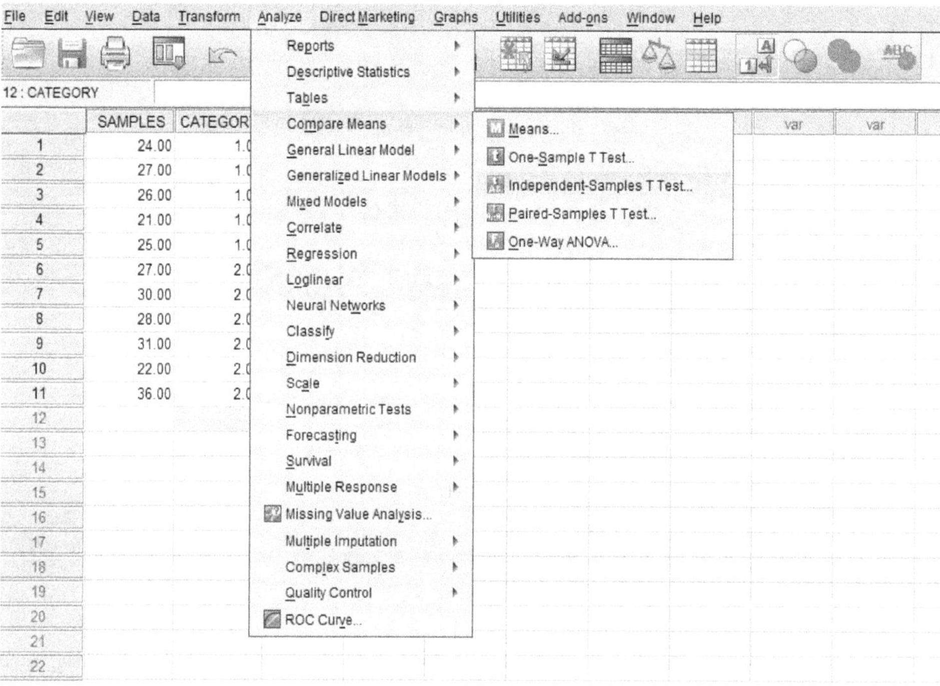

Then the **Independent-Samples T-Test** dialogue box will be displayed as shown below:

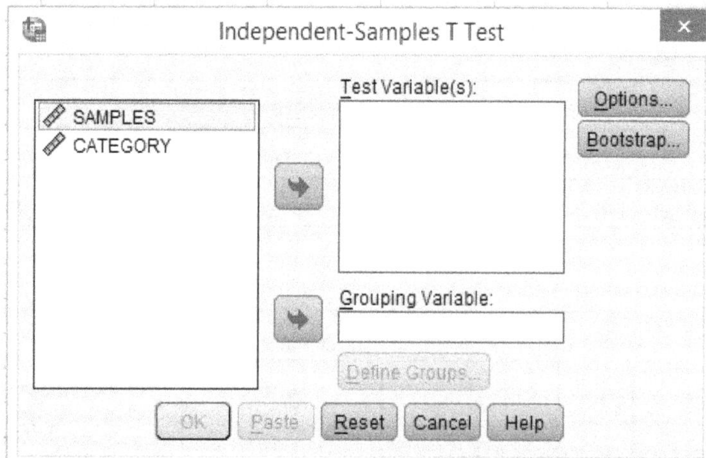

Transfer the dependent variable, into the test variable(s) box and transfer the independent variable, into the grouping variable box by highlighting the relevant variables and pressing the 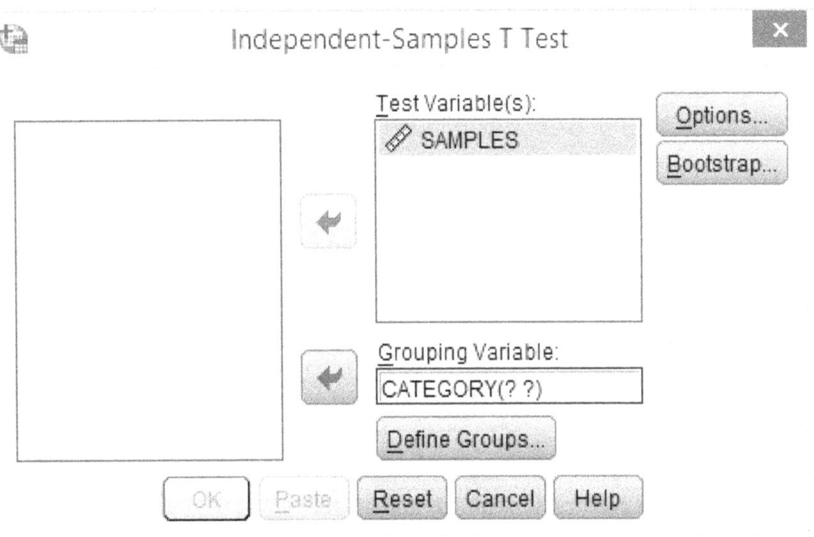 buttons, then the following screen will appear:

Then one has to define the groups. There Click on the Define Group button, then the **Define Groups** dialogue box will appear, as shown below:

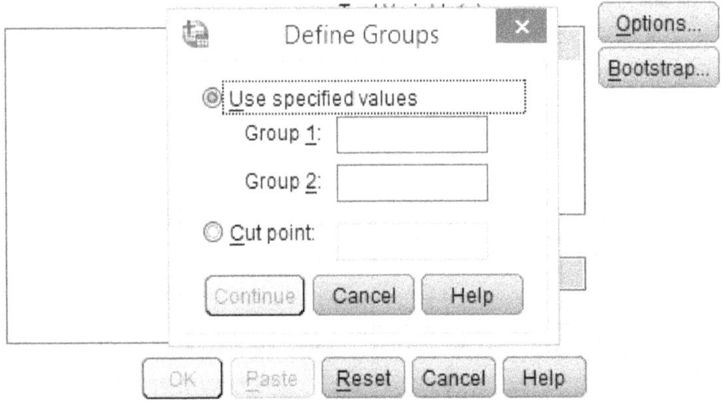

Enter "**1**" into the Group1 box box and enter "**2**" into the Group 2 box. Here group 1 is first sample1 and group 2 is Sample2.

Click the Continue button.

If you need to change the confidence level limits or change how to exclude cases, click the Option button. You will be presented with the following:

Click the Continue button. You will be returned to the **Independent-Samples T Test** dialogue box.

Click the ok button and result obtained will displayed in different tables as shown below

<table>
<tr><th colspan="6">Group Statistics</th></tr>
<tr><td></td><td>CATEGORY</td><td>N</td><td>Mean</td><td>Std. Deviation</td><td>Std. Error Mean</td></tr>
<tr><td rowspan="2">SAMPLES</td><td>1.00</td><td>5</td><td>24.6000</td><td>2.30217</td><td>1.02956</td></tr>
<tr><td>2.00</td><td>6</td><td>29.0000</td><td>4.64758</td><td>1.89737</td></tr>
</table>

<table>
<tr><th colspan="10">Independent Samples Test</th></tr>
<tr><td rowspan="3"></td><td rowspan="3"></td><td colspan="2">Levene's Test for Equality of Variances</td><td colspan="6">t-test for Equality of Means</td></tr>
<tr><td rowspan="2">F</td><td rowspan="2">Sig.</td><td rowspan="2">t</td><td rowspan="2">df</td><td rowspan="2">Sig. (2-tailed)</td><td rowspan="2">Mean Difference</td><td rowspan="2">Std. Error Difference</td><td colspan="2">95% Confidence Interval of the Difference</td></tr>
<tr><td>Lower</td><td>Upper</td></tr>
<tr><td rowspan="2">SAMPLES</td><td>Equal variances assumed</td><td>1.386</td><td>.269</td><td>-1.918</td><td>9</td><td>.087</td><td>-4.40000</td><td>2.29428</td><td>-9.59001</td><td>.79001</td></tr>
<tr><td>Equal variances not assumed</td><td></td><td></td><td>-2.038</td><td>7.559</td><td>.078</td><td>-4.40000</td><td>2.15870</td><td>-9.42901</td><td>.62901</td></tr>
</table>

COMPUTATION of T-value using Paired T-Test

If a investigator wants to study the effect of particular drug on the basis of number of hours participants sleep. Investigator should have two conditions while performing clinical trial experiment, One group is administered drug to the participants and another group administered placebo. Each participant participates in both groups are in same condition. Paired Samples T-Test is applied to know the level of significance using SPSS and the procedure is as explained below..

TREATMENT	CONTROL	var
6.00	9.00	
5.00	10.00	
4.00	8.00	
7.00	9.00	
5.00	11.00	

Click **Analyze > Compare Means > Paired Sample t-test...** on the top menu, as shown below.

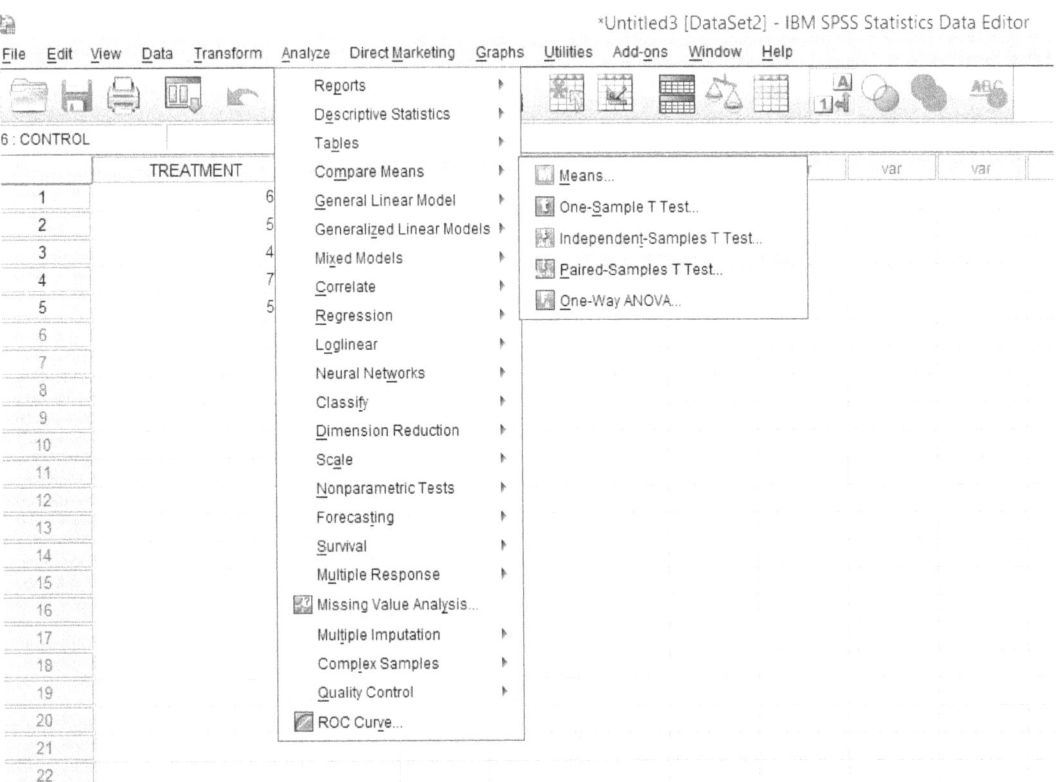

Transfer the variables into particular group using the appropriate ➡ symbol

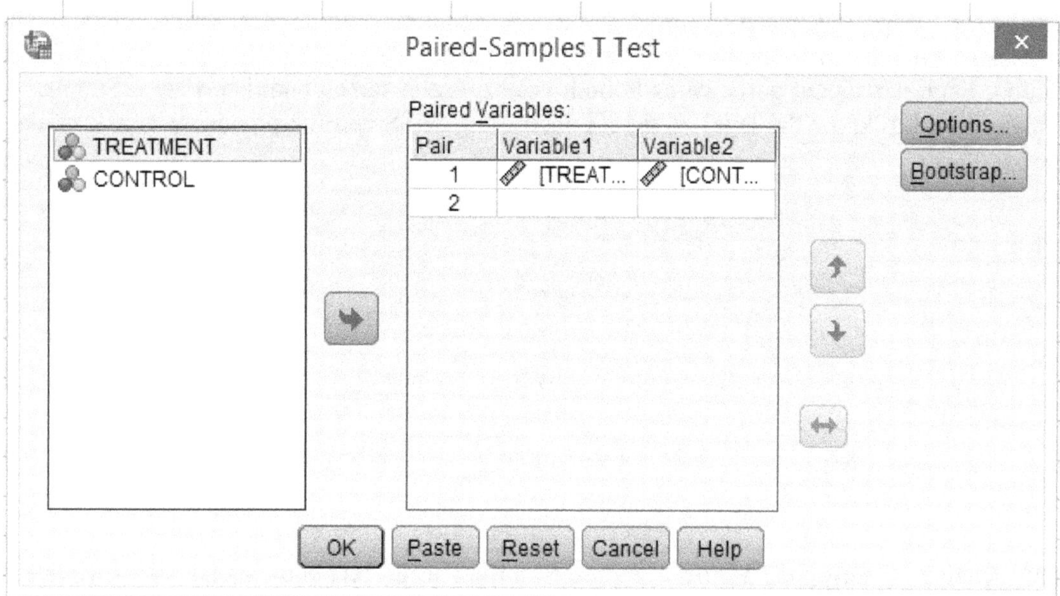

Click OK and the result will be obtained and obtained data will be recorded in a table as shown below.

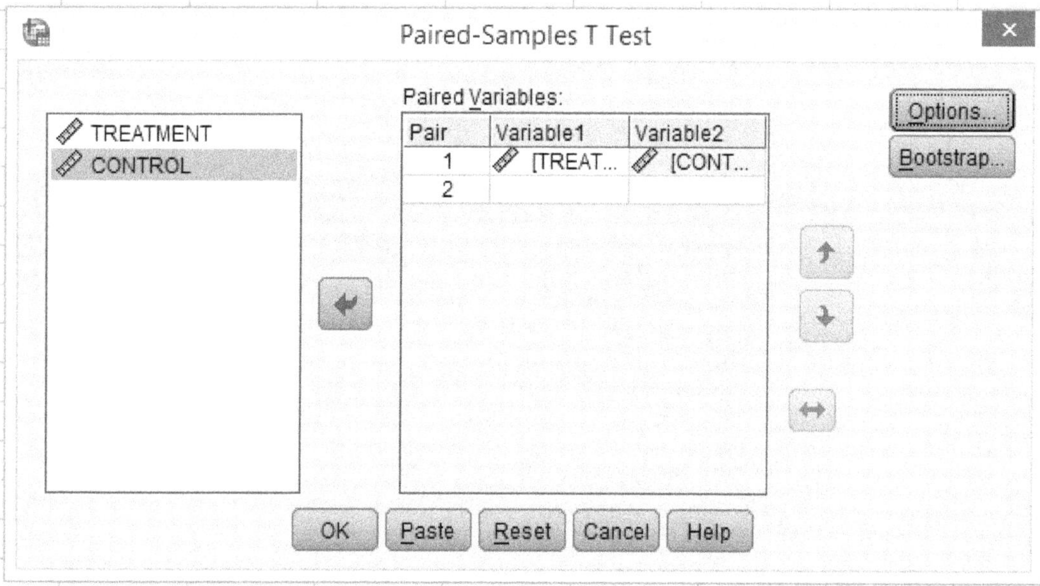

Paired Samples Statistics

		Mean	N	Std. Deviation	Std. Error Mean
Pair 1	TREATMENT	5.4000	5	1.14018	.50990
	CONTROL	9.4000	5	1.14018	.50990

Paired Samples Test

		Paired Differences					t	df	Sig. (2-tailed)
		Mean	Std. Deviation	Std. Error Mean	95% Confidence Interval of the Difference				
					Lower	Upper			
Pair 1	TREATMENT - CONTROL	-4.00000	1.58114	.70711	-5.96324	-2.03676	-5.657	4	.005

COMPUTATION of ONE-WAY ANOVA

The one-way analysis of variance (ANOVA) is used to determine whether there is any statistically significant differences between the means of more than two independent (unrelated) groups. For example, you could use a one-way ANOVA to verify the level of significance between different treatment which are used to treat three different groups of patients who are suffering from same type of disease. Since you may have three, four, five or more groups in your study design, determining which of these groups differ from each other is important. You can do this using a post hoc test.

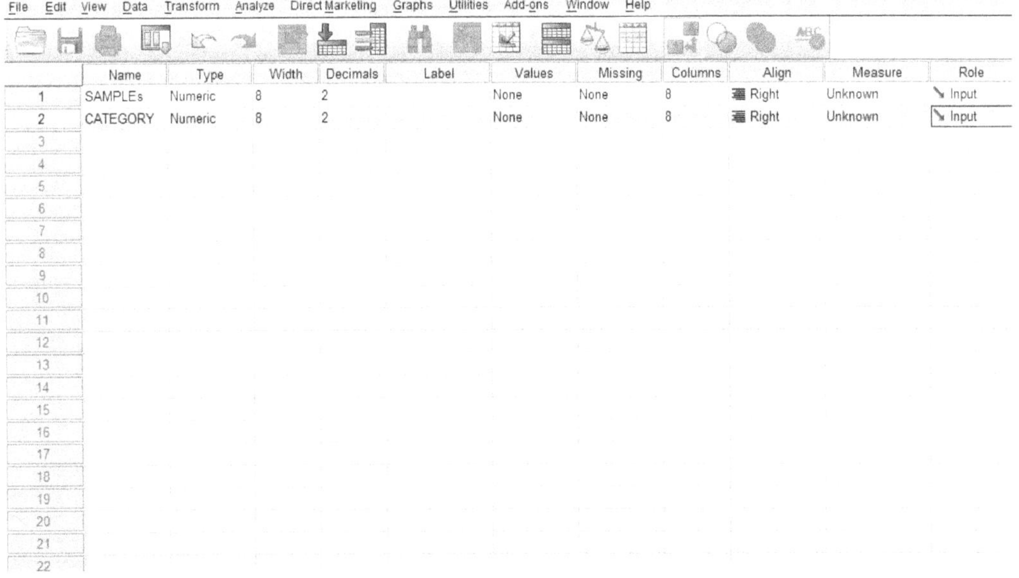

Click **Analyze** > **Compare Means** > **One-Way ANOVA...** on the top menu, as shown below.

	SAMPLEs	CATEGORY
1	25.00	1.00
2	30.00	1.00
3	36.00	1.00
4	38.00	1.00
5	31.00	1.00
6	31.00	2.00
7	39.00	2.00
8	38.00	2.00
9	42.00	2.00
10	35.00	2.00
11	24.00	3.00
12	30.00	3.00
13	28.00	3.00
14	25.00	3.00
15	28.00	3.00

Data View sheet

Click **Analyze** > **Compare Means** > **One-Way ANOVA...** on the top menu, as shown below.

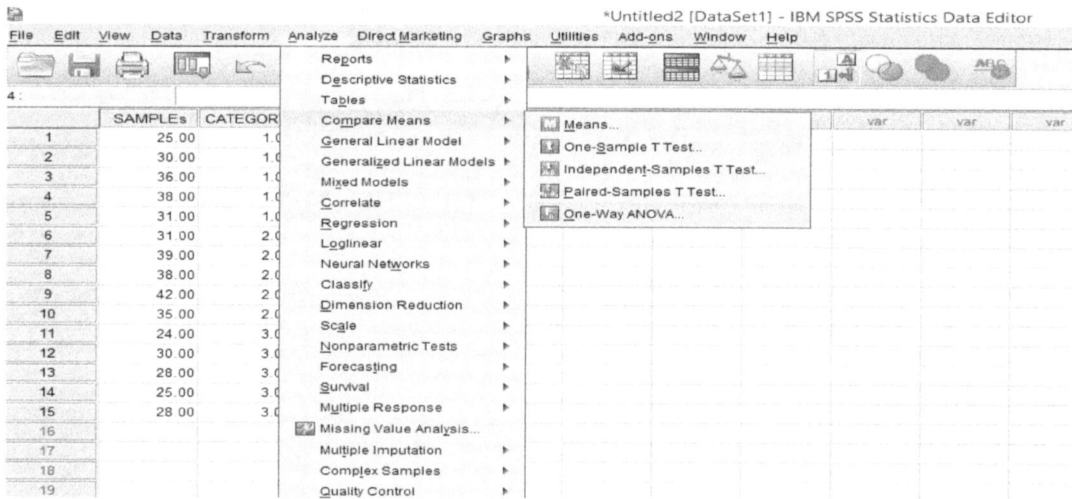

Then the **One-Way ANOVA** dialogue box will appear:

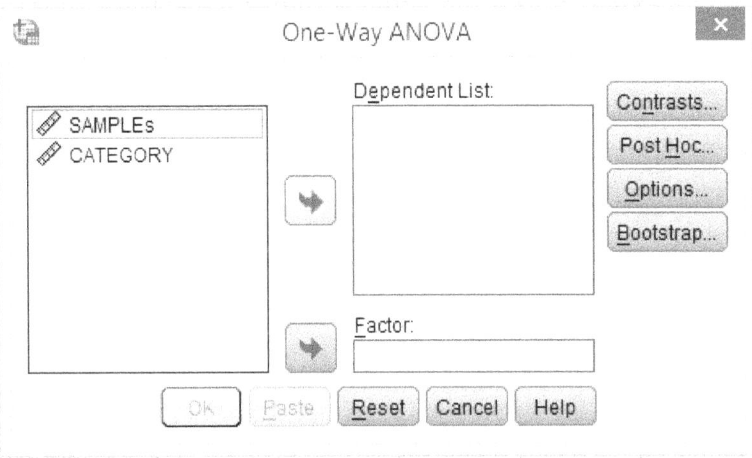

Transfer the dependent variable or sample in dependent list box and category into factor box, appropriate buttons (or drag-and-drop the variables into the boxes), as shown below:

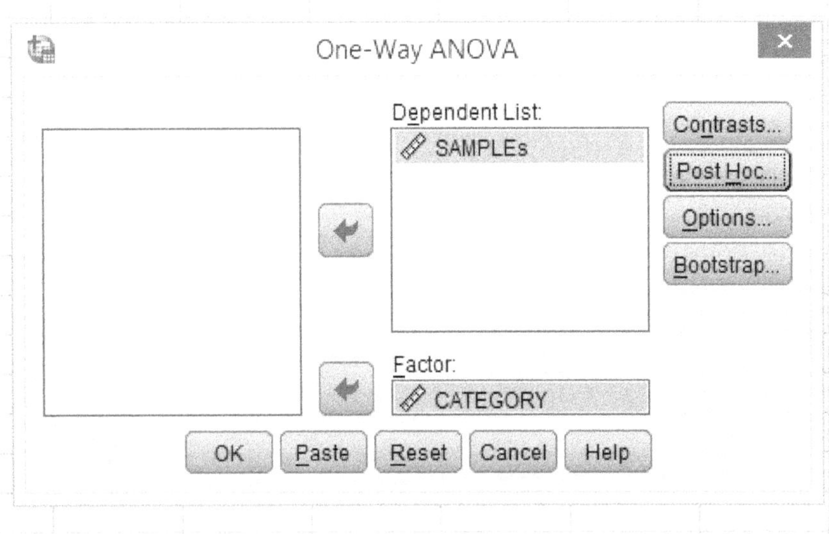

Click the POST HOCK button press Continue

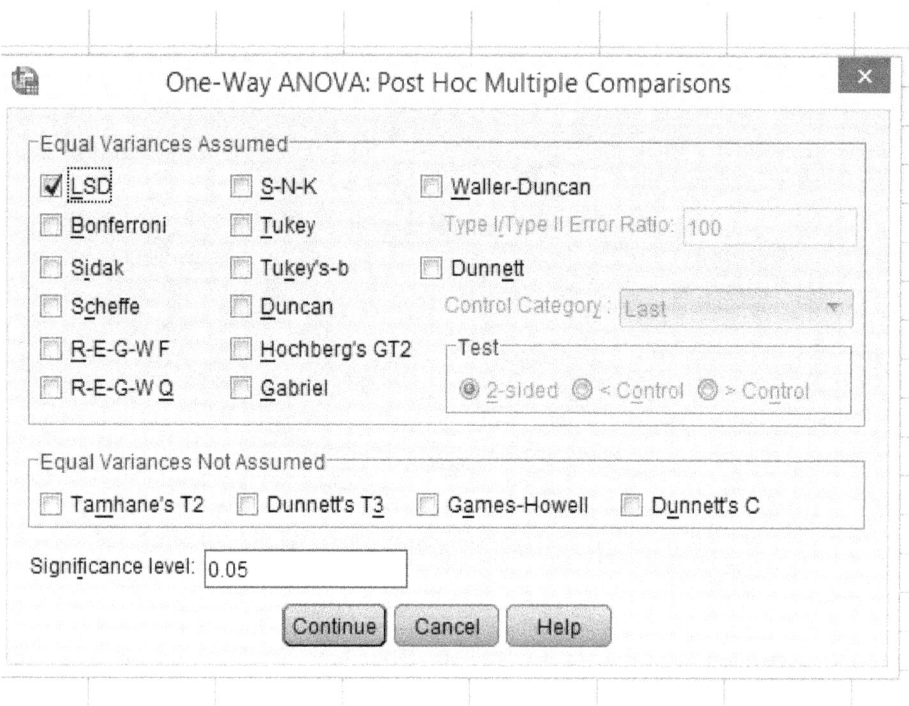

Click the OK button and desired result will be obtained and result will be recorded in a table, as shown below.

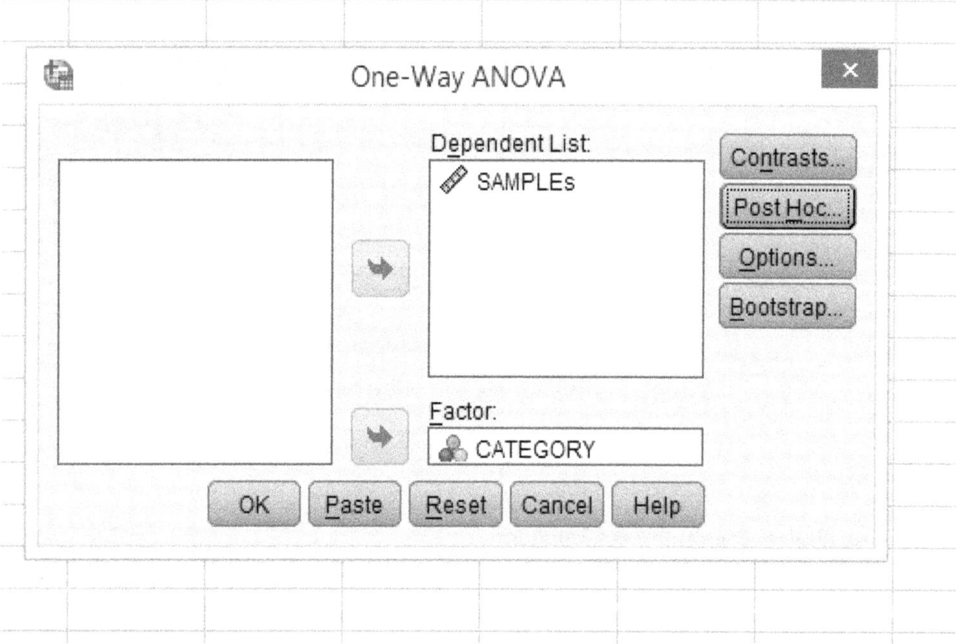

ANOVA

SAMPLEs

	Sum of Squares	df	Mean Square	F	Sig.
Between Groups	250.000	2	125.000	7.500	.008
Within Groups	200.000	12	16.667		
Total	450.000	14			

Multiple Comparisons

Dependent Variable: SAMPLEs

LSD

(I) CATEGORY	(J) CATEGORY	Mean Difference (I-J)	Std. Error	Sig.	95% Confidence Interval	
					Lower Bound	Upper Bound
1.00	2.00	-5.00000	2.58199	.077	-10.6257	.6257
	3.00	5.00000	2.58199	.077	-.6257	10.6257
2.00	1.00	5.00000	2.58199	.077	-.6257	10.6257
	3.00	10.00000*	2.58199	.002	4.3743	15.6257
3.00	1.00	-5.00000	2.58199	.077	-10.6257	.6257
	2.00	-10.00000*	2.58199	.002	-15.6257	-4.3743

*. The mean difference is significant at 0.05 level. The sample three found to be more significant than other two samples.

COMPUTATION OF TWO_WAY ANOVA

The two-way ANOVA will compares the mean differences between groups that have been split on two independent variables or factors. The primary purpose of a two-way ANOVA is to verify the interaction effect of two independent variables on a dependent variable. For example, you could use a two-way ANOVA to understand whether there is an interaction between Treatment given and the doctors who will treat the patients using different drugs. You may want to determine whether there is any interaction between physical activity level and gender on blood cholesterol concentration in children, where physical activity (low/moderate/high) and gender (male/female) are your independent variables, and cholesterol concentration is your dependent variable.

The interaction term in a two-way ANOVA informs you whether the effect of one of your independent variables on the dependent variable is the same for all values of your independent variable (and vice versa).

To compute the mean and standard deviation data should be entered in the data view sheet Click "Analyze" on the toolbar and then move mouse over "General linear model." Click General linear model" to open the variables dialog box. Then select the variables you want to perform Two-ANOVA calculation. The detail of the calculation procedure is explained below.

First the data view spreadsheet needs to be set up as shown below

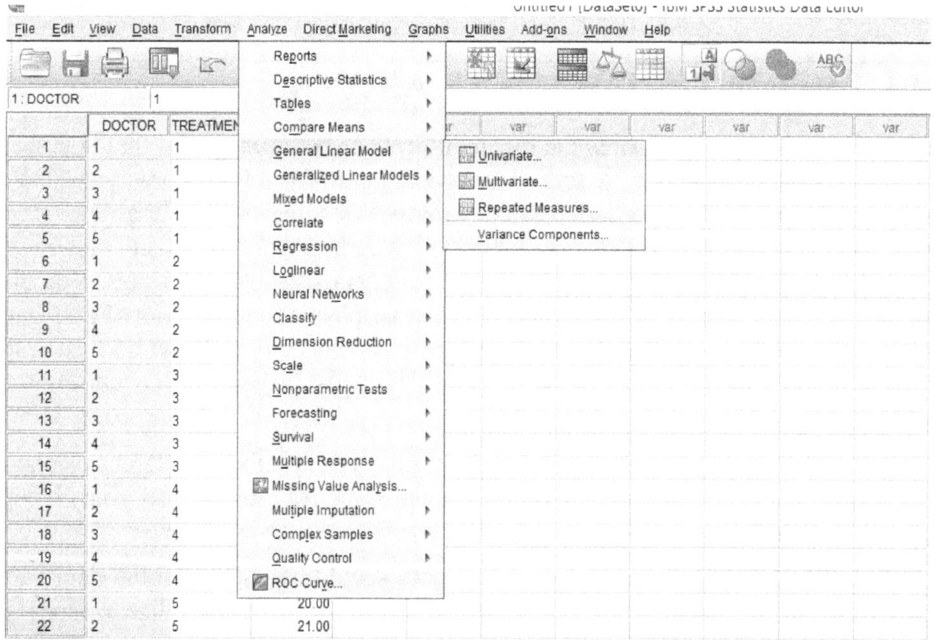

Data View spread sheet

To analyze the data select Analyze-→ General linear model → Univariate → Then click the Univariate dialogue box

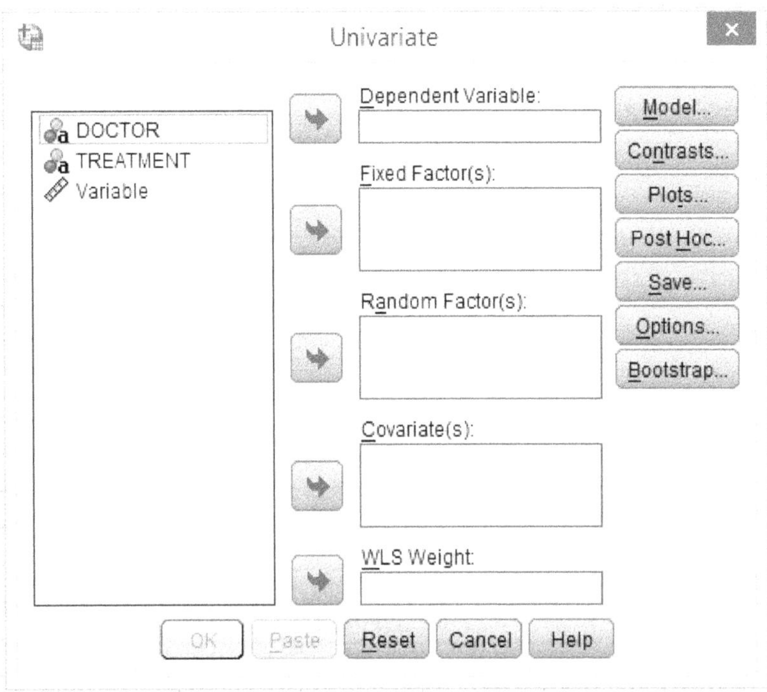

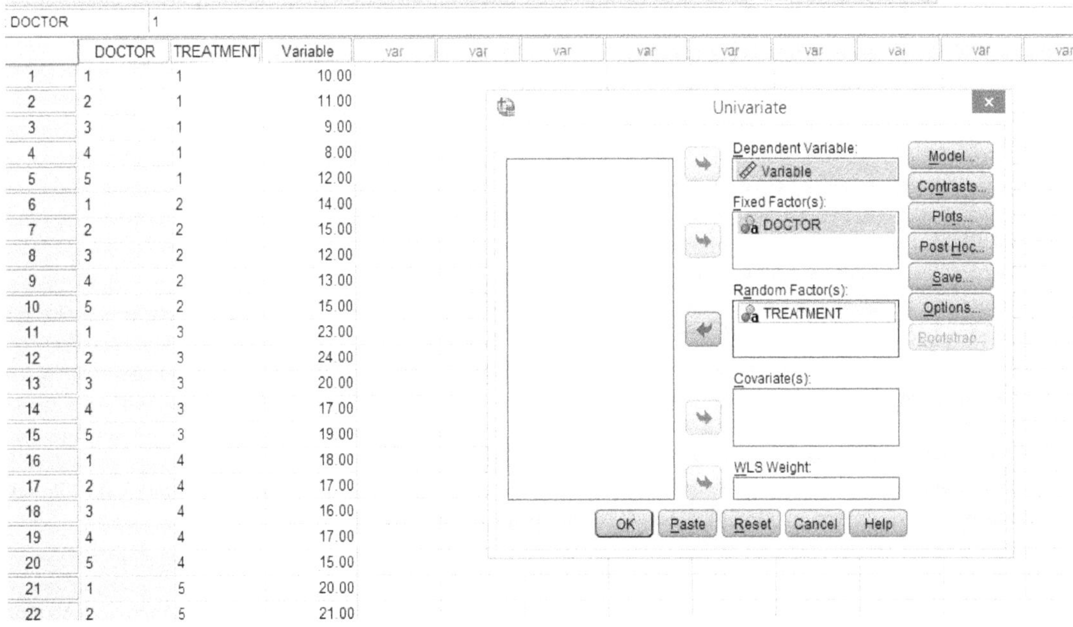

	DOCTOR	TREATMENT	Variable
1	1	1	10.00
2	2	1	11.00
3	3	1	9.00
4	4	1	8.00
5	5	1	12.00
6	1	2	14.00
7	2	2	15.00
8	3	2	12.00
9	4	2	13.00
10	5	2	15.00
11	1	3	23.00
12	2	3	24.00
13	3	3	20.00
14	4	3	17.00
15	5	3	19.00
16	1	4	18.00
17	2	4	17.00
18	3	4	16.00
19	4	4	17.00
20	5	4	15.00
21	1	5	20.00
22	2	5	21.00

Between-Subjects Factors

		N
DOCTOR	1	5
	2	5
	3	5
	4	5
	5	5
TREATMENT	1	5
	2	5
	3	5
	4	5
	5	5

Tests of Between-Subjects Effects

Dependent Variable: Variable

Source		Type III Sum of Squares	df	Mean Square	F	Sig.
Intercept	Hypothesis	6625.960	1	6625.960	65.178	.001
	Error	406.640	4	101.660[a]		
DOCTOR	Hypothesis	25.840	4	6.460	2.991	.051
	Error	34.560	16	2.160[b]		
TREATMENT	Hypothesis	406.640	4	101.660	47.065	.000
	Error	34.560	16	2.160[b]		
DOCTOR * TREATMENT	Hypothesis	34.560	16	2.160	.	.
	Error	.000	0	.[c]		

a. MS(TREATMENT)

b. MS(DOCTOR * TREATMENT)

c. MS(Error)

THE WILCOXON SIGNED-RANK TEST

Procedure in SPSS Statistics

The Wilcoxon signed-rank test is a nonparametric test equivalent to the dependent t-test. As the Wilcoxon signed-rank test does not assume normality in the data, it can be used when this assumption has been violated and the use of the paired t-test is inappropriate.

For example, you could use a Wilcoxon signed-rank test to understand whether there is any significance improvement in decreasing the weight before following the diet and after following the diet for a period of after a 6 weeks, from the day when they were advised to follow the diet.

To perform statistical calculation using Wilcoxon signed-rank test in SPSS statistical software, user has to enter the data in data sheet as shown below

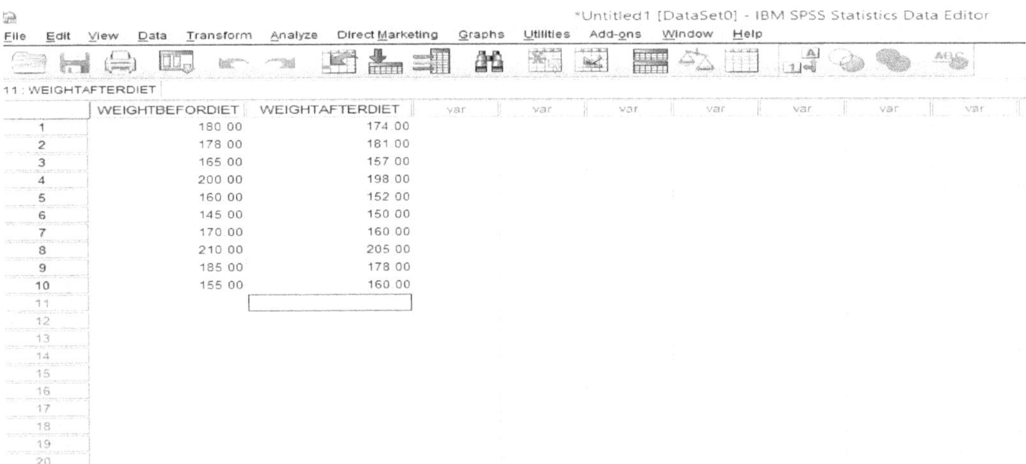

To analyze the data Click **Analyze > Nonparametric Tests > Legacy Dialogs > 2 Related Samples...** on the top menu, as shown below:

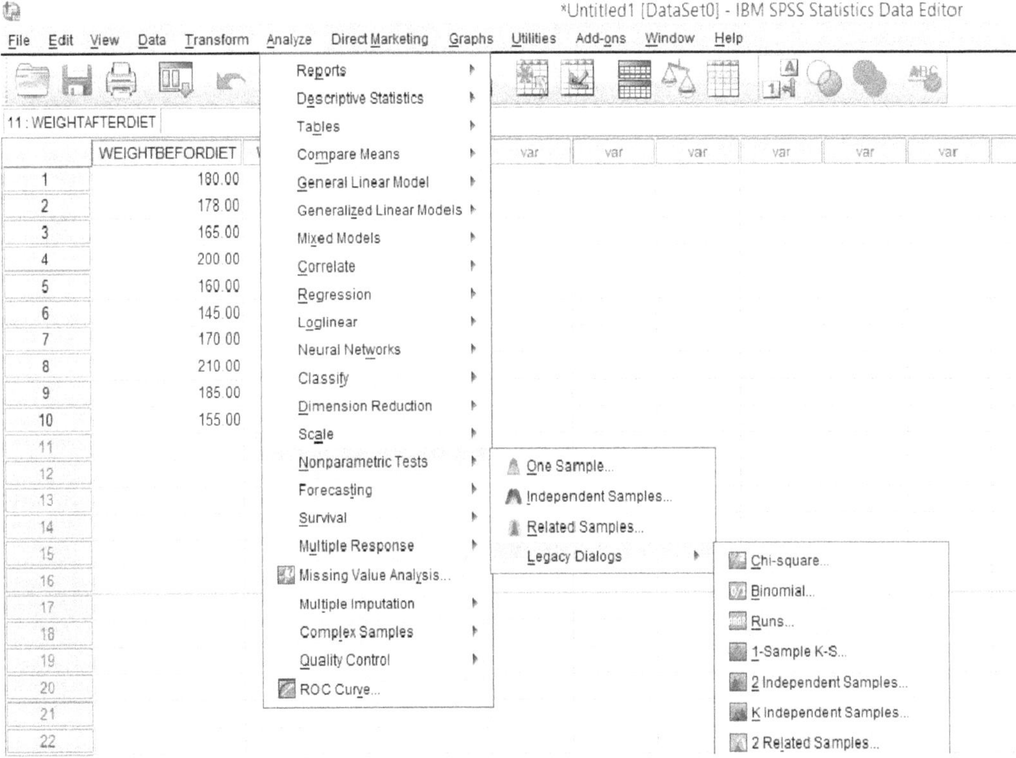

- You will be presented with the Two-Related-Samples **Tests** dialogue box, as shown below

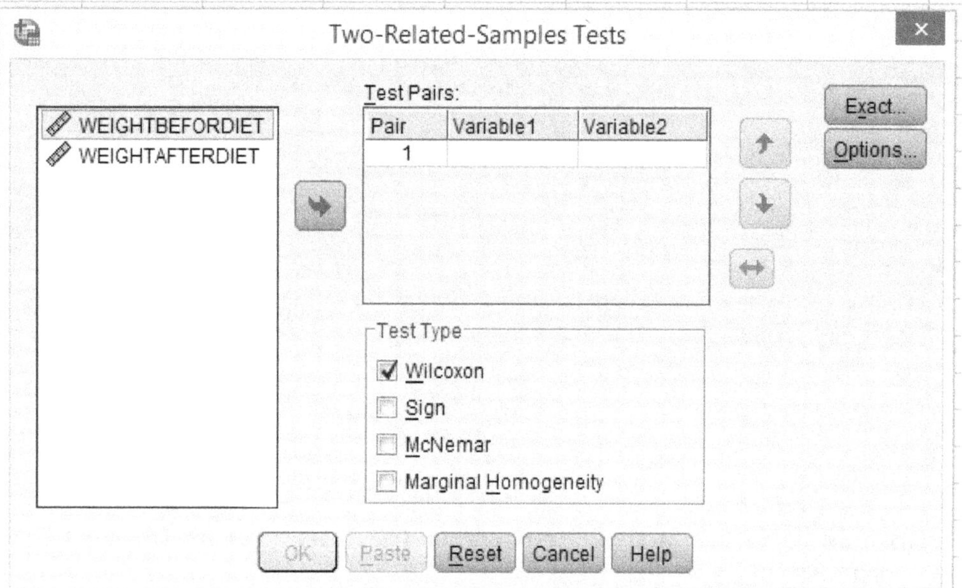

- Transfer the variables you are interested in analysing into the **Test** Pairs: box.

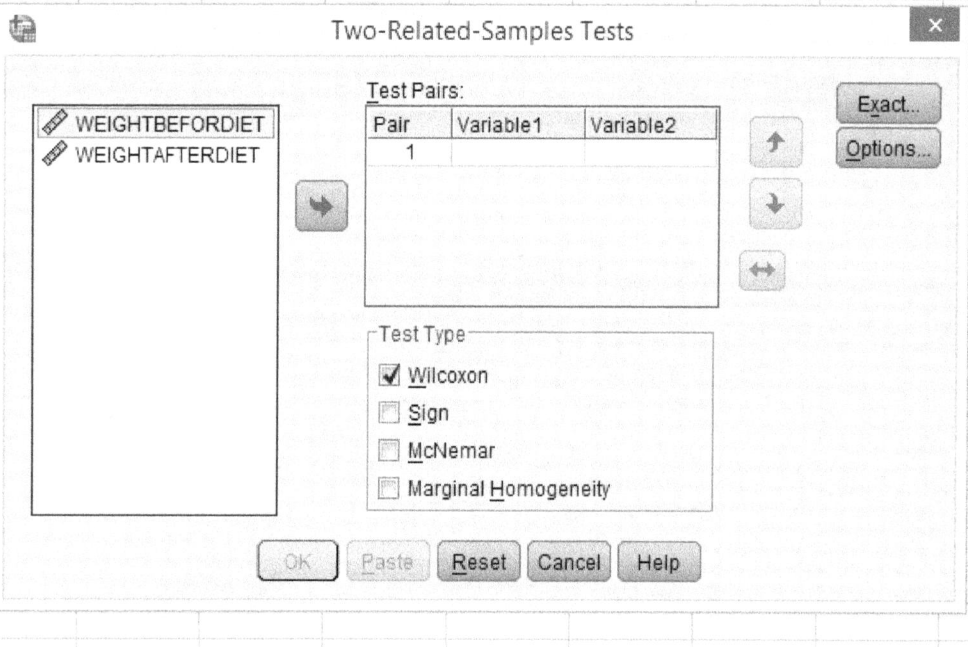

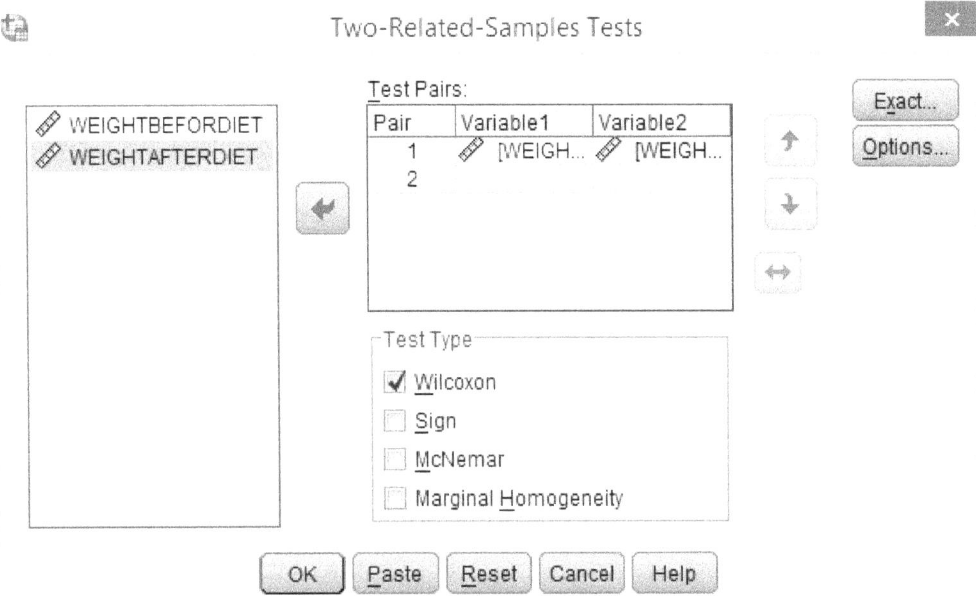

If user wants to generate descriptive or quartiles for your variables, he has to select them by clicking the option button and ticking the descriptive and quartiles checkboxes in the statistics area, you can decide how to deal with missing values. You will end up with a screen similar to the one below:

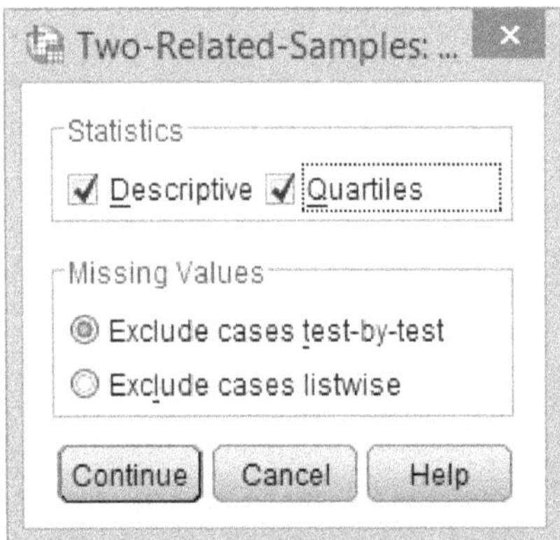

Then Click the continue button, then the **Two-Related-Samples Tests** dialogue box will appear back on the screen then click OK and desired result will be obtained

Ranks				
		N	Mean Rank	Sum of Ranks
WEIGHTAFTERDIET - WEIGHTBEFORDIET	Negative Ranks	7[a]	6.43	45.00
	Positive Ranks	3[b]	3.33	10.00
	Ties	0[c]		
	Total	10		

a. WEIGHTAFTERDIET < WEIGHTBEFORDIET

b. WEIGHTAFTERDIET > WEIGHTBEFORDIET

c. WEIGHTAFTERDIET = WEIGHTBEFORDIET

Test Statistics[a]

	WEIGHTAFTERDIET - WEIGHTBEFORDIET
Z	-1.790^{b}
Asymp. Sig. (2-tailed)	.074

a. Wilcoxon Signed Ranks Test

b. Based on positive ranks.

17 Statistical Software R

R – AS A STATISTICAL SOFTWARE AND

TREATED AS LANGUAGE

According to a statistics R is one of the online statistical software, which can be used for data analysis, to do some statistical calculation and to construct graphs using some built in command. This is used for most of the statistical procedures, which begins with descriptive statistics along with correlation, regression, ANOVA, MANOVA etc. This R is a object oriented, but it is simpler than C^{++}. Here also, user write program using in built R-Commands to solve problems.

The facilities, that can get from R become liabilities, if we do not understand them sufficiently well to use them efficiently.

Use of statistical software is almost becoming must for handling or analyzing large data and complex procedure of analysis.

Along with several software packages like SPSS, SAS MINITAB, R has been strongly advocated for the reasons, which are listed below

1. R has very good computing performance. It takes little time for the evaluation of commands.

2. The statistical software R is one of the free software, which will be used by college, University and other settings like R & D in Pharmaceutical industries.

3. It has got an excellent built-in-help system.

4. This is most useful for some graphical analysis

5. R is very much similar to a computer programming language, hence for those who are good or familiar in writing the program in different languages like C+, C++ , FORTRAN, will be very easy and not too hard for new user.

6. It will become very easy to extend with user written functions. In fact, this R can be modified by the user and its development is open to contributors. Original source cannot be modified by user, but that can be modified only by R-core team.

7. It provides scripting and interfacing facilities for the user.

ARITHMETIC OPERATORS

The usual operator modes of data that are available in R are logical (Boolean True/False), numeric (Integer/Real), complex (Real + imaginary number).

The data analysis in R proceeds as an interactive dialogue, with the integers. As soon as the user type command at the prompt (>) and press the enter key, then the interpreter responds after executing the command.

The commonly used mathematical operators to perform arithmetic operations are as listed below.

Operation with corresponding function

+	-----	Addition operator
−	-----	Subtraction Operator
*	------	Multiplication Operator
/	------	Division Operator
^	-------	Exponential Operator

Example 1: When two numbers 3 and 5 are added 3+5, then the output will be [1] 8, when they are subtracted 3-5, then the output is [1] -2. Similarly user can do all type of operations using remaining operators.

ASSIGN OPERATOR

The commonly used assignment operator in R is <- to give a data object (or any other object) its value. Here the operator -> may also be used. Here with -> operator, the assignment is from left to right.

Example: x <- 3, In this example the assignment operator will assign the value to the object x. x^2 -> y, here the assignment operator will assign the square of x to the object y.

COMPARISION OPERATOR

The comparison operators which are used in R – software are

>	-----	Greater than operator
<	----	Less than operator
>=	------	Greater or equal
<=	------	less or equal
==	------	equal to
!=	-----	is not equal to
!	------	logical not
&	-------	logical and
|	-------	logical or

VECTOR BASE OF R

R contains data structures vector base is one of the most useful data structure in R. A vector can be defined as a series of elements that are of the same type. This series of observations can be stored in R.

Example: c(3, 7, 8, 5)

[1] 3 7 8 5

FUNCTION

There are different mathematical and statistical functions which are defined in R. The function will have a name which is typed and that is then followed by a pair of parentheses (open and closed parentheses).

C- Function

To enter small data very quickly, the commonly used R – command is the c ("combine") function. This function combines all the terms together.

Example:

x<-c(1,2,4,7,9);

[1] 1 2 4 7 9

This function can also be used to construct a vector of character strings

Example: <-c("SUNDAY","MANDAY");

SCAN FUNCTION

When an investigator wants to record the height of 10 patients. Here one has to create a data object ht using scan function, that is written as ht = scan(), then response for this command will be obtained as 1:

Then the data is entered are separated by spaces. After inputting all the 10 values, press the enter key two times, then the output will appear as

1: 64 65 63 66 67 68 70 72 70 71

11;

Read 10 items.

rep Function

rep function is a R – Command , that will be used to enter the data containing repeated values.

Example: If one wish to enter the following small data set : 2 2 2 3 3 3 5 5 5 5 9 9, then the R-Command is written as x < -c(rep(2,3), rep(3,3),rep(5,4), rep(9,2));. The first argument to rep()function is the number to be repeated and the second argument is the number of times that the number to repeated.

If one wish to have a vector(x) and want to repeat each of its element equal number of times, say 5 times, then the command can be written as rep(x, each=4)

Example:

> x<-1:5; rep(x,each=4)

[1] 1 1 1 1 2 2 2 2 3 3 3 3 4 4 4 4 5 5 5 5

Data.frame function:

To write the data in a table (columns and rows,) the data frame function is used. The vectors which are included in the data frame must be of same length or if one of them is shorter, it is recycled an appropriate number of times.

Example:

Suppose the vector x=(1,2,3,4) , y=(2,3,5), z=(10,12) and w =(15), then create a data frame table.

> x<-c(1,2,3,4);

> y<-c(2,3,5);

> z<-c(10,12);

> w<-c(15);

> d<-data.frame(x,w)

> d

  x w

1 1 15

2 2 15

3 3 15

4 4 15

Since the length z is 1, therefore 15 is repeated 4-times to create the data frame of (x,z).

COMMAND FOR MATRIX

Here one can input the data either column wise or row wise using the matrix function.

Example:

> fr.dist<-matrix(c(seq(10,60, by=10),5,10,120,22,13,5), nrow=6);

> fr.dist;

    [,1] [,2]

[1,] 10   5

[2,] 20 10

[3,] 30 120

[4,] 40 22

[5,] 50 13

[6,] 60 5

The column of data set are combined by c function. This is the first argument for the matrix function. The second argument explains about number of rows. Either we have to give the number of rows or columns (ncol=2).

> fr.dist<-matrix(c(seq(10,60, by=10),5,10,120,22,13,5), nrow=6);

> rownames(fr.dist)<-c("1","2","3","4","5","6");

> colnames(fr.dist)<-c("Age", "Frequency");

> fr.dist; then the output will be as written below

```
  Age  Frequency
1  10      5
2  20      10
3  30      120
4  40      22
5  50      13
6  60      5
```

BUILT – IN FUNCTIONS

Commonly used built in functions are

Length(x), max(x), min(x), range(x), sum(x), cumsum(x), mean(x), median(x) and var(x).

Length function - length(x): Total number of elements of data x will be obtained using this function

Example: >

x<-c(4,6,8,12,7);

> length(x);

[1] 5

Maximum function - max(x):

What is the maximum value of the data x, that can be obtained using max(x)

> x<-c(4,6,8,12,7);

> max(x);

[1] 12

Minimum function - min(x):

What is the minimum value of the data x, that can be obtained using min(x)

```
> x<-c(4,6,8,12,7,2);
> min(x);
[1] 2
```

Range function – range(x)

```
> x<-c(4,6,8,12,7);
> range(x);
[1]  4 12
>
```

Sum function – sum(x):

The sum of the values of x can be obtained using sum function, that is defined as sum(x);

```
> x<-c(4,6,8,12,7);
> sum(x);
[1] 37
>
```

Cumulative Frequency Function – Cumsum Function – Cumsum(x):

The cumsum function is used to obtain the cumulative sum of the values of the series x or data x and defined as cumsum(x).

```
> x<-c(4,6,8,12,7);
> cumsum(x);
[1]  4 10 18 30 37
>
```

Mean function – mean(x):

The mean of the series x can be obtained using the function mean(x).

```
> x<-c(4,6,8,12,7);
> mean(x)
[1] 7.4
>
```

Median function – median(x):

The median of the series x can be obtained using the function mean(x).

> x<-c(4,6,8,12,7);

> median(x)

[1] 7

>

Variance function – var(x):

To obtain the variance of the series x, the R command is defined as var(x)

> x<-c(4,6,8,12,7);

> var(x)

[1] 8.8

   After obtaining the variance, standard deviation can be obtained using the square root function as explained below.

> sd<-sqrt(var(x));

> sd

[1] 2.96

Worked Examples

1. Obtain the arithmetic mean of the given distribution using R – commands (Discrete series)

Height– In inches X	Number of Patients f
67	3
68	6
66	12
70	20
72	10
71	5
69	3

Solution:

> x<-c(67,68,66,70,72,71,69);

> f<-c(3,6,12,20,10,5,3);

> n<-sum(f);

> n

[1] 59

```
> fx<-(f*x);
> fx
[1]  201  408  792 1400  720  355  207
> sum<-sum(fx);
> sum
[1] 4083
> mean<-sum/n;
> mean
[1] 69.20339
```

2. Obtain the arithmetic mean of the given distribution using R – commands (Continuous series)

Age of Patient	Number of Patients
10-20	8
20-30	12
30-40	20
40-50	30
50-60	15
60-70	14
70-80	05

```
> l₁<-seq(10,70, by=10);
> l1
[1] 10 20 30 40 50 60 70
> l₂<-seq(20,80,by=10);
> l₂
[1] 20 30 40 50 60 70 80
> mid<-(l₁+l₂)/2;
> mid
[1] 15 25 35 45 55 65 75
> f<-c(8,12,20,30,15,14,5);
> f
[1]  8 12 20 30 15 14  5
> prd<-(mid*f);
> prd
[1]  120  300  700 1350  825  910  375
```

```
> s<-sum(prd);
> s
[1] 4580
> n<-sum(f);
> n
[1] 104
> mean<-s/n
> mean
[1] 44.03846
>
```

COMPUTATION OF STANDARD DEVIATION OF DISCRETE AND CONTINUOUS SERIES

Example 1: Compute the standard deviation for the given distribution

Weight in KG (X)	04	06	08	10	12	14	16	18	20
Number of Patients f	5	10	18	22	30	10	08	05	03

Solution:

```
> weight<-c(4,6,8,10,12,14,16,18,20)
> f<-c(5,10,18,22,30,10,8,5,3);
> n<-sum(f)
> fx<-f*weight;
> sum<-sum(fx);
> mean<-sum/n;
> devn<-weight-mean;
> devn;
[1] -7.009009 -5.009009 -3.009009 -1.009009  0.990991  2.990991  4.990991
[8]  6.990991  8.990991
> d²<-devn^2
> d²*f
[1] 245.63104 250.90171 162.97443  22.39818  29.46189  89.46027 199.27993
[8] 244.36978 242.51376
> d2*f;
```

```
[1] 245.63104 250.90171 162.97443  22.39818  29.46189  89.46027 199.27993
[8] 244.36978 242.51376
> SUM<-sum(d2*f)
> SUM
[1] 1486.991
> sd<-sqrt(SUM/n);
> sd
[1] 3.660098
>
> fr.dist<-data.frame(weight, f, devn, d^2); fr.dist;
     weight    f   d=weight -Mean          d^2
1     4       5     -7.009009         49.1262073
2     6       10    -5.009009         25.0901713
3     8       18    -3.009009          9.0541352
4     10      22    -1.009009          1.0180992
5     12      30     0.990991          0.9820631
6     14      10     2.990991          8.9460271
7     16      8      4.990991         24.9099911
8     18      5      6.990991         48.8739550
9     20      3      8.990991         80.8379190
>
```

 Standard deviation = 3.660098

R – Command to Calculate the Coefficient of Correlation between Two Variables

If x and y are two groups of variables, then R – command or function used to calculate coefficient of correlation between these two variables is > <-cor(x,y)

Example:

```
> x<-c(23,24,26,27,29);
> y<-c(18,20,22,24,25);
> r<-cor(x,y);
> r
[1] 0.9800099
>
```

1. Compute coefficient of correlation between age and Bilirubin level of 10 patients.

AGE X	Bilirubin (mg/dl) Y
70	11
68	12.3
81	14.7
59	9.1
64	7.8
48	6
50	9
44	7
50	8
42	8

```
> x<-c(70,68,81,59,64,48,50,44,50,42);

> y<-c(11,12.3,14.7,9.1,7.8,6,9,7,8,8);

> r<-cor(x,y);

> r
```

[1] 0.8627299.

2. A single dose of 500 mg drug was administered by a rapid IV injection to the patient who is weighing 75 kg. Plasma sample were obtained from 0 hour to 7 hours and assay of the drug as tabulated below. Compute coefficient of correlation between time and concentration

Time(t)	Concentration (mg/L) (X)
0	69
0.25	54.8
0.5	43.2
0.75	35.1
1	29
1.5	21.3
2	17
2.5	14.2
3	12.7
4	10.5
5	9
6	8.2
7	7

```
> time<-c(0,0.25,0.5,0.75,1,1.5,2,2.5,3,4,5,6,7);
```

> con<-c(69,54.8,43.2,35.1,29,21.3,17,14.2,12.7,10.5,9,8.2,7);

> cor(time,con)

[1] -0.8048316

>

R-Command to Fit the Line of Regression

The R-command fit the line of regression y on x and x on y. The command used fit is

FIT Y on X

fit<- lm(y~x);

Here the values of X and Y are stored in the objects x and y respectively. Then the intercept and regression coefficient are obtained using the R-Command fit$ coefficient;

X	5	8	7	6	4
Y	3	4	5	2	1

> x<-c(5,8,7,6,4);

> y<-c(3,4,5,2,1);

> fit<-lm(y~x);

> fit$coefficients;

(Intercept)   x

     -1.8   0.8

>

Then the equation Y on X is written as Y = -1.8+0.8X

FIT X on Y

> x<-c(5,8,7,6,4);

> y<-c(3,4,5,2,1);

> fit<-lm(x~y);

> fit$coefficients;

(Intercept)   y

      3.6   0.8

>

Then the equation can be written as X=3.6+0.8Y

R-Command to find t-test value

1. Sample t-test

The R-command for sample t-test is defined as t.test(x, mu,alt,conf. level), where x is a vector of observations, mu is the defined population mean.

One Sample t-test

Example:

> x<-c(65,66,69,64,68,60)

> t.test(x,mu‾64);

data: x

t = 1.0193, df = 5, p-value = 0.3548

alternative hypothesis: true mean is not equal to 64

95 percent confidence interval:

 61.97077 68.69590

sample estimates:

mean of x

 65.33333

>

2. Two Sample t-test – Pooled t-test

The R-command used for computation of t-value between means of two samples x and y to know or verify the level of significance is defined as **t.test(x,y,alt="less", var.equal=T).**

Example

X	12	16	17	15	19	20	14	16	12	
Y	13	18	19	18	20	19	16	20	18	17

> x<-c(12,16,17,15,19,20,14,16,12);

> y<-c(13,18,19,18,20,19,16,20,18,17);

> t.test(x,y,alt="less",var.equal = T);

 Two Sample t-test

data: x and y

t = -1.8992, df = 17, p-value = 0.03732

alternative hypothesis: true difference in means is less than 0

95 percent confidence interval:

 -Inf -0.1793133

sample estimates:

mean of x mean of y

 15.66667 17.80000

Non-parametric test alternative to pooled t-test or two sample t-test

Wilcoxon Rank Sum Test

X	12	16	17	15	19	20	14	16	12	
Y	13	18	19	18	20	19	16	20	18	17

Here two sided test is performed using R-Command, which is defined as Wilcox.test(x,y);

x<-c(12,16,17,15,19,20,14,1612);

> y<-c(13,18,19,18,20,19,16,20,18,17);

> wilcox.test(x,y);

Wilcoxon rank sum test with continuity correction

data: x and y

W = 32, p-value = 0.5021

alternative hypothesis: true location shift is not equal to 0

3. Paired t-test (Student t-test, Comparison test, difference test)

The R-command used for computation of t-value to know the level of significance between before and after treatment, between Placebo and treatment groups is defined as

t.test(d, mu=0). Where d difference between before and after treatment or difference between placebo and treatment group.

Example

> x<-c(21,23,25,27,22,25);

> y<-c(18,19,20,24,20,24);

> d<-x-y

> d

[1] 3 4 5 3 2 1

> t.test(d,mu=0);

    Paired t-test

data: d

t = 5.1962, df = 5, p-value = 0.003478

alternative hypothesis: true mean is not equal to 0

95 percent confidence interval:

1.515874 4.484126

sample estimates:

mean of x

3

Non-parametric test as alternative to Paired t-test:

Wilcoxon signed Rank test:

This test is an alternative to paired t-test. In this case both the data need not be symmetric distributions, but the difference d need to be symmetric and continuous. The R-command to test this hypothesis is defined as **Wilcox.test(x,y,paired=T);**

Example:

> pre<-c(7,6,10,16,8,13,8,14,16,11,12,13,9,10,17,8,5)

> post<-c(11,14,16,17,9,15,9,17,20,12,14,15,14,15,18,15,9);

> **wilcox.test(pre,post,mu=0, paired =t,alt = "less");**

   Wilcoxon signed rank test with continuity correction

data: pre and post

V = 0, p-value = 0.0001517

alternative hypothesis: true location shift is less than 0

Parametric one-way analysis of Variance:

One way ANOVA is statistical tool, which will be used to verify the level of significance between means of more than two samples or for the comparison of means of more two populations. If X_1, X_2 and X_3 are three samples taken from three different populations, then to verify the level of significance between them, the investigator has to assume that the parent populations are normal with mean μ_i and standard deviation σi for $i = 1,2,3 ...k..$. For testing the problem, H0: $\mu_1 = \mu_2 = \mu_3 = \mu_k$ against $H_1 : \mu i \neq \mu j$ for at least one pair (i, j), $i \neq j$.

The R – Command which will be used carry out one way ANOVA id defined as

Oneway.test (values~ind, data=d, var.equal=T);

Example:

X1	X2	X3
15	12	10
12	13	12
8	11	9
11	14	10
9	14	8

> x1<-c(15,12,8,11,9);

> x2<-c(12,13,11,14,14);

> x3<-c(10,12,9,10,8);

> d<-stack(list("x1"=x1,"x2"=x2,"x3"=x3));

> names(d);

[1] "values" "ind"

> **oneway.test(values~ind,data=d,var.equal=T);**

   One-way analysis of means

data: values and ind

F = 3, num df = 2, denom df = 12, p-value = 0.08779

>

CHISQUARE TEST

Chi-square test is a non-parametric test will be applied to know level of significance between the observed and expected values when data are tabulated in category form.

R-command which will be used to verify the level of significance between the observed and expected is defined as chisq.test(x,); or chisq.test (x, correct=FALSE);

```
> x<-matrix(c(28,20,289,276), nrow=2,byrow=T);
> x
     [,1] [,2]
[1,]  28   20
[2,] 289  276
> chisq.test(x);
```

      Pearson's Chi-squared test with Yates' continuity correction

data: x

X-squared = 0.64909, df = 1, p-value = 0.4204

> chisq.test(x, correct=FALSE);

  Pearson's Chi-squared test

data: x

X-squared = 0.91411, df = 1, p-value = 0.339

Example 2: A certain drug is claimed to be effective in curing in cold. Experiment was conducted with a group 114 people who were suffering from cold, 60 were treated with drug and 54 were treated with sugar pills. Results obtained as listed below. Use R-chisq command and verify the level of significance.

Solution:

```
> x<-matrix(c(50,10,42,22),nrow=2,byrow=T);
> x
     [1] [2]
[1]  50  10
[2]  42  22
> chisq.test(x, correct=FALSE);
```

  Pearson's Chi-squared test

data: x

X-squared = 5.0719, df = 1, p-value = 0.02432

>

Index

R

S

T

U

V

W

Z